# Pediatric Cardiology

*Editors*

PEI-NI JONE
D. DUNBAR IVY
STEPHEN R. DANIELS

# PEDIATRIC CLINICS
# OF NORTH AMERICA

www.pediatric.theclinics.com

*Consulting Editor*
BONITA F. STANTON

October 2020 • Volume 67 • Number 5

**ELSEVIER**

1600 John F. Kennedy Boulevard • Suite 1800 • Philadelphia, Pennsylvania, 19103-2899

http://www.theclinics.com

**THE PEDIATRIC CLINICS OF NORTH AMERICA Volume 67, Number 5**
**October 2020 ISSN 0031-3955, ISBN-13: 978-0-323-75586-3**

Editor: Kerry Holland
Developmental Editor: Casey Potter

The Pediatric Clinics of North America (ISSN 0031-3955) is published bimonthly by Elsevier Inc., 360 Park Avenue South, New York, NY 10010-1710. Months of issue are February, April, June, August, October, and December. Periodicals postage paid at New York, NY and additional mailing offices. Subscription prices are $240.00 per year (US individuals), $695.00 per year (US institutions), $315.00 per year (Canadian individuals), $924.00 per year (Canadian institutions), $362.00 per year (international individuals), $924.00 per year (international institutions), $100.00 per year (US students and residents), $100.00 per year (Canadian students and residents), and $165.00 per year (international residents and students). To receive students/resident rare, orders must be accompanied by name of affiliated institution, date of term, and the signature of program/residency coordinator on institution letterhead. Orders will be billed at individual rate until proof of status is received. Foreign air speed delivery is included in all Clinics subscription prices. All prices are subject to change without notice. **POSTMASTER:** Send address changes to The Pediatric Clinics of North America, Elsevier Health Sciences Division, Subscription Customer Service, 3251 Riverport Lane, Maryland Heights, MO 63043. **Customer Service: 1-800-654-2452 (US and Canada). From outside of the US and Canada: 1-314-447-8871. Fax: 1-314-447-8029. For print support, E-mail: JournalsCustomerService-usa@elsevier.com. For online support, E-mail: JournalsOnlineSupport-usa@elsevier.com.**

Reprints. For copies of 100 or more, of articles in this publication, please contact the Commercial Reprints Department, Elsevier Inc., 360 Park Avenue South, New York, NY 10010-1710. Tel.: 212-633-3874; Fax: 212-633-3820; E-mail: reprints@elsevier.com.

The Pediatric Clinics of North America is also published in Spanish by McGraw-Hill Inter-americana Editores S.A., Mexico City, Mexico; in Portuguese by Riechmann and Affonso Editores, Rua Comandante Coelho 1085, CEP 21250, Rio de Janeiro, Brazil; and in Greek by Althayia SA, Athens, Greece.

The Pediatric Clinics of North America is covered in MEDLINE/PubMed (Index Medicus), Excerpta Medica, Current Contents, Current Contents/Clinical Medicine, Science Citation Index, ASCA, ISI/BIOMED, and BIOSIS.

## PROGRAM OBJECTIVE

The goal of the *Pediatric Clinics of North America* is to keep practicing physicians and residents up to date with current clinical practice in pediatrics by providing timely articles reviewing the state-of-the-art in patient care.

## TARGET AUDIENCE

All practicing pediatricians, physicians and healthcare professionals who provide patient care to pediatric patients.

## LEARNING OBJECTIVES

Upon completion of this activity, participants will be able to:

1. Review the basic evaluation of heart murmur, chest pain, syncope, and palpitations in the pediatric population.
2. Discuss revolutions in preventive cardiology, technological advances and the development of artificial intelligence for managing big data and the impact on automated imaging.
3. Recognize advances in pediatric heart failure and pediatric pulmonary hypertension impacting improved survival rates in this special population.

## ACCREDITATIONS

### *Physician Credit*

The Elsevier Office of Continuing Medical Education (EOCME) is accredited by the Accreditation Council for Continuing Medical Education (ACCME) to provide continuing medical education for physicians.

The EOCME designates this journal-based activity for a maximum of 14 *AMA PRA Category 1 Credit*(s)™. Physicians should claim only the credit commensurate with the extent of their participation in the activity.

All other healthcare professionals requesting continuing education credit for this this journal-based activity will be issued a certificate of participation.

### *ABP Maintenance of Certification Credit*

Successful completion of this CME activity, which includes participation in the activity and individual assessment of and feedback to the learner, enables the learner to earn up to 14 MOC points in the American Board of Pediatrics' (ABP) Maintenance of Certification (MOC) program. It is the CME activity provider's responsibility to submit learner completion information to ACCME for the purpose of granting ABP MOC credit.

## DISCLOSURE OF CONFLICTS OF INTEREST

The EOCME assesses conflict of interest with its instructors, faculty, planners, and other individuals who are in a position to control the content of CME activities. All relevant conflicts of interest that are identified are thoroughly vetted by EOCME for fair balance, scientific objectivity, and patient care recommendations. EOCME is committed to providing its learners with CME activities that promote improvements or quality in healthcare and not a specific proprietary business or a commercial interest.

**The planning committee, staff, authors and editors listed below have identified no financial relationships or relationships to products or devices they or their spouse/life partner have with commercial interest related to the content of this CME activity:**

Scott Auerbach, MD; Dale A. Burkett, MD; Anthony C. Chang, MD, MBA, MPH, MS; Sarah B. Clauss, MD; Daniel A. Cox, DO; Stephen R. Daniels, MD, PhD; Sarah D. de Ferranti, MD; Laura Fisher; Benjamin S. Frank, MD; Kevin G. Friedman, MD; Sharib Gaffar, MD; Addison S. Gearhart, MD; Benjamin H. Goot, MD; Kerry Holland; D. Dunbar Ivy, MD; Roni M. Jacobsen, MD; Pei-Ni Jone, MD; Marilu Kelly, MSN, RN, CNE, CHCP; Meghan Kiley Metcalf, MD; Rajkumar Mayakrishnann; Adam Putschoegl, DO; Jack Rychik, MD; Craig Sable, MD; Renata Shih, MD; Christopher A. Sumski, DO; Lloyd Y. Tani, MD; Johannes von Alvensleben, MD; Kae Watanabe, MD.

**The planning committee, staff, authors and editors listed below have identified financial relationships or relationships to products or devices they or their spouse/life partner have with commercial interest related to the content of this CME activity:**

Gareth J. Morgan, MD: speaker's bureau and consultant/advisor for Abbott, Edwards Lifesciences Corporation, Medtronic, and Occlutech.

Jenny E. Zablah, MD: speaker's bureau and consultant/advisor for Abbott.

## UNAPPROVED/OFF-LABEL USE DISCLOSURE

The EOCME requires CME faculty to disclose to the participants:

1. When products or procedures being discussed are off-label, unlabelled, experimental, and/or investigational (not US Food and Drug Administration [FDA] approved); and
2. Any limitations on the information presented, such as data that are preliminary or that represent ongoing research, interim analyses, and/or unsupported opinions. Faculty may discuss information about pharmaceutical agents that is outside of FDA-approved labelling. This information is intended solely for CME and is not intended to promote off-label use of these medications. If you have any questions, contact the medical affairs department of the manufacturer for the most recent prescribing information.

## TO ENROLL

To enroll in the *Pediatric Clinics of North America* Continuing Medical Education program, call customer service at 1-800-654-2452 or sign up online at http://www.theclinics.com/home/cme. The CME program is available to subscribers for an additional annual fee of USD 300.00.

## METHOD OF PARTICIPATION

In order to claim credit, participants must complete the following:

1. Complete enrolment as indicated above.
2. Read the activity.
3. Complete the CME Test and Evaluation. Participants must achieve a score of 70% on the test. All CME Tests and Evaluations must be completed online.

In order to claim MOC points, participants must complete the following:

1. Complete steps listed above for claiming CME credit.
2. Provide your specialty board ID#, birth date (MM/DD), and attestation.
3. Online MOC submission is only available for the American Board of pediatrics' (ABP) Maintenance of Certification (MOC) program.

## CME INQUIRIES/SPECIAL NEEDS

For all CME inquiries or special needs, please contact elsevierCME@elsevier.com.

# Contributors

## CONSULTING EDITOR

**BONITA F. STANTON, MD**
Founding Dean, and Robert C. and Laura C. Garrett Endowed Chair, Hackensack
Meridian School of Medicine, President, Academic Enterprise, Hackensack Meridian
Health, Nutley, New Jersey

## EDITORS

**PEI-NI JONE, MD**
Associate Professor of Pediatrics, Pediatric Cardiology, Children's Hospital
Colorado, Department of Pediatrics, University of Colorado School of Medicine, Aurora,
Colorado

**D. DUNBAR IVY, MD**
Chief and Selby's Chair of Pediatric Cardiology, Professor, Department of Pediatrics,
University of Colorado School of Medicine, Director, Pediatric Pulmonary Hypertension
Program, Children's Hospital Colorado, Aurora, Colorado

**STEPHEN R. DANIELS, MD, PhD**
Professor and Chair of Pediatrics, Pediatrician-in-Chief, Department of Pediatrics,
University of Colorado School of Medicine, Children's Hospital Colorado, Aurora,
Colorado

## AUTHORS

**SCOTT AUERBACH, MD**
Pediatric Cardiologist, Department of Pediatrics, Children's Hospital Colorado, Aurora,
Colorado

**DALE A. BURKETT, MD**
Assistant Professor, Division of Pediatric Cardiology, Heart Institute, Children's Hospital
Colorado, University of Colorado, Aurora, Colorado

**ANTHONY C. CHANG, MD, MBA, MPH, MS**
Chief Intelligence and Innovation Officer, Medical Director, The Sharon Disney Lund
Medical Intelligence and Innovation Institute (MI3), Children's Hospital of Orange County,
Orange, California

**SARAH B. CLAUSS, MD**
Associate Professor of Pediatrics, Children's National Medical Center, George
Washington School of Medicine, Washington, DC

**DANIEL A. COX, DO**
Assistant Professor of Pediatrics, Adjunct Assistant Professor of Internal Medicine,
University of Utah School of Medicine, Salt Lake City, Utah

**SARAH D. DE FERRANTI, MD, MPH**
Associate Professor of Pediatrics, Boston Children's Hospital, Harvard School of Medicine, Boston, Massachusetts

**BENJAMIN S. FRANK, MD**
Assistant Professor, Department of Pediatrics, Section of Cardiology, University of Colorado School of Medicine, Aurora, Colorado

**KEVIN G. FRIEDMAN, MD**
Department of Cardiology, Boston Children's Hospital, Harvard Medical School, Boston, Massachusetts

**SHARIB GAFFAR, MD**
Pediatrics Resident, PGY-3, UC Irvine Pediatrics Residency Program, Choc Children's Hospital of Orange County, Orange, California

**ADDISON S. GEARHART, MD**
Pediatric Cardiology Fellow, PGY-4, Boston Children's Hospital Heart Center, Boston, Massachusetts

**BENJAMIN H. GOOT, MD**
Herma Heart Institute, Children's Wisconsin, Medical College of Wisconsin, Milwaukee, Wisconsin

**D. DUNBAR IVY, MD**
Chief and Selby's Chair of Pediatric Cardiology, Professor, Department of Pediatrics, University of Colorado School of Medicine, Director, Pediatric Pulmonary Hypertension Program, Children's Hospital Colorado, Aurora, Colorado

**RONI M. JACOBSEN, MD, FACC**
Assistant Professor of Medicine and Pediatrics, Pediatric and Adult Congenital Cardiology, University of Colorado School of Medicine, Children's Hospital Colorado, University of Colorado Hospital, Aurora, Colorado

**PEI-NI JONE, MD**
Associate Professor of Pediatrics, Pediatric Cardiology, Children's Hospital Colorado, Department of Pediatrics, University of Colorado School of Medicine, Aurora, Colorado

**MEGHAN KILEY METCALF, MD**
Pediatric Cardiology Fellow, Division of Cardiology, The Children's Hospital of Philadelphia, Instructor, Department of Pediatrics, Perelman School of Medicine at the University of Pennsylvania, Philadelphia, Pennsylvania

**GARETH J. MORGAN, MBBaO, BCH, MRCPCH, MPhil, MSCAI**
Associate Professor of Pediatrics, University of Colorado School of Medicine, Congenital Interventional Cardiologist, Children's Hospital Colorado, Aurora, Colorado

**ADAM PUTSCHOEGL, DO**
Pediatric Cardiologist, Department of Pediatrics, Children's Hospital & Medical Center/ University of Nebraska Medical Center, Omaha, Nebraska

**JACK RYCHIK, MD**
Robert and Dolores Harrington Endowed Chair in Pediatric Cardiology, Division of Cardiology, The Children's Hospital of Philadelphia, Professor, Department of Pediatrics, Perelman School of Medicine at the University of Pennsylvania, Philadelphia, Pennsylvania

**CRAIG SABLE, MD**
Associate Chief, Cardiology, Children's National Hospital, Northwest, Washington, DC

**RENATA SHIH, MD**
Assistant Professor, University of Florida, Gainesville, Florida

**CHRISTOPHER A. SUMSKI, DO**
Herma Heart Institute, Children's Wisconsin, Medical College of Wisconsin, Milwaukee, Wisconsin

**LLOYD Y. TANI, MD**
Professor of Pediatrics, University of Utah School of Medicine, Salt Lake City, Utah

**JOHANNES C. VON ALVENSLEBEN, MD**
Children's Hospital Colorado, University of Colorado School of Medicine, Aurora, Colorado

**KAE WATANABE, MD**
Assistant Professor, Northwestern University, Chicago, Illinois

**JENNY E. ZABLAH, MD, FSCAI, FACC, FAAP**
Assistant Professor of Pediatrics, University of Colorado School of Medicine, Congenital Interventional Cardiologist, Children's Hospital Colorado, Aurora, Colorado

# Contents

Chest pain and heart murmurs are common issues primary care providers
must evaluate and manage. Both are a source of anxiety for patients, parents, and providers, necessitating evaluation and understanding to ensure
appropriate management. Most pediatric chest pain can be treated symp-
tomatically and with reassurance. This article examines the approach to
pediatric chest pain including identification of key historical points, common causes of chest pain, and when to refer. The article also delineates
our approach to auscultation, describes common benign murmurs, and offers suggestions on when to refer for further evaluation.

Syncope and palpitations are common complaints for patients presenting
to their primary care provider. They represent symptoms that most often
have a benign etiology but rarely can be the first warning sign of a serious
condition, such as arrhythmias, structural heart disease, or noncardiac
disease. The history, physical examination, and noninvasive testing can,
in most cases, distinguish benign from pathologic causes. This article in-
troduces syncope and palpitations, with emphasis on the differential diagnoses, initial presentation, diagnostic strategy, and various management
strategies.

Treatment of Kawasaki disease (KD) with intravenous immunoglobulin
(IVIG) administered within the initial 10 days of fever onset decreases the
risk of coronary artery aneurysms (CAAs) from ~ 25% to less than 5%.
However, patients with IVIG resistance, young infants, men, highly inflamed patients, and/or those with coronary changes at diagnosis remain
at high risk for CAA. High-risk patients may benefit from acute, adjunctive
antiinflammatory treatment in addition to IVIG. Optimal therapy remains
unknown. This article reviews the acute pharmacologic management of
patients with KD, focusing on adjunctive primary therapy options and
treatment of patients with IVIG resistance.

delayed because initial symptoms are similar to common pediatric illnesses. Disease progression is tracked by symptoms, echocardiogram,
and biomarkers. Treatment is extrapolated from mostly adult heart failure
(HF) literature. Recent studies demonstrate differences between pediatric
and adult HF pathophysiology. Increased collaboration among PHF programs is advancing the management of PHF. Unfortunately, there are patients who ultimately require heart transplantation, with increasing
numbers supported by a ventricular assist device as a bridge to
transplantation.

Pulmonary hypertension (PH), the syndrome of increased pressure in the
pulmonary arteries, is associated with significant morbidity and mortality
for affected children and is associated with a variety of potential underlying
causes. Several pulmonary arterial hypertension–targeted therapies have
become available to reduce pulmonary artery pressure and improve
outcome, but there is still no cure for most patients. This review provides
a description of select causes of PH encountered in pediatrics and an update on the most recent data pertaining to evaluation and management of
children with PH. Available evidence for specific classes of PH-targeted
therapies in pediatrics is discussed.

Although progress had been made in reducing cardiovascular disease
(CVD) mortality, the positive trend has reversed in recent years, and
CVD remains the most common cause of mortality in US women and
men. Youth represent the future of CVD prevention; emerging evidence
suggests exposure to risk factors in children contributes to atherosclerosis
and results in vascular changes and increased CVD events. The contributors to CVD include those commonly seen in adults. This article reviews
hypercholesterolemia, hypertension, obesity, diabetes, and smoking. It
discusses the prevalence of each disease, diagnosis, treatment, and cardiovascular complications.

Hypoplastic left heart syndrome (HLHS) is a complex form of congenital
heart disease defined by anatomic and functional inadequacy of the left
side of the heart with nonviability of the left ventricle to perform systemic
perfusion. Lethal if not treated, a strategy for survival currently is well established, with continuing improvement in outcomes over the past 30
years. Prenatal diagnosis, good newborn care, improved surgical skills,
specialized postoperative care, and unique strategies for interstage monitoring all have contributed to increasing likelihood of survival. The unique
life with a single right ventricle and a Fontan circulation is a focused area
of investigation.

There is a growing population of patients living with congenital heart disease (CHD), now with more adults living with CHD than children. Adults with CHD have unique health care needs, requiring a thoughtful approach to cardiac, neurocognitive, mental, and physical health issues. They have increased risk of anxiety, depression, pragmatic language impairment, limited social cognition, worse educational attainment and unemployment, and delayed progression into independent adulthood. As a result, it is important to establish an individualized approach to obtain successful transition and transfer of care from the pediatric to adult health care world in this patient population.

This article aims to summarize some of the key advances in congenital interventional cardiology over the past few years, from novel imaging technologies, such as virtual reality, fusion imaging, and 3-dimensional printed models, to newly available devices and techniques to facilitate complex procedures including percutaneous pulmonary valve replacement and hybrid procedures. It is an exciting time for the field, with rapid development of techniques, devices, and imaging tools that allow a minimally invasive approach for many congenital cardiac defects with progressively less radiation and contrast doses.

Artificial intelligence (AI) in the last decade centered primarily around digitizing and incorporating the large volumes of patient data from electronic health records. AI is now poised to make the next step in health care integration, with precision medicine, imaging support, and development of individual health trends with the popularization of wearable devices. Future clinical pediatric cardiologists will use AI as an adjunct in delivering optimum patient care, with the help of accurate predictive risk calculators, continual health monitoring from wearables, and precision medicine. Physicians must also protect their patients' health information from monetization or exploitation.

# PEDIATRIC CLINICS OF NORTH AMERICA

**SERIES OF RELATED INTEREST**

Clinics in Perinatology
http://www.perinatology.theclinics.com/
Advances in Pediatrics
http://www.advancesinpediatrics.com/

**THE CLINICS ARE AVAILABLE ONLINE!**
Access your subscription at:
www.theclinics.com

# Foreword

# Generations of Dedicated Researchers Resulting in Generations of Constant Progress: Pediatric Cardiology

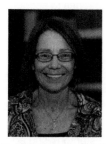

Bonita F. Stanton, MD
*Consulting Editor*

Each issue of *Pediatric Clinics of North America* addresses a different issue or set of related issues designed to continually update child health care providers as to the most current approaches to eliminate and/or mitigate the effects of illness on children and child health. Rarely, however, are readers given the opportunity to view developments across multiple domains within a specific field—in this case pediatric cardiology—from a historical perspective. The approach employed in this issue allows the reader to acquire the knowledge of the changes that are occurring and have occurred, the impact of the changes on the overall cardiac disorders, and expectations for the future of the specific disorder.

This issue of *Pediatric Clinics of North America* specifically and deliberately examines the evolution of the role of the cardiac physical exam; the ongoing revolution in the technological options for diagnosis and treatment; the impact of Big Data on diagnosis and management of cardiac disorders from childhood to adulthood; emerging recognition and understanding of the cardiac manifestations of medical problems ascribed to other organs; and the emergence of new pediatric heart-related disorders. The breadth and depth of this substantial update of our understanding and treatment of pediatric cardiac disorders reflect the substantial investment of senior pediatric cardiologists across the nation—and the world. As a profession, pediatric cardiologists actively engage in research to push the frontiers of our knowledge and understanding of pediatric heart disorders, thereby setting the expectation to carry on the research tradition to the next generation of pediatric cardiologists beginning during their training. Reflected in the articles within this issue is the recognition not only of technical

Pediatr Clin N Am 67 (2020) xv–xvi
https://doi.org/10.1016/j.pcl.2020.07.008
0031-3955/20/© 2020 Published by Elsevier Inc.

and research advances but also of the importance of maintaining an ethical perspective in the care, education, and research endeavors regarding children with heart disease. The training efforts for pediatric cardiologists focused on research certainly include pediatric cardiology fellowships but also special research programs in collaboration with the National Institutes of Health (particularly the National Heart, Lung, and Blood Institute), the pharmaceutical industry, the Food and Drug Administration, and numerous other state, federal, and international organizations concerned with research, child health, cardiology, innovation, technology, and pharmacology.[1,2]

Throughout this issue the reader will be reminded of the similarities but also the differences in the manifestations and the treatment of cardiac-related problems between children and adults. Always important, understanding why these differences exist and how to both recognize them and adapt treatment and research approaches to account for and better understand them, has become urgent as more and more children with significant heart disease are now living into adulthood.[2,3]

Bonita F. Stanton, MD
Hackensack Meridian School of Medicine
340 Kingsland Street, Building 123
Nutley, NJ 07110, USA

*E-mail address:*
bonita.stanton@shu.edu

## REFERENCES

1. Lai WW, Vetter VL, Richmond M, et al. Clinical research careers: reports from a NHLBI Pediatric Heart Network Clinical Research Skills Development Conference. Am Heart J 2011;161(1):13–67.
2. Pasquali SK, Jacobs JP, Farber GK, et al. Report of the National Heart, Lung, and Blood Institute working group: an integrated network for congenital heart disease research. Circulation 2016;133(14):1410–8.
3. Benjamin DK Jr, Smith PB, Jadhav P, et al. Pediatric antihypertensive trial failures: analysis of endpoints and dose range. Hypertension 2008;51:834–40.

# Preface

# Pediatric Cardiology: From Basics to Innovation

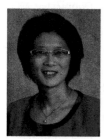
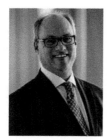
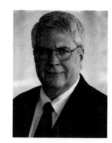

Pei-Ni Jone, MD    D. Dunbar Ivy, MD    Stephen R. Daniels, MD, PhD

*Editors*

We are honored to be the guest editors of this special issue of *Pediatric Clinics of North America* devoted to Pediatric Cardiology: From Basics to Innovation. This issue starts with the basic evaluation of heart murmur, chest pain, syncope, and palpitations and then progresses to the latest update on treatment of Kawasaki disease, myocarditis, and infective endocarditis. Tremendous progress has been made in pediatric heart failure and pediatric pulmonary hypertension with better survival in these patient populations. Preventive cardiology describes the growing population of obesity and how pediatricians and pediatric cardiologists may help in these public health issues. Surveillance of rheumatic heart disease worldwide is explored. Then the most common lesions in congenital heart disease to the most complex single-ventricle patients are discussed in detail with better surgical outcomes in single-ventricle patients. With better surgical outcomes, children with congenital heart disease are surviving into adulthood with challenging issues, such as transitioning from pediatric to adult cardiologists and neurocognitive issues. Rapid development of technology in the last decade has led to innovations of 3D echocardiography and devices that can be used in interventional cardiology without sending patients to surgery. Last, technology has revolutionized the development of artificial intelligence to manage and handle big data for pediatric cardiology with eventual automation of imaging as an example. We hope you will enjoy this exciting journey of pediatric cardiology as it has evolved over the

Pediatr Clin N Am 67 (2020) xvii–xviii
https://doi.org/10.1016/j.pcl.2020.07.009
0031-3955/20/© 2020 Published by Elsevier Inc.

pediatric.theclinics.com

last 20 years with better treatment and management of children with cardiovascular health.

Pei-Ni Jone, MD
Children's Hospital Colorado
13123 East 16th Avenue
Aurora, CO 80045, USA

D. Dunbar Ivy, MD
Children's Hospital Colorado
13123 East 16th Avenue
Aurora, CO 80045, USA

Stephen R. Daniels, MD, PhD
Children's Hospital Colorado
13123 East 16th Avenue
Aurora, CO 80045, USA

*E-mail addresses:*
pei-ni.jone@childrenscolorado.org (P.-N. Jone)
dunbar.ivy@childrenscolorado.org (D.D. Ivy)
stephen.daniels@childrenscolorado.org (S.R. Daniels)

# Evaluating Chest Pain and Heart Murmurs in Pediatric and Adolescent Patients

Christopher A. Sumski, DO*, Benjamin H. Goot, MD

## KEYWORDS

- Chest pain • Pediatrics • Heart murmur • Auscultation • Innocent murmurs

## KEY POINTS

- History and physical often identify the cause of chest pain in pediatrics, which is rarely cardiac in origin.
- Chest pain associated with exercise, syncope, or palpitations should be further evaluated.
- Vibratory, quiet, intermittent systolic murmurs in otherwise healthy children rarely need further evaluation.
- Loud, harsh, or diastolic murmurs, murmurs accompanied by a thrill, or other abnormal findings should be evaluated by pediatric cardiology.

## CHEST PAIN

### Introduction

Chest pain accounts for 0.3% to 0.6% of pediatric visits to the emergency department or outpatient clinic.[1,2] There are many etiologies, but cardiac pathology typically remains the primary concern.[1,3] Distress and fear regarding chest pain is likely caused by public awareness of the relationship between this symptom and heart disease, and the publicity of rare cases of pediatric sudden cardiac death.[1,4–6] Additionally, with the popularity of activity monitors tracking health statistics, people are more keenly aware of their heart. This confluence leads to concerns that affect quality of life and can lead to missing school and self-limitation from exercise.[1]

Chest pain in pediatrics is rarely cardiac in nature. Saleeb and colleagues[6] reviewed 3700 patients without previously known cardiovascular disease, representing nearly 18,000 patient-years, and found low incidence of cardiac pathology (1%) and no mortality secondary to cardiac disease following assessment. Conversely, in a separate

Herma Heart Institute, Children's Wisconsin & Medical College of Wisconsin, 9000 West Wisconsin Avenue, Milwaukee, WI 53226, USA
* Corresponding author.
E-mail address: csumski@wustl.edu

Pediatr Clin N Am 67 (2020) 783–799
https://doi.org/10.1016/j.pcl.2020.05.003
0031-3955/20/© 2020 Elsevier Inc. All rights reserved.

---

**Box 1**
**Common noncardiac differential diagnosis**

Musculoskeletal
- Idiopathic
- Muscle strain
- Costochondritis
- Slipped rib
- Chest wall abnormalities
- Trauma
- Precordial catch syndrome

Pulmonary
- Pneumonia
- Pleuritis
- Pneumothorax
- Asthma
- Pulmonary embolus
- Pulmonary contusion
- Pleural effusion
- Chronic cough

Gastrointestinal
- Gastroesophageal reflux disease
- Peptic ulcer disease
- Gastritis
- Esophageal spasm
- Esophagitis

Psychogenic
- Anxiety
- Depression
- Bullying

Miscellaneous
- Herpes zoster
- Toxin/drug exposure
- Breast tenderness

---

study by the same group evaluating those with proven cardiac disease, most patients with serious cardiac pathology presented with chest pain with exertion, suggesting this complaint is not one to take lightly.[3]

### Differential Diagnosis

Practitioners evaluating a young patient with chest pain should remain open-minded. Considerations cover many systems (**Box 1**) including cardiac, gastrointestinal, musculoskeletal, pulmonary, and psychogenic sources.[6,7] This section provides an overview of some common sources and diagnostic clues.

### Musculoskeletal

Musculoskeletal causes of chest pain are common and can arise from bone, cartilage, muscles, tendons, or ligaments.[1,7,8] Often the answer is found in the history alone. For example, excessive exercise, asthma, or a recent coughing illness suggests a muscular strain, whereas a boney abnormality is a consideration with recent trauma.

Idiopathic chest pain is common and presents as sharp, unilateral pain lasting several seconds to minutes. It is usually left sided and not reproducible on palpation. The pain is intermittent and usually without any clear triggers. No treatment is required other than reassurance. Idiopathic chest pain often self-resolves in weeks to months.[1,9]

Costochondritis represents inflammation of costochondral joints. Pain occurs at the joints and involves multiple costal cartilages. The cause is not always known, but inflammation is often preceded by respiratory illness. There rarely is redness, warmth, or induration but the pain is usually reproducible with palpation. Costochondritis is often self-limited; however, treatment with nonsteroidal anti-inflammatory drugs may be necessary.

Very brief, sharp, stabbing pain worse by deep inspiration is suggestive of precordial catch. The cause is not understood. Pain is usually over the left sternal border and can be intense. Usually patients report needing to take shallow breaths while awaiting resolution. The pain usually self-resolves, requiring only reassurance.

Slipping rib syndrome is caused by increased mobility of the floating ribs. This hypermobility allows the ribs to slip upward putting pressure on the intercostal nerve.[10] There may be a history of trauma, and pain is worse with coughing, stretching, or activity. The hooking maneuver, where the provider elicits a slipping of the ribs by retracting the costal margin anteriorly and superiorly, is diagnostic. Treatment is usually symptomatic, but could require surgery for relief.

### Pulmonary

Respiratory illnesses or bronchospasm can lead to strain or overuse of the accessory muscles of respiration and pain. Wiens and colleagues[11] reported a higher than anticipated incidence of exercise-induced asthma in patients with chest pain. Physical examination may be normal, but history of shortness of breath, coughing, chest tightness, or wheezing would be present. With exercise-induced bronchospasm, symptoms could be replicated with exercise testing and improved with β-agonists.

Pneumonia may present with chest pain from muscle strain or pleural irritation. Although not universally present, fever, cough, and respiratory symptoms may be concurrent with the chest pain. Supporting physical examination findings include focal decreased breath sounds, crackles, and tachypnea. Chest radiograph may be useful in the diagnosis.

Pneumothorax represents air between the chest wall and lung parenchyma. Multiple mechanisms can cause pneumothorax. Common etiologies include trauma or spontaneous pneumothorax in those with connective tissue disease. Symptoms include sudden onset chest pain, shortness of breath, and/or increased work of breathing. Evaluation demonstrates decreased breath sounds and associated absence of lung markings on radiograph. It is important to evaluate for respiratory compromise in patients presenting with pneumothorax.

Pulmonary embolism is a rare cause of chest pain in children; however, because of its serious nature, at-risk patients who present with chest pain, shortness of breath, and cyanosis should prompt assessment.[12] Risk factors include patient or family history of clotting disorder, malignancy, recent surgery, period of immobilization, or oral contraceptive use.

### Gastrointestinal

The most common gastrointestinal cause of chest pain is gastroesophageal reflux, but other considerations include peptic ulcer disease, esophageal spasm, esophageal or gastric inflammation, or cholecystitis. Diagnosis is primarily made by history, based on relationships to eating, diet, and pain quality (eg, burning pain associated with reflux). Treatment is typically conservative with diet adjustment and, if necessary, medication.

### Psychogenic

A diagnosis of exclusion, psychogenic chest pain should be a consideration once other causes are ruled out.[1,7] History may identify an acute stressor at home or school. With increasing concerns over cyberbullying and school violence one must be vigilant to assess for this.[13] Once identified, treatment is largely conservative and includes reassurance and coping strategies. Psychiatric evaluation, counseling, and directed therapy may be necessary.

### Miscellaneous

Miscellaneous causes include pain associated with breast development or abnormal thoracic shape, such as pectus abnormalities or scoliosis. Herpes zoster of the chest wall may cause pain or burning before a rash develops. Toxin ingestion should be considered, especially if the patient has a positive history or clinical signs of abuse. Drug abuse with amphetamines and cocaine has been linked to chest pain and acute myocardial infarction.[14,15]

### Cardiac

Cardiac chest pain is divided into anatomic abnormalities, myocardial/pericardial abnormalities, and arrhythmias. Potential causes are listed in **Box 2**.

Hypertrophic cardiomyopathy causes asymmetric myocardial hypertrophy and affects 1:500 individuals in the United States. According to Maron and colleagues[4] it is the most common cardiac cause of sudden death among young competitive athletes.[16] Hypertrophy can cause left ventricular outflow obstruction.[17] Furthermore, the increased mass increases oxygen demand, especially with exercise, whereas the obstruction can cause decreases (instead of the normal increase) in blood pressure and coronary perfusion. This can lead to ischemia, arrhythmia, and death. Chest pain is not the typical presenting symptom, but has been described, along with palpitations, syncope, and sudden death.[1] Because of increased screening practices, patients may also be identified due to an affected family member.[18] On examination patients have a systolic ejection murmur if there is obstruction, louder with standing or Valsalva. The electrocardiogram (EKG) can be normal, or findings including increased voltages and ischemic changes may be present.

Aortic stenosis can also lead to left ventricular outflow tract obstruction and cause chest pain. Stenosis can occur below, at the level of, or above the aortic valve.

---

**Box 2**
**Common cardiac causes of chest pain**

Anatomic abnormalities
- Anomalous coronaries
- Coronary insufficiency secondary to narrowing or compression
- Coronary aneurysm
- Left ventricular outflow obstruction (aortic stenosis, hypertrophic cardiomyopathy)
- Aortic dissection

Myocardial/pericardial
- Cardiomyopathy
- Myocarditis
- Pericarditis
- Pericardial effusion

Arrhythmogenic
- Supraventricular tachycardia
- Ventricular tachyarrhythmia
- Frequent ectopy (often described as pain by younger patients)

Obstruction leads to increased workload for the left ventricle, resulting in hypertrophy, increased oxygen demand, and diminished coronary reserve. These changes (in addition to limited cardiac output during exercise) can lead to ischemia and arrhythmia.[19,20] Aortic stenosis is often progressive, and symptoms may be absent until late in the disease. If present they include dyspnea with exertion, angina, and syncope. A systolic ejection murmur that radiates to the carotids and a laterally displaced point of maximum impulse because of hypertrophy may be found on examination.

If pain occurs during times of increased myocardial oxygen demand, such as exertion, coronary insufficiency should be a consideration. Repeat ischemic events can lead to myocardial scar, a nidus for potentially dangerous arrhythmias. This insufficiency can be caused by anatomic abnormalities of the coronaries, such as an abnormal vessel origin or an atypical course that results in intraluminal narrowing.[21,22] Autopsy studies have suggested anomalous aortic origin of the coronary artery accounts for approximately 15% of all sudden death in young competitive athletes but true incidence is unknown because not all patients are symptomatic.[4,21,22] Furthermore, coronary vasospasm, congenital heart disease related anomalies, and stenosis or aneurysm following vasculitis (ie, Kawasaki disease) should also be considered.[8,22–24] Exertional symptoms, palpitations, presyncope, or syncope associated with chest pain should all prompt assessment of the coronaries.

Inflammatory processes of the myocardium or pericardium can cause chest pain. Etiologies include viral, bacterial, and autoimmune causes. The extent of inflammation exists on a spectrum involving the pericardium, myocardium, or both (myopericarditis). Typically myopericarditis is a pericardial process extending into the myocardium, whereas myocarditis is primarily within the myocardium, although this is not always clearly defined.[25,26] Importantly, myocarditis should be treated aggressively because there is potential for further sequelae including cardiac arrest.[4] Inflammatory disease most often presents with acute, sharp or squeezing, substernal chest pain. With pericardial involvement the pain is worse with supine positioning leading patients to lean forward. Pain can be worse with inspiration or movement. On auscultation a pericardial friction rub may be appreciated. Effusion, if present, can lead to tamponade and hemodynamic compromise, therefore pulsus paradoxus, jugular venous distention, or profound tachycardia should prompt echocardiography. Pericarditis treatment is typically conservative with nonsteroidal anti-inflammatory drugs unless there is a large effusion or myocardial involvement because these scenarios may require admission and expert consultation.

Evaluation for an arrhythmia may be warranted when assessing chest pain in a pediatric patient. Tachyarrhythmias, such as supraventricular tachycardia, can be interpreted as pain, especially in younger children.[1] Ventricular arrhythmias can present with chest pain, although these patients are likely to also report syncope, exercise intolerance, or aborted sudden cardiac death. Tachycardia itself can cause demand ischemia and/or ventricular dysfunction, but this is rare, depends on type of arrhythmia, and usually requires prolonged episodes. More typically symptoms include self-limited palpitations alongside chest discomfort. If arrhythmia is ongoing or there is predisposition to arrhythmia, EKG will be diagnostic.

### Approach to the Patient with Chest Pain

The evaluation of a patient with chest pain should focus on a detailed history and physical examination because these frequently determine cause.[1,6] It is unusual for a patient with isolated chest pain to present as critically ill, therefore there is often time for investigation.

---

**Box 3**
**Important questions**

- What were you doing when the pain started/stopped?
- How long did the pain last?
- Where did the pain hurt the most?
- Could you do anything to make the pain worse or better?
- Did you pass out when the chest pain happened?
- Did you have pain anywhere else?
- Did you experience trouble breathing associated with the pain?
- Did you feel like your heart was skipping beats when you were having pain?
- How often do you have the pain?

---

*History*

**Box 3** highlights some important historical features. Of primary importance is identifying entities needing acute management. **Box 4** identifies features suggesting cardiac disease. Such features as chronicity or reproducibility argue against cardiac ischemia or acute phenomena, such as pneumothorax or pulmonary embolus. Symptoms of palpitations or shortness of breath are often described as chest pain in children, therefore clarification of this point is necessary. Identifying association with activities (eg, eating, exertion, or stress) is important, as is what follows the pain (eg, vomiting, syncope, headache). History should include a review of systems with attention to symptoms of indigestion, cough or dyspnea, fatigue, activity tolerance, joint pains or redness, edema, fevers, associated illnesses, or recent trauma.

It is important to obtain family, social, medication, and personal medical histories when investigating chest pain. Family history of frequent syncope, sudden cardiac death (including sudden death during exercise or sudden infant death syndrome), congenital heart disease, cardiomyopathy, and arrhythmia are important because entities may be familial.[4] Social history could uncover drug abuse or use of e-cigarettes, which has been associated with lung injury and chest pain.[27–30] A medical history including connective tissue disease, autoimmune disease, or Kawasaki disease may direct one to rule out coronary insufficiency, aortic dissection, pericardial effusion, or pneumothorax.

---

**Box 4**
**Cardiac "red flags"**

- Chest pain with exercise or associated with physical activity
- Chest pain associated with palpitations
- Chest pain associated with syncope
- Family history (first degree) of sudden cardiac death or cardiomyopathy
- Known history of congenital heart disease
- Known history of Kawasaki disease
- Known history of connective tissue disease
- Chest pain associated with EKG abnormalities

---

## Physical examination

Physical examination is always indicated when assessing chest pain, but most pediatric cases have normal examinations.[6] Fever may support an infectious or inflammatory process, whereas desaturation or tachypnea should prompt urgent assessment for an intrapulmonary process, such as pneumonia or pulmonary embolus. Tachycardia is associated with a noncardiac cause, such as anxiety, or more serious pathology, such as arrhythmia, myocarditis, or compensated heart failure. The general appearance of a patient lends information including degree of current distress or features of chronic disease. The chest should be examined for deformity or trauma, including palpation of the costochondral joints, sternum, and ribs. Tenderness of breast tissue, regardless of gender, can occur, especially in adolescents. Lung examination helps evaluate for pulmonary etiologies. Cardiac examination should include palpation for a hyperdynamic precordium or displacement of the PMI. Patients with chest pain and a heart murmur should prompt consideration for referral to a pediatric cardiologist. Systolic ejection quality murmurs may be consistent with aortic valve stenosis, whereas systolic murmurs that disappear when the patient is supine or become louder with Valsalva can occur in hypertrophic cardiomyopathy. Heart sounds should be evaluated for clicks, gallops, rubs, or for accentuated $P_2$ suggesting pulmonary hypertension. Depending on clinical history and examination findings, one should consider connective tissue disease, such as Marfan syndrome.[31]

## Diagnostic testing

Studies have shown that in the absence of specific indications, testing beyond the history and physical is often not helpful.[1,32] There are some patients, however, in whom further testing is indicated.

**Chest radiograph** A chest radiograph is useful to evaluate for pneumonia, pneumothorax, or skeletal abnormality. Cardiomegaly should be further evaluated, but because pericardial effusion or enlarged thymus masquerades as cardiomegaly, two views should be obtained.

**Electrocardiogram** EKG is useful because ST-segment changes in a specific coronary distribution suggest myocardial ischemia, whereas diffuse ST-segment abnormalities are suspicious for pericarditis. Nonspecific repolarization abnormalities may be seen in cardiomyopathy or myocarditis. Lastly, hypertrophy is present in some cardiomyopathies or structural abnormalities. An EKG may also provide evidence of heritable arrhythmias (eg, long QT syndrome) or predisposition to arrhythmia (eg, Wolff-Parkinson-White syndrome), although pediatric EKG interpretation requires caution because findings can be nonspecific and related to age, body habitus, or lead placement.

**Exercise stress test** An exercise stress test allows for dynamic assessment of heart rhythm and evaluation for ischemia during exercise. Exercise stress test is used for patients with exertional symptoms and is most useful when patients are old enough to cooperate while providing maximal effort and symptoms are reproduced during the test.

**Echocardiogram** Echocardiography allows for visualization of the myocardium, ventricular size and function, and anatomic abnormalities. Echocardiography can also be expensive, low yield, and identify incidental findings that lead to clinical dilemmas,[6,33] such as identifying an anomalous right coronary artery arising from the left sinus of Valsalva (it is unclear if anatomy always presents a nidus for ischemia).[21] We therefore highly recommend that echocardiography be obtained in consultation with a cardiologist.

**Laboratory examination** Laboratory tests are infrequently useful in the work-up of chest pain. Troponin testing should be used judiciously given false-positive rates, but is helpful when myocarditis or ischemia are primary concerns.[34]

### Management

Patients with isolated chest pain and an unremarkable history and physical examination often require reassurance only. Initial evaluation is important, because an extensive work-up and referrals leads to increased patient anxiety. Kaden and colleagues[35] reported that in their survey 37% of the adolescents with chest pain were more anxious after visiting their primary doctor. For patients referred to cardiology only about half were then reassured despite no pathology. Patients with an identified organic cause to their pain require appropriate medical treatment and referral as necessary. In particular patients with a red flag for cardiac disease (see **Box 4**) should prompt cardiac evaluation.

## AUSCULTATION AND HEART MURMURS
### Introduction

Advances in diagnostic testing have de-emphasized examination skills and many providers are not confident in their auscultation skills.[36] Early ultrasound education and the expansion of point-of-care ultrasound has made it easy for learners to bypass the intricacies of physical examination.[37–41] The result is the mystification of auscultation. Furthermore, in health care today expensive testing is highly scrutinized, and there is pressure to use medical resources in a responsible manner while avoiding anxiety created by referral to subspecialists.[42–44] Physical examination and auscultation are cost-effective, safe, and accurate in the hands of a skilled practitioner.[45,46] Here we review the skills and practice of cardiac auscultation with emphasis on the evaluation of murmurs.

### Sound

Sounds represent pressure changes transmitted through a medium and organized in a sinusoidal wave (**Fig. 1**) that is described in terms of wavelength and amplitude. Shorter wavelength causes higher pitch and higher amplitude causes louder volume.[47] When waves of sound cause vibration of the tympanic membrane, they are summated and interpreted by the brain as sound.[47] Sound waves that accompany the primary wave are referred to as overtones or undertones. If these tones are related in a predictable pattern, the result is "musical" or "harmonic." If they are chaotic, then you hear "harsh" sound.[47]

### The cardiac cycle

Interpretation of auscultatory findings requires an understanding of the cardiac cycle (**Fig. 2**). The cycle begins with depolarization and action potential propagation through

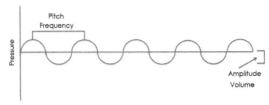

**Fig. 1.** Sound is pressure change over time. Increased amplitude relates to volume, whereas shorter wavelength to higher pitch. (*Courtesy of* Christopher A. Sumski, DO, Milwaukee, WI.)

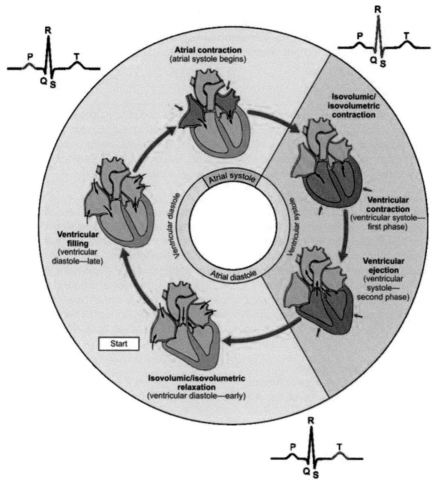

**Fig. 2.** The cardiac cycle. (*From* OpenStax College. Anatomy & physiology – cardiac cycle. Available at: https://openstax.org/books/anatomy-and-physiology/pages/19-3-cardiac-cycle. License: https://creativecommons.org/licenses/by/4.0/legalcode)

the myocardium, causing contraction. This increases the pressure in the ventricular cavity causing atrioventricular valve closure and then semilunar valve opening and ventricular ejection. After ejection, relaxation begins with a decrease in ventricular pressure. When pressure falls lower than that of the great arteries the semilunar valves close. Diastole begins with atrioventricular valves opening and the ventricular filling. After the "atrial kick" at the end of diastole the cycle repeats.

### Heart sounds
Heart sounds result from vibrations in the blood resonating throughout the chest. The first heart sound ($S_1$) occurs with atrioventricular valve closure. Generally $S_1$ is single, because mitral and tricuspid valve closure occurs coincidentally.

The second heart sound ($S_2$) represents the closure of the aortic and pulmonary valves. Higher pressure in the aorta causes the first component of $S_2$ (aortic valve closure, $A_2$) to be earlier and louder than the second component (pulmonary valve closure, $P_2$). This is known as "splitting" of $S_2$. Splitting is widened or accentuated under some circumstances (**Fig. 3**). Increased pulmonary blood flow, such as with atrial septal defects with left to right shunting, produces splitting that does not vary (fixed split $S_2$).

### Approach to Murmurs

Murmurs are the most common reason for referral to pediatric cardiology.[47–49] They are largely benign, only approximately 1% representing pathology.[47] Evaluation should include complete history, including personal, family, and social history. History, in addition to patient age, presence of symptoms, and examination findings, has been helpful in predicting the presence of heart disease without imaging.[45]

### Auscultation method

There are four classic "listening posts" (**Fig. 4**) that correspond to locations where the cardiac valves are best heard. These distinctions are less helpful in children, in particular children with congenital heart disease. Therefore when evaluating patients with murmurs, practitioners should listen throughout the precordium.

Auscultation should be performed with the stethoscope's diaphragm (high frequency sounds) and the bell (low frequency sounds). Listen for one sound at a time. Just as it is difficult to characterize a single instrument in a symphony, it is difficult to interpret a single murmur or sound in the context of many. Abnormal findings should be characterized with the patient supine, sitting, and standing to evaluate changes with position.

### Description of heart sounds

Description is a crucial task in murmur evaluation. It allows for better communication with others and accurate serial evaluation. Complete description includes seven characteristics.

1. Timing: Refers to timing within the cardiac cycle; systolic or diastolic, and early, mid, or late. A murmur is continuous if appreciated throughout the cardiac cycle.
2. Volume: Systolic murmurs are graded 1 to 6. Diastolic murmurs are graded 1 to 4 (**Box 5**).
3. Location: Where a murmur is loudest and where it radiates. Common places for radiation include the back, axillae, or neck.
4. Duration: Murmurs can be short or long, or heard throughout the cycle.
5. Shape: The "shape" of a murmur is a description of the sound. Common shapes include ejection (crescendo-decrescendo), crescendo, decrescendo, and holosystolic (**Fig. 5**).

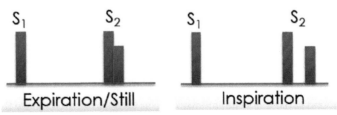

**Fig. 3.** Splitting of $S_2$ with inspiration represents an increase of venous return and an increase in the blood ejected through the pulmonary valve, delaying closure. (*Courtesy of* Christopher A. Sumski, DO, Milwaukee, WI.)

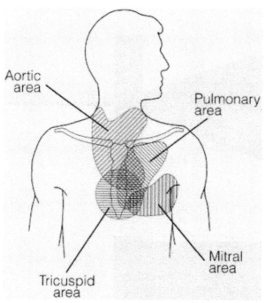

**Fig. 4.** Primary auscultating areas are best thought of as general areas, and not specific discrete locations. (*From* Pelech AN. The cardiac murmur. when to refer? Pediatr Clin North Am 1998;45(1):114; with permission.)

6. Pitch: Pitch is generally high or low. This is related to the pressure gradient causing the turbulence and therefore murmur.
7. Quality: Examples of murmur quality include musical/vibratory, harsh, and machinery-like.

### Common Innocent Murmurs

### Still murmur

A Still murmur is a systolic murmur often noted in children ages 2 to 6 years; however, it has been described in infants and adolescents.[47] The cause is debated but thought to be related to vibration of chordae, relative narrowing of the outflow tracts during

---

**Box 5**
**Murmur grading**

- Systolic murmurs
  - 1/6 – quieter than $S_1$ and $S_2$
  - 2/6 – about the same volume as $S_1$ and $S_2$
  - 3/6 – louder than $S_1$ and $S_2$
  - 4/6 – thrill present, audible with only stethoscope fully on the chest
  - 5/6 – thrill present, audible with stethoscope partially lifted off chest
  - 6/6 – thrill present, audible with stethoscope off chest

- Diastolic murmurs
  - 1/4 – quiet, barely audible
  - 2/4 – quiet but audible
  - 3/4 – clearly audible
  - 4/4 – loud

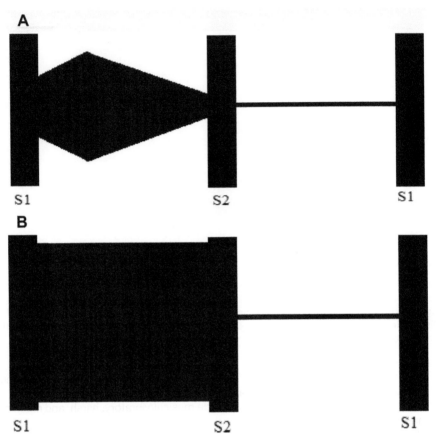

**Fig. 5.** Examples of the shapes of a systolic ejection murmur (*A*) and holosystolic murmur (*B*). (*Courtesy of* Christopher A. Sumski, DO, Milwaukee, WI.)

systole, or semilunar valve leaflet vibration.[47,48,50–53] A Still murmur is vibratory, low frequency, and systolic, loudest at the left lower sternal border and apex. Generally graded 1 to 2/6 and without radiation, it is louder with moving from standing or sitting to supine, whereas lessening or disappearing with Valsalva.[51]

### Peripheral pulmonary stenosis
Peripheral pulmonary stenosis (PPS) typically occurs in infants until 6 to 9 months of age. PPS is secondary to turbulent blood flow in the branch pulmonary arteries. In utero, there is less blood flow to the lungs secondary to the ductus arteriosus and foramen ovale. Given the reduced flow, the branch pulmonary arteries are often small. They are also angled acutely in neonates. With the increase in pulmonary blood flow after birth, turbulence can occur.[54] A PPS murmur is graded 1 to 2/6, systolic ejection quality, and moderately pitched. It is loudest over the left upper sternal border (LUSB) and radiates to the axillae and back. Persistence past 1 year or a murmur that gets louder on re-examination should prompt referral to pediatric cardiology.

### Pulmonary flow murmurs
A benign pulmonary flow murmur is heard in many infants, children, and adolescents. The murmur is similar to that of PPS without much radiation. Typically it is heard over

the LUSB and is loudest when supine, diminishing when holding inspiration or upright positioning. The murmur is differentiated from pulmonary valve stenosis because valvar stenosis is higher pitch, louder, and often accompanied by a click. The pulmonary flow murmur is louder when there is a higher output state, such as with fever, anemia, or recent β-agonist therapy.

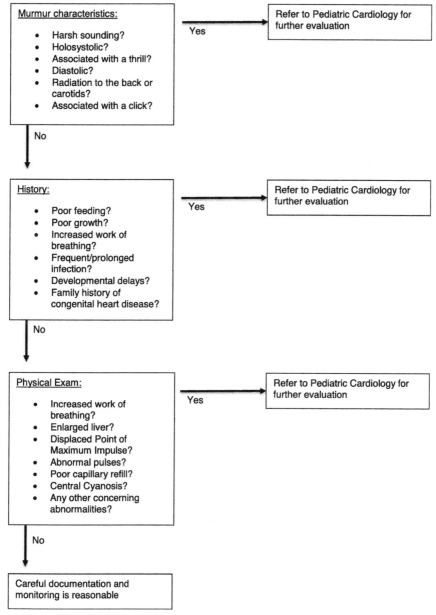

**Fig. 6.** Decision-making algorithm for murmur evaluation.

### Venous hum

A venous hum is a low-pitched, continuous murmur in children located over the anterior neck extending to just inferior to the clavicle. Usually it is loudest on the patient's right side. It is thought to be caused by the convergence of venous streams from the internal jugular and subclavian veins.[55] The murmur is louder with the patient sitting upright, looking away from the examiner and diminished with jugular compression or turning the head toward the side with the murmur.

### Pathologic Murmurs

When putting abnormal murmur features together, one can create a differential. A holosystolic shape typically represents atrioventricular valve insufficiency or a ventricular septal defect. If accompanied by a thrill then this may represent a ventricular septal defect with significant pressure gradient. Early decrescendo systolic murmurs may represent tiny muscular ventricular septal defects. A crescendo-decrescendo systolic murmur represents systolic ejection, and may reflect pathology in the outflow tracts or semilunar valves. Murmurs of semilunar valve stenosis often include a click, a sharp noise during systole caused by stenotic leaflet motion. Furthermore, an associated thrill suggests advanced stenosis. Lower frequency machinery-like, continuous murmurs are often associated with a patent ductus arteriosus.

### Management

Evaluation of any child with a heart murmur should include a thorough history and physical examination. Decision-making should be done in a holistic context. Thriving children are less likely to have cardiac disease. Murmurs that are musical, vibratory, systolic ejection, vary with position, and 1 to 2/6 are likely innocent and generally need only reassessment at all visits.[43,47,56] A concerning history, such as failure to thrive, poor feeding, or frequent respiratory infections, should lower the threshold for referral.

Concerning murmurs (**Fig. 6**) include harsh, higher grade, diastolic, or murmurs that radiate to the neck/carotids. Murmurs quieter with supine positioning and louder with standing are abnormal. Murmurs (even innocent murmurs) occurring in the setting of other abnormal examination findings warrant further evaluation.

### DISCLOSURE

The authors have nothing to disclose.
Funding: None.

### REFERENCES

1. Cava JR, Sayger PL. Chest pain in children and adolescents. Pediatr Clin North Am 2004;51(6):1553–68.

2. Gesuete V, Fregolent D, Contorno S, et al. Follow-up study of patients admitted to the pediatric emergency department for chest pain. Eur J Pediatr 2019. https://doi.org/10.1007/s00431-019-03495-5.

3. Kane DA, Fulton DR, Saleeb S, et al. Needles in hay: chest pain as the presenting symptom in children with serious underlying cardiac pathology: chest pain as presenting symptom in children. Congenit Heart Dis 2010;5(4):366–73.

4. Maron BJ, Haas TS, Ahluwalia A, et al. Demographics and epidemiology of sudden deaths in young competitive athletes: from the United States National Registry. Am J Med 2016;129(11):1170–7.

5. Harmon KG, Asif IM, Klossner D, et al. Incidence of sudden cardiac death in National Collegiate Athletic Association athletes. Circulation 2011;123(15): 1594–600.

6. Saleeb SF, Li WYV, Warren SZ, et al. Effectiveness of screening for life-threatening chest pain in children. Pediatrics 2011;128(5):e1062–8.

7. Pantell RH, Goodman BW. Adolescent chest pain: a prospective study. J Am Acad Child Psychiatry 1983;22(5):510.

8. Veeram Reddy SR, Singh H. Chest pain in children and adolescents. Pediatr Rev 2010;31(1):e1–9.

9. Driscoll DJ, Glicklich L, Gallen W. Chest pain in children: a prospective study. Pediatrics 1976;57(5):648–51.

10. McMahon LE. Slipping rib syndrome: a review of evaluation, diagnosis and treatment. Semin Pediatr Surg 2018;27(3):183–8.

11. Wiens L, Portnoy J, Sabath R, et al. Chest pain in otherwise healthy children and adolescents is frequently caused by exercise-induced asthma. Pediatrics 1992; 90(3):350–3.

12. Di Nisio M, van Es N, Büller HR. Deep vein thrombosis and pulmonary embolism. Lancet 2016;388(10063):3060–73.

13. Nixon C. Current perspectives: the impact of cyberbullying on adolescent health. Adolesc Health Med Ther 2014;143. https://doi.org/10.2147/AHMT.S36456.

14. Westover AN, Nakonezny PA, Haley RW. Acute myocardial infarction in young adults who abuse amphetamines. Drug Alcohol Depend 2008;96(1–2):49–56.

15. Qureshi AI, Suri MFK, Guterman LR, et al. Cocaine use and the likelihood of nonfatal myocardial infarction and stroke: data from the third national health and nutrition examination survey. Circulation 2001;103(4):502–6.

16. Shah M. Hypertrophic cardiomyopathy. Cardiol Young 2017;27(S1):S25–30.

17. Klues HG, Schiffers A, Maron BJ. Phenotypic spectrum and patterns of left ventricular hypertrophy in hypertrophic cardiomyopathy: morphologic observations and significance as assessed by two-dimensional echocardiography in 600 patients. J Am Coll Cardiol 1995;26(7):1699–708.

18. Geske JB, Ommen SR, Gersh BJ. Hypertrophic cardiomyopathy. JACC Heart Fail 2018;6(5):364–75.

19. Carabello B, Paulus W. Aortic stenosis. Lancet 2009;373:956–66.

20. Frank S, Johnson A, Ross J. Natural history of valvular aortic stenosis. Heart 1973;35(1):41–6.

21. Angelini P. Coronary artery anomalies: an entity in search of an identity. Circulation 2007;115(10):1296–305.

22. Molossi S, Sachdeva S. Anomalous coronary arteries: what is known and what still remains to be learned? Curr Opin Cardiol 2020;35(1):42–51.

23. Takahashi M. Cardiac ischemia in pediatric patients. Pediatr Clin North Am 2010; 57(6):1261–80.

24. Picard F, Sayah N, Spagnoli V, et al. Vasospastic angina: A literature review of current evidence. Arch Cardiovasc Dis 2019;112(1):44–55.

25. Kobayashi D, Aggarwal S, Kheiwa A, et al. Myopericarditis in children: elevated troponin I level does not predict outcome. Pediatr Cardiol 2012;33(7):1040–5.

26. Imazio M, Trinchero R. Myopericarditis: etiology, management, and prognosis. Int J Cardiol 2008;127(1):17–26.

27. Sommerfeld CG, Weiner DJ, Nowalk A, et al. Hypersensitivity pneumonitis and acute respiratory distress syndrome from E-cigarette use. Pediatrics 2018; 141(6):e20163927.

28. Siegel DA, Jatlaoui TC, Koumans EH, et al. Update: interim guidance for health care providers evaluating and caring for patients with suspected e-cigarette, or vaping, product use associated lung injury—United States, October 2019. MMWR Morb Mortal Wkly Rep 2019;68(41):9.

29. Thakrar PD, Boyd KP, Swanson CP, et al. E-cigarette, or vaping, product use-associated lung injury in adolescents: a review of imaging features. Pediatr Radiol 2020. https://doi.org/10.1007/s00247-019-04572-5.

30. Kalininskiy A, Bach CT, Nacca NE, et al. E-cigarette, or vaping, product use associated lung injury (EVALI): case series and diagnostic approach. Lancet Respir Med 2019;7(12):1017–26.

31. Loeys BL, Dietz HC, Braverman AC, et al. The revised Ghent nosology for the Marfan syndrome. J Med Genet 2010;47(7):476–85.

32. Driscoll DJ, Glicklich L, Gallen W. Chest pain in children: A prospective Study. Pediatrics 1976;57(5):648–51.

33. Epstein S, Gerber L, Borer J. Chest wall syndrome: a common cause of unexplained cardiac pain. J Am Med Assoc 1979;241(26):2793–7.

34. Harris TH, Gossett JG. Diagnosis and diagnostic modalities in pediatric patients with elevated troponin. Pediatr Cardiol 2016;37(8):1469–74.

35. Kaden G, Shenker R, Gootman N. Chest pain in adolescents. J Adolesc Health 1991;12(3):251–5.

36. Mangione S. The teaching and practice of cardiac auscultation during internal medicine and cardiology training: a nationwide survey. Ann Intern Med 1993; 119(1):47.

37. Kimura BJ. Point-of-care cardiac ultrasound techniques in the physical examination: better at the bedside. Heart 2017;103(13):987–94.

38. Patel SG, Benninger B, Mirjalili SA. Integrating ultrasound into modern medical curricula. Clin Anat 2017;30(4):452–60.

39. Dolara A. The decline of cardiac auscultation: 'the ball of the match point is poised on the net'. J Cardiovasc Med 2008;9(11):1173–4.

40. Cardim N, Fernandez Golfin C, Ferreira D, et al. Usefulness of a new miniaturized echocardiographic system in outpatient cardiology consultations as an extension of physical examination. J Am Soc Echocardiogr 2011;24(2):117–24.

41. Mehta M, Jacobson T, Peters D, et al. Handheld ultrasound versus physical examination in patients referred for transthoracic echocardiography for a suspected cardiac condition. JACC Cardiovasc Imaging 2014;7(10):983–90.

42. Geggel RL, Horowitz LM, Brown EA, et al. Parental anxiety associated with referral of a child to a pediatric cardiologist for evaluation of a Still's murmur. J Pediatr 2002;140(6):747–52.

43. Campbell RM, Douglas PS, Eidem BW, et al. ACC/AAP/AHA/ASE/HRS/SCAI/SCCT/SCMR/SOPE 2014 Appropriate use criteria for initial transthoracic echocardiography in outpatient pediatric cardiology. J Am Soc Echocardiogr 2014; 27(12):1247–66.

44. Danford DA, Nasir A, Gumbiner C. Cost assessment of the evaluation of heart murmurs in children. Pediatrics 1993;91(2):365–8.

45. Newburger J, Rosenthal A, Williams R, et al. Noninvasive tests in the initial evaluation of heart murmurs in children. N Engl J Med 1983;308(2):61–4.

46. Fuster V. The stethoscope's prognosis. J Am Coll Cardiol 2016;67(9):1118–9.

47. Pelech AN. The physiology of cardiac auscultation. Pediatr Clin North Am 2004; 51(6):1515–35.

48. Smythe JF, Teixeira OHP, Demers P. Initial evaluation of heart murmurs: are laboratory tests necessary? Pediatrics 1990;86(4):497–500.

49. McCrindle BW. Factors prompting referral for cardiology evaluation of heart murmurs in children. Arch Pediatr Adolesc Med 1995;149(11):1277.
50. Fogel D. The innocent systolic murmur in children: a clinical study of its incidence and characteristics. Am Heart J 1960;59(6):844–55.
51. Biancaniello T. Innocent murmurs. Circulation 2005;111(3). https://doi.org/10.1161/01.CIR.0000153388.41229.CB.
52. Schwartz ML, Goldberg SJ, Wilson N, et al. Relation of Still's murmur, small aortic diameter and high aortic velocity. Am J Cardiol 1986;57(15):1344–8.
53. Stein PD, Sabbah HN. Aortic origin of innocent murmurs. Am J Cardiol 1977;39(5):665–71.
54. Danilowicz DA, Rudolph AM, Hoffman JIE, et al. Physiologic pressure differences between main and branch pulmonary arteries in infants. Circulation 1972;45(2):410–9.
55. Cutforth R, Wiseman J, Sutherland RD. The genesis of the cervical venous hum. Am Heart J 1970;80(4):488–92.
56. Rosenthal A. How to distinguish between innocent and pathologic murmurs in childhood. Pediatr Clin North Am 1984;31(6):1229–40.

# Syncope and Palpitations
## A Review

Johannes C. von Alvensleben, MD

## KEYWORDS

- Syncope • Palpitations • Vasovagal • Supraventricular tachycardia
- Wolff-Parkinson-White • Ectopy

## KEY POINTS

- Syncope and palpitations are some of the most common referrals to pediatric cardiology and frequently have a benign etiology.
- A carefully planned approach to syncope is preferred to avoid an involved and expensive diagnosis evaluation.
- Vasovagal syncope, although benign, can cause a major impact on lifestyle but frequently can be treated successfully with nonpharmacologic interventions.
- Patient history often can distinguish nonarrhythmogenic palpitations from those caused by supraventricular tachycardia accurately.

## SYNCOPE

### Introduction

Syncope is defined as the transient loss of consciousness and postural tone resulting from an abrupt, temporary decrease in cerebral blood flow. It is one of the most common referrals to pediatric cardiology.[1-3] There is an estimated 30% lifetime risk.[1] A majority of episodes are self-limited and benign and are known as vasovagal syncope, or simple fainting. It is a disorder of heart rate and blood pressure control by the autonomic nervous system that causes hypotension or bradycardia. Rarely, syncope can be the first warning sign of a serious condition, such as arrhythmia, structural heart disease, or noncardiac disease.[4] Even vasovagal syncope, if recurrent, can cause a major impact on lifestyle, interfering with school and/or sports. Many states impose driving restrictions following syncope.[5] Therefore, accurate diagnosis and counseling are important.

### Diagnostic Evaluation

Given the many possible causes of syncope, a carefully planned approach is preferred to avoid an involved and expensive diagnostic evaluation. The patient history, family

Funding: None.

Children's Hospital Colorado, University of Colorado School of Medicine, 13123 East 16th Avenue, B100, Aurora, CO 80045, USA

*E-mail address:* Johannes.vonAlvensleben@childrenscolorado.org

history, physical examination, and an electrocardiogram (EKG) are fundamental and direct the remainder of the evaluation. Important historical details include the age of the patient (syncope is rare before 10 years of age except for breathing holding syncope),[4,6,7] time of day (early morning is typical), state of hydration and nutrition at the time of the event (last fluid or food intake), environmental conditions (ambient temperature), patient's activity or body position immediately prior to the syncope episode, frequency and duration of the episodes, and any aura, prodrome, or specific symptoms prior to the episode. Witnesses should provide details regarding the patient's condition prior to syncope, duration of loss of consciousness, any injuries or seizure-like movements, loss of bowel or bladder function, heart rate during episode, and duration and nature of recovery. Medication history (prescription and over-the-counter supplements) is critical and may point to proarrhythmic potential. Additionally, a history of severe viral illness, such as infectious mononucleosis, frequently precedes the development of vasovagal syncope. Pertinent positives of the past medical history include neurologic disorders, traumatic brain injury, and neurosurgical interventions.

It is not uncommon to elicit a history of multiple family members who experienced syncope during adolescence that subsequently resolved. If the family history is positive for recurrent syncope, however, it also is important to consider familial disorders and question about the presence of hypertrophic or dilated cardiomyopathy, long QT syndrome, Brugada syndrome, exertional syncope (to consider catecholaminergic polymorphic ventricular tachycardia [CPVT]), primary pulmonary hypertension, or arrhythmogenic right ventricular cardiomyopathy (ARVC).[4,5,8–15] Additionally, families should be asked about sudden unexplained death in children or young adults (drownings, single-car accidents, sudden cardiac death, and sudden infant death syndrome), seizures, and congenital deafness. A genetic counselor frequently can be helpful in organizing the family history.

On physical examination, the general condition should be noted, with particular emphasis on hydration, nutritional status (evidence of eating disorders), and manifestations of thyroid disease. Orthostatic vital signs should be obtained, but care must be taken to follow a strict protocol to avoid false-positive results. Orthostatic hypotension is defined as a decrease in systolic blood pressure of 20 mm Hg or a decrease in diastolic blood pressure of 10 mm Hg after 3 minutes of standing compared with blood pressure in the supine or sitting position. Pulse strength, rate, and any differences between upper and lower extremities should be noted. The presence of heart murmurs suggesting anatomic disease should prompt an echocardiogram. Finally, a phenotype of inherited connective tissue disorders (ie, Marfan syndrome) should be considered.

An EKG should be obtained, particularly if syncope is recurrent or occurs with exercise. It should be evaluated for heart rate, corrected QT interval, T-wave abnormalities (including T-wave alternans), or any ventricular arrhythmias as well as for ventricular preexcitation, atrioventricular (AV) conduction disturbances, or features consistent with Brugada syndrome.[9–12] All patients with exertional syncope, even those with positive orthostatic vital signs, should undergo additional evaluation with an echocardiogram and exercise stress testing. Echocardiograms are necessary to examine for cardiomyopathy, myocarditis, anomalous coronary arteries, pulmonary arterial hypertension, and ARVC. An exercise test is necessary for CPVT. Additional testing may include a signal averaged EKG, Holter monitor, magnetic resonance imaging (MRI), cardiac catheterization, and invasive electrophysiologic testing. Tilt table testing is performed less commonly in pediatric patients because a diagnosis of vasovagal syncope does not require a positive tilt test and results of unclear significance (ie, prolonged asystolic pauses) are common.

### Vasovagal/Neurocardiogenic Syncope

#### Pathophysiology/clinical presentation

By far the most common etiology for syncope in pediatrics is vasovagal or neurocardiogenic syncope. Although the pathophysiologic mechanisms are heterogenous and not completely understood, it is thought to be primarily a response of the cardiac–central nervous system reflex.[16–18] The most common initiating event is prolonged or rapid assumption of an upright position, which results in gravitationally mediated venous pooling in the lower extremities. This causes central hypovolemia leading to decreased venous return and stroke volume. Alternatively, an emotional or physical stress (pain or fright) or a reflex mechanism related to hair grooming, deglutition syncope (swallowing), or micturition can trigger this sequence by creating a sympathetic response characterized by tachycardia and vasoconstriction. This increased sympathetic output may result in a subsequent parasympathetic response characterized by bradycardia or asystole. Additionally, the abrupt withdrawal of sympathetically mediated tachycardia despite persistent peripheral vasodilation causes a decrease in systemic blood pressure and venous return/stroke volume.[19,20]

As a result of loss of consciousness, the patient falls into a supine state, which restores venous return and central blood volume. The loss of consciousness is short (<1–2 min), with rapid return to baseline behavior. Bowel or bladder incontinence is uncommon and, although seizures rarely occur, myoclonic jerks are common. A prodrome, consisting of nausea, epigastric pain, clammy sensation, pallor, dizziness, lightheadedness, tunnel vision, and weakness, is very characteristic of vasovagal or neurocardiogenic syncope. Some patients with profound bradycardia or asystole may have little to no warning and typically require additional evaluation to confirm the diagnosis. If the prodrome is of sufficient duration, patients may learn to recognize it and lie down to prevent complete loss of consciousness.[20]

#### Therapy

Maintaining adequate intravascular volume is the mainstay of treatment of vasovagal syncope.[1,17,20–22] Although choosing a fluid volume goal is acceptable, having patients target clear urine at least 5 times per day ensures appropriate intake. Increased salt intake with salt tablets or simply increased dietary sources (a handful of salted peanuts or crackers) also is recommended. Counter-regulatory maneuvers, such as leg pumping, leg crossing, and squatting, can ameliorate the presyncopal symptoms and frequently avoid complete loss of consciousness. Finally, regular aerobic exercise should be encouraged because it strengthens the muscles of the lower extremities and improves vascular tone. Medications can be useful although these frequently rely on adequate hydration for effectiveness.

There are only limited randomized studies of medications in pediatric patients.[23–28] Fludrocortisone is a mineralocorticoid that results in renal salt resorption and thus increases intravascular volume. Nonrandomized and nonblinded studies in pediatric patients demonstrated a decrease in the frequency and severity of syncopal events. The fluid resorption effect of fludrocortisone comes at the expense of urinary potassium and serum electrolytes must be followed to prevent excessive hypokalemia. Although uncommon, hypertension can occur, especially when fludrocortisone is combined with other agents, such as α-agonists.

α-Agonists act through their vasoconstrictor effects with venoconstriction maintaining preload and arterial constriction preventing reflex hypotension. The primary oral α-agonist is midodrine but its utility is limited by the necessity for 3-times daily administration. Randomized studies have revealed that midodrine, even as monotherapy, was effective in vasovagal syncope, although supine hypertension may be more common than previously suspected. Patients should be advised not to take midodrine just prior to sleeping.

Although β-blockers have been used for treatment of syncope by targeting the increased sympathetic output with resultant parasympathetic response, the side effects may mask the therapeutic benefits and there is a paucity of data regarding their effectiveness. Mood suppression, particularly in adolescent patients, is a known and potentially serious adverse effect. Cardioselective β-blockers may have a reduced incidence of noncardiac effects though the most effective agent for the prevention of syncope (propranolol) is nonselective and is most beneficial in its short-acting form.

Vagolytic agents (disopyramide) help control hypervagotonia, and the selective serotonin reuptake inhibitors also have been effective in alleviating symptoms in select patients.

## PALPITATIONS
### Introduction

The complaint of palpitations is a common presenting concern that patients bring to their primary care provider. Although a vast majority of patients have no life-threatening cause for their symptoms, it can present a diagnostic challenge to providers and frequently results in a referral to other specialists.[29–31] Understanding the most common causes for palpitations or syncope, as well as the red flags that should prompt a more intensive work-up or referral, can make the evaluation of these complaints more manageable.[32–34]

Palpitations are the perceived abnormality of the heartbeat characterized by awareness of cardiac muscle contractions in the chest: hard, fast, and/or irregular beats. They are both symptoms reported by the patient and a medical diagnosis but do not necessarily imply a structural or functional abnormality of the heart. In general, the provider is attempting to determine whether the palpitations are secondary to an arrhythmia, with the most common diagnoses being supraventricular tachycardia (SVT), premature atrial contractions (PACs), and premature ventricular contractions (PVCs).

### Diagnosis: History

When determining whether palpitations likely are secondary to an arrhythmia, the history can be helpful. Several important aspects include

- Onset and termination: Are they abrupt or gradual?
- Rate: Can the rate be counted or is it "too fast to count"?
- Association with rest or exercise
- Association with chest pain, shortness of breath, dizziness, or syncope
- Duration: Do palpitations last for seconds or hours?
- Frequency: Do they occur daily (or several times per day) or less often?

SVT, with the different subcategories described later, typically has an abrupt onset and termination and may be described by younger patients as "heart beeping."[35] The rate usually is too fast to count and has the sensation of "buzzing" under the fingertips. It commonly is associated with chest discomfort, shortness of breath, and occasionally dizziness. Syncope is quite rare. Younger patients frequently experience SVT while at rest, whereas adolescent patients develop SVT during exercise. This presentation is secondary to the differing SVT mechanisms that are more common in these age groups; younger patients are far more likely to have accessory pathway–mediated SVT and adolescent patients developing AV nodal reentrant tachycardia (AVNRT). Daily symptoms that last for only a few seconds are much less likely to be SVT.

Extrasystoles, PACs and PVCs, commonly are asymptomatic in pediatric patients. When sensed, they frequently are the pause after the premature beat and the more forceful subsequent sinus beat that causes the most discomfort. Patients describe distinct and hard beats that are in contrast to the rapid and less forceful beats of SVT.[36,37]

### Diagnosis: Other History and Physical Examination

In general, family history is less helpful to determine whether an arrhythmia is to blame for palpitations.[29] Although PVCs tend to run in families, their overall prevalence is so high that a positive family history rarely is predictive. Family members requiring cardiac interventions at a young age, either in childhood or young adulthood, should be noted.

Like family history, the physical examination also is unlikely to assist in the diagnosis. Although extrasystoles or an irregular rhythm may suggest atrial or ventricular ectopy, sinus arrhythmia presents similarly and is a normal finding. A murmur can point to specific structural heart abnormalities, which may or may not be related.

### Diagnosis: Testing

Providers can determine whether an arrhythmia is occurring with an EKG, Holter monitor, and/or transient event monitor. Knowing the clinical utility of each can assist the provider in selecting the correct test.

- An EKG is best used to assess the presence of an ongoing arrhythmia (PACs or PVCs) or potential risk of arrhythmia (ventricular preexcitation suggesting Wolff-Parkinson-White syndrome).
- A Holter monitor is used to determine the overall frequency of ectopy or to assess heart variability in the setting of baseline bradycardia or tachycardia. It typically is not useful in the evaluation of episodic palpitations.
- A transient event monitor is usually the most useful in assessing episodic palpitations, particularly for the documentation of SVT.

### Specific Diagnoses

#### Premature atrial contractions

In a vast majority of patients, the diagnosis of isolated PACs is an incidental finding and not related specifically to palpitations. In these circumstances, PACs do not contribute to symptoms, do not cause cardiac pathology (myopathy), and do not require ongoing follow-up.[30,31]

Referral is indicated in the setting of an ectopic atrial tachycardia, which is detected most commonly on a Holter monitor or transient event monitor. In this case, a baseline echocardiogram is obtained to rule out structural heart disease or the development of a tachycardia-induced cardiomyopathy. Medications, most frequently a β-blocker, can be used to control the ectopic focus, although many patients eventually undergo an electrophysiologic study and ablation. Exercise restrictions typically are not necessary unless a known structural abnormality or cardiomyopathy is present.

#### Premature ventricular contractions

As with PACs, PVCs most commonly are an incidental finding during routine evaluations. Unlike PACs, however, even isolated or asymptomatic PVCs should prompt a referral to cardiology because there is a risk of ectopy-induced cardiomyopathies.

PVCs may arise from almost any location in the ventricles, although a right ventricular or left ventricular outflow tract origin accounts for the vast majority, particularly in otherwise healthy individuals. Providers can use a 12-lead EKG to predict this, with a positive PVC deflection in limb leads I, II, and aVF and a negative PVC deflection in the precordial lead V1.[38,39] Locations other than the outflow tracts typically prompt a more intensive evaluation. All patients should have an EKG and a baseline 24-hour Holter monitor. In those cases where PVC origin is the outflow tract, the EKG is reassuring, and the 24-hour ectopic burden is less than 10%, no additional follow-up typically is necessary. Patients are not restricted from athletic participation from a cardiac perspective. When the ectopic burden is greater than 10%, some degree of follow-up typically is recommended, with the most common annual evaluations with a repeat EKG. As before, athletic participation is not restricted.[40]

Exercise stress tests typically are reserved for patients with atypical PVC morphologies (nonoutflow tract origin) or if there is a potential association with symptoms and/or syncope. Outflow tract–mediated PVCs typically are suppressed by exercise. A history of exertional symptoms, in particular syncope, necessitates a stress test to evaluate for CPVT. Increasing PVC frequency, the development of nonsustained ventricular tachycardia, and evidence of ischemia (repolarization abnormalities, such as ST segment elevation/depression or T-wave changes) all are strongly suggestive of a pathologic PVC etiology. Additional evaluation tools include cardiac MRI to assess for cardiac fibrosis or morphologic predictors for ARVC and a signal-averaged EKG.[41]

As with PACs, a majority of patients with PVCs do not require intervention, although providers can utilize β-blockade for symptomatic ectopy. Ablation procedures are reserved for symptomatic patients not controlled with medications or those with the development of cardiomyopathies.

### Supraventricular tachycardia

SVT is the most common tachyarrhythmia in pediatrics (excluding sinus tachycardia), with an incidence of approximately 1:1000. Many patients present in the first year of life and 90% of pediatric SVTs involve a reentrant circuit between the atria and ventricles.[42,43]

As described previously, the mechanism of SVT can vary in the younger versus older pediatric patients with accessory pathways (either concealed or Wolff-Parkinson-White syndrome) more common in younger patients. AVNRT is the most likely cause of SVT in adolescents and young adults. Also included within the category of SVT is atrial flutter, ectopic atrial tachycardia, and atrial fibrillation. With the exception of ectopic atrial tachycardia, these other mechanisms are uncommon in pediatric patients in the absence of congenital heart disease.[44,45]

Accessory pathways are anomalous strands of myocardium that bridge the groove between atria and ventricles, supporting a reentrant tachycardia.[46–49] In the typical baseline state, electrical activation of the ventricular myocardium proceeds from the atrium via the AV node and His-Purkinje system. The AV valves (tricuspid and mitral) provide an electrically insulating buffer that directs activation from the atria to the AV node. Antegrade activation of the ventricular myocardium through an accessory fiber results in early depolarization as conduction reaches the ventricles in advance of activation through the AV node–His-Purkinje system (ventricular preexcitation). On an EKG, this can be observed as manifest accessory pathway conduction as evidenced by a short PR interval, delta wave, and a widened QRS complex. Concealed accessory pathways allow only for retrograde conduction (ventricles to atria) are not evident on a baseline EKG.

Although common, the percentage of children with SVT having accessory pathway-mediated SVT diminishes with age: 85% in children less than 1 year, 82% in children between 1 year and 5 years, and 56% in children between 6 years and 10 years.

Despite the frequency of the arrhythmia in children, between 15% and 40% of infants under 6 months of age having documented SVT do not have recurrence beyond the first year of life.[43]

There are few estimates of the incidence of AVNRT in children. Although it is the most common mechanism of regular SVT in adults, AVNRT is uncommon in small children, comprising up to 3% to 13% of infant SVTs. Its relative incidence increases across the pediatric age range, equaling and then exceeding that of accessory pathway–mediated SVT during the teenage years. In addition to the sensation of palpitations and association with activity, patients may complain of pulsations in the neck, often visible to parents or other observers, due to oscillations in central venous pressure caused by simultaneous contraction of atria and ventricles. This presentation may be more common in AVNRT although formal studies have not been performed.

*Diagnosis and initial evaluation*
A baseline EKG is necessary to evaluate for ventricular preexcitation (described previously) but intermittent preexcitation also may be seen on a Holter monitor or transient event monitor. A diagnosis of SVT relies on documentation of the arrhythmia, either on a transient event monitor or a 12-lead EKG during active palpitations. A Holter monitor is much less useful in this case because of the transient and episodic nature of SVT. Prior to diagnosis, providers can review vagal maneuvers with patients for whom a strong suspicion of SVT is suggested by the history.

A screening echocardiogram should be performed to assess for structural abnormalities. Although most patients with SVT structurally have normal hearts, the presence of congenital heart disease, in particular Ebstein anomaly, and L-transposition of the great arteries, predisposes to accessory pathways. Patients with Wolff-Parkinson-White syndrome and congenital heart disease tend to have multiple pathways.[44]

*Management*
In the absence of Wolff-Parkinson-White syndrome, SVT is rarely a life-threatening condition and management options include observation with vagal maneuvers, antiarrhythmics for rhythm control, and electrophysiologic study/ablation. All pediatric patients with ventricular preexcitation are recommended to undergo invasive testing, given the risk of preexcited atrial fibrillation and sudden death.

The decision regarding treatment is governed largely by the features of each individual patient. They include the frequency of episodes, duration of symptoms, severity of symptoms with episodes, response to prior medications, and the patient's and family's understanding and views regarding the various options.[45,50–55] Patients who have minimal symptoms with episodes that are short and self-terminating or respond to vagal maneuvers may pursue no further treatment.

Episodes of SVT may be responsive to antiarrhythmic agents and their selection is guided by underlying substrate and patient age. β-Blockers are a common first-line agent, with their effect mediated by a reduction in SVT triggers (premature beats) or by slowing accessory pathway or AV nodal conduction. Fatigue, mood suppression, and exercise limitations can occur, particularly in adolescent patients. Digoxin remains in wide use, although should be avoided in patients with ventricular preexcitation because it may precipitate enhanced antegrade conduction via the accessory pathway. For this same reason, calcium channel blocking agents also are contraindicated in Wolff-Parkinson-White syndrome. Class I medications, such as flecainide, often are effective in refractory cases of SVT. Amiodarone and sotalol, both class III agents, also are second-line or third-line medications, primarily reserved for after multiple other agents fail or for those with congenital heart disease.

Ablation of the SVT substrate, using transcatheter radiofrequency current or cryo-therapy, now is performed regularly for the elimination of symptomatic SVT in children.[50,52] For many pediatric electrophysiologists, ablation is offered as first-line therapy in those deemed low risk for complications. In the current era, patients weighing greater than 15 kg have a similar complication profile as adolescents and young adults. Those with congenital heart disease, in particular complex or single ventricle disease, have a significantly higher complication and recurrence risks. In otherwise healthy patients, the overall long-term success rate is greater than 90%, with some substrates, in particular left-sided accessory pathways, approaching 100% SVT elimination.

## DISCLOSURE

The author has nothing to disclose.

## REFERENCES

1. Kapoor WN. Syncope. N Engl J Med 2000;343:1856.
2. Lewis DA, Dhala A. Syncope in the pediatric patient. The cardiologist's perspective. Pediatr Clin North Am 1999;46:205.
3. Friedman KG, Alexander ME. Chest pain and syncope in children: a practical approach to the diagnosis of cardiac disease. J Pediatr 2013;163:896.
4. Gillette PC, Garson A Jr. Sudden cardiac death in the pediatric population. Circulation 1992;85:164.
5. Strickberger SA, Benson DW, Biaggioni I, et al. AHA/ACCF Scientific Statement on the evaluation of syncope: from the American Heart Association Councils on Clinical Cardiology, Cardiovascular Nursing, Cardiovascular Disease in the Young, and Stroke, and the Quality of Care and Outcomes Research Interdisciplinary Working Group; and the American College of Cardiology Foundation: in collaboration with the Heart Rhythm Society: endorsed by the American Autonomic Society. Circulation 2006;113:316.
6. Pratt JL, Fleisher GR. Syncope in children and adolescents. Pediatr Emerg Care 1989;5:80.
7. Massin MM, Bourguignont A, Coremans C, et al. Syncope in pediatric patients presenting to an emergency department. J Pediatr 2004;145:223.
8. Alexander ME, Berul CI. Ventricular arrhythmias: when to worry. Pediatr Cardiol 2000;21:532.
9. Mivelaz Y, Di Bernardo S, Pruvot E, et al. Brugada syndrome in childhood: a potential fatal arrhythmia not always recognised by paediatricians. A case report and review of the literature. Eur J Pediatr 2006;165:507.
10. Probst V, Evain S, Gournay V, et al. Monomorphic ventricular tachycardia due to Brugada syndrome successfully treated by hydroquinidine therapy in a 3-year-old child. J Cardiovasc Electrophysiol 2006;17:97.
11. Probst V, Denjoy I, Meregalli PG, et al. Clinical aspects and prognosis of Brugada syndrome in children. Circulation 2007;115:2042.
12. Skinner JR, Chung SK, Nel CA, et al. Brugada syndrome masquerading as febrile seizures. Pediatrics 2007;119:e1206.
13. Basso C, Corrado D, Rossi L, et al. Ventricular preexcitation in children and young adults: atrial myocarditis as a possible trigger of sudden death. Circulation 2001;103:269.
14. Schimpf R, Wolpert C, Gaita F, et al. Short QT syndrome. Cardiovasc Res 2005; 67:357.

15. Maron BJ. Sudden death in young athletes. N Engl J Med 2003;349:1064.
16. Igarashi M, Boehm RM Jr, May WN, et al. Syncope associated with hair-grooming. Brain Dev 1988;10:249.
17. DiMario FJ Jr. Prospective study of children with cyanotic and pallid breath-holding spells. Pediatrics 2001;107:265.
18. DiMario FJ Jr, Burleson JA. Autonomic nervous system function in severe breath-holding spells. Pediatr Neurol 1993;9:268.
19. DiMario FJ Jr, Bauer L, Baxter D. Respiratory sinus arrhythmia in children with severe cyanotic and pallid breath-holding spells. J Child Neurol 1998;13:440.
20. Scott WA. Evaluating the child with syncope. Pediatr Ann 1991;20:350.
21. Singer W, Sletten DM, Opfer-Gehrking TL, et al. Postural tachycardia in children and adolescents: what is abnormal? J Pediatr 2012;160:222–6.
22. Winker R, Barth A, Bidmon D, et al. Endurance exercise training in orthostatic intolerance: a randomized, controlled trial. Hypertension 2005;45:391–8.
23. Rowe PC, Calkins H, DeBusk K, et al. Fludrocortisone acetate to treat neurally mediated hypotension in chronic fatigue syndrome: a randomized controlled trial. JAMA 2001;285:52–9.
24. Jacob G, Shannon JR, Black B, et al. Effects of volume loading and pressor agents in idiopathic orthostatic tachycardia. Circulation 1997;96:575–80.
25. Gordon VM, Opfer-Gehrking TL, Novak V, et al. Hemodynamic and symptomatic effects of acute interventions on tilt in patients with postural tachycardia syndrome. Clin Auton Res 2000;10:29–33.
26. Raj SR, Black BK, Biaggioni I, et al. Propranolol decreases tachycardia and improves symptoms in the postural tachycardia syndrome: less is more. Circulation 2009;120:725–34.
27. Fu Q, Vangundy TB, Shibata S, et al. Exercise training versus propranolol in the treatment of the postural orthostatic tachycardia syndrome. Hypertension 2011; 58:167–75.
28. Gaffney FA, Lane LB, Pettinger W, et al. Effects of long-term clonidine administration on the hemodynamic and neuroendocrine postural responses of patients with dysautonomia. Chest 1983;83:436–8.
29. Weber BE, Kapoor WN. Evaluation and outcomes of patients with palpitations. Am J Med 1996;100:138.
30. Doniger SJ, Sharieff GQ. Pediatric dysrhythmias. Pediatr Clin North Am 2006; 53:85.
31. Kaltman J, Shah M. Evaluation of the child with an arrhythmia. Pediatr Clin North Am 2004;51:1537.
32. Wisten A, Messner T. Symptoms preceding sudden cardiac death in the young are common but often misinterpreted. Scand Cardiovasc J 2005;39:143.
33. Amital H, Glikson M, Burstein M, et al. Clinical characteristics of unexpected death among young enlisted military personnel: results of a three-decade retrospective surveillance. Chest 2004;126:528.
34. Woods WA, McCulloch MA. Cardiovascular emergencies in the pediatric patient. Emerg Med Clin North Am 2005;23:1233.
35. Vos P, Pulles-Heintzberger CF, Delhaas T. Supraventricular tachycardia: an incidental diagnosis in infants and difficult to prove in children. Acta Paediatr 2003;92:1058.
36. Ginsburg GS, Riddle MA, Davies M. Somatic symptoms in children and adolescents with anxiety disorders. J Am Acad Child Adolesc Psychiatry 2006;45:1179.
37. Gardner WN. The pathophysiology of hyperventilation disorders. Chest 1996; 109:516.

38. Park MK, Guntheroth WG. How to read pediatric ECG's. 3rd edition. St Louis (MO): Mosby Yearbook; 1992.
39. Wathen JE, Rewers AB, Yetman AT, et al. Accuracy of ECG interpretation in the pediatric emergency department. Ann Emerg Med 2005;46:507.
40. Drago F, Leoni L, Bronzetti G, et al. Premature ventricular complexes in children with structurally normal hearts: clinical review and recommendations for diagnosis and treatment. Minerva Pediatr 2017;69:427–33.
41. Porcedda G, Brambilla A, Favilli S, et al. Frequent ventricular premature beats in children and adolescents: natural history and relationship with sport activity in a long-term follow-up. Pediatr Cardiol 2020;41:123–8.
42. Tripathi A, Black GB, Park YM, et al. Factors associated with the occurrence and treatment of supraventricular tachycardia in a pediatric congenital heart disease cohort. Pediatr Cardiol 2014;35:368.
43. Ko JK, Deal BJ, Strasburger JF, et al. Supraventricular tachycardia mechanisms and their age distribution in pediatric patients. Am J Cardiol 1992;69:1028.
44. Josephson ME, Wellens HJ. Differential diagnosis of supraventricular tachycardia. Cardiol Clin 1990;8:411.
45. Perry JC. Supraventricular tachycardia. In: Garson A Jr, Bricker JT, Fisher DJ, et al, editors. Science and practice of pediatric cardiology. 2nd edition. Baltimore: Williams and Wilkins; 1998. p. 2059.
46. Krahn AD, Manfreda J, Tate RB, et al. The natural history of electrocardiographic preexcitation in men. The Manitoba Follow-up Study. Ann Intern Med 1992;116:456.
47. Sano S, Komori S, Amano T, et al. Prevalence of ventricular preexcitation in Japanese schoolchildren. Heart 1998;79:374.
48. Perry JC, Garson A Jr. Supraventricular tachycardia due to Wolff-Parkinson-White syndrome in children: early disappearance and late recurrence. J Am Coll Cardiol 1990;16:1215.
49. Deal BJ, Keane JF, Gillette PC, et al. Wolff-Parkinson-White syndrome and supraventricular tachycardia during infancy: management and follow-up. J Am Coll Cardiol 1985;5:130.
50. Tanel RE, Walsh EP, Triedman JK, et al. Five-year experience with radiofrequency catheter ablation: implications for management of arrhythmias in pediatric and young adult patients. J Pediatr 1997;131:878.
51. Weindling SN, Saul JP, Walsh EP. Efficacy and risks of medical therapy for supraventricular tachycardia in neonates and infants. Am Heart J 1996;131:66.
52. Van Hare GF, Chiesa NA, Campbell RM, et al. Atrioventricular nodal reentrant tachycardia in children: effect of slow pathway ablation on fast pathway function. J Cardiovasc Electrophysiol 2002;13:203.
53. Kugler JD, Danford DA. Management of infants, children, and adolescents with paroxysmal supraventricular tachycardia. J Pediatr 1996;129:324.
54. Silka MJ, Kron J, Halperin BD, et al. Mechanisms of AV node reentrant tachycardia in young patients with and without dual AV node physiology. Pacing Clin Electrophysiol 1994;17:2129.
55. Gilljam T, Jaeggi E, Gow RM. Neonatal supraventricular tachycardia: outcomes over a 27-year period at a single institution. Acta Paediatr 2008;97:1035.

# Update on the Management of Kawasaki Disease

Kevin G. Friedman, MD[a],*, Pei-Ni Jone, MD[b]

## KEYWORDS

- Kawasaki disease • Coronary artery aneurysms • Corticosteroids
- Intravenous immunoglobulin

## KEY POINTS

- Treatment with intravenous immunoglobulin (IVIG) within the first 10 days of illness reduces incidence of coronary artery aneurysms.
- IVIG resistance, male patients, young infants, coronary artery changes at diagnosis, and highly inflamed patients are risk factors for coronary artery aneurysm development.
- High-risk patients may benefit from acute, adjunctive antiinflammatory treatment in addition to IVIG.

## BACKGROUND

Kawasaki disease (KD) is a self-limited vasculitis of unknown cause that is the most common cause of acquired heart disease in children in the developed world.[1,2] Coronary artery aneurysms (CAAs) are the most serious complication of Kawasaki disease. Treatment in the acute phase is designed to reduce inflammation, prevent CAA; and, in cases where CAA is present, prevent coronary thrombosis. CAAs occur in 15% to 25% of patients who are not treated in the acute phase of the disease with high-dose intravenous immunoglobulin (IVIG).[3] IVIG is well established as first-line therapy for KD and decreases CAA incidence ~5-fold.[3] However, despite appropriate therapy with IVIG, ~5% of patients still develop CAA and ~25% of children and more than 50% of infants less than 6 months old develop coronary artery (CA) abnormalities based on the 2017 American Heart Association (AHA) KD guidelines.[2,4,5] Long-term coronary outcomes are largely related to the extent of enlargement of the CAA in the first month of illness.[2,6,7] Mildly dilated CAAs typically remodel to a normal internal lumen diameter.[6,8] However, large CAAs that have lost their intimal and medial layers cannot remodel to normal, rarely regress, and are prone

[a] Department of Cardiology, Boston Children's Hospital, Harvard Medical School, Boston, MA 02115, USA; [b] Department of Pediatrics, Pediatric Cardiology, Children's Hospital Colorado, University of Colorado School of Medicine, Aurora, CO, USA
* Corresponding author.
*E-mail address:* Kevin.Friedman@cardio.chboston.org

Pediatr Clin N Am 67 (2020) 811–819
https://doi.org/10.1016/j.pcl.2020.06.002
0031-3955/20/© 2020 Elsevier Inc. All rights reserved.

to thrombosis and stenosis, which lead to risk for myocardial ischemia, infarction, and major adverse cardiac events.[2,6,8,9] In order to further improve outcomes, adjunctive antiinflammatory therapies are frequently used in the acute phase in patients considered at high risk for CAA and/or patients refractory to initial IVIG treatment. The 2017 AHA KD guidelines recommend consideration of primary adjunctive antiinflammatory therapy for patients at high risk for CAA, but they do not specify criteria for defining high risk nor which antiinflammatory agent to use, because of lack of evidence.[2] This knowledge gap leads to wide practice variation in indications for adjunctive therapy and choice of agent.

Identification of patients at the time of presentation who are at high risk for persistent CAA and adverse cardiac sequelae is vital, because these are the patients who are most likely to benefit from primary adjunctive therapy. In Japan, clinical risk scores accurately predict patients who are at high risk for IVIG resistance and CAA.[10,11] However in the diverse North American population, Japanese clinical risk scores lack adequate sensitivity and specificity for identifying high-risk patients, and are not routinely used in clinical practice.[12,13] In the absence of useful clinical risk scoring systems, the strongest predictor of both CAA persistence and major adverse cardiac events is CA z score at diagnosis.[6,8] Baseline maximum z score greater than or equal to 2.0 is strongly associated with persistent CAA at 4 to 6 weeks compared with a baseline maximum z score less than 2.0 (16% vs 2%, $P<.001$).[14] Thus, baseline coronary changes, young age (<1 year), and high markers of inflammation constitute criteria for selecting patients with KD at highest risk for adverse cardiac outcome who might benefit from primary adjunctive therapy. Son and colleagues[14] recently developed and validated a scoring system that primarily relies on baseline CA z score, C-reactive protein (CRP), and age to accurately identify patients at high risk for CAA at 4 to 6 weeks.

This article describes the current pharmacologic options for (1) primary adjunctive treatment of the high-risk patients with KD and (2) second-line/rescue therapy for IVIG-resistant patients.

## THERAPIES
### Aspirin

Aspirin has been a mainstay of therapy for KD, for both its antiinflammatory and antithrombotic effects. Most clinicians use high or medium dose aspirin (80–100 mg/kg/d or 30 to 50 mg/kg/d) divided into 4 daily doses until defervescence occurs and then reduce the dosage to 3 to 5 mg/kg/d, administered once daily until the end of the subacute phase. Meta-analysis has shown that medium-dose or high-dose aspirin regimens in conjunction with IVIG have a similar incidence of coronary abnormalities at 30 and 60 days from onset of illness.[15] In patients with aneurysms, low-dose aspirin therapy is continued, sometimes in combination with anticoagulants or other antiplatelet agents.

### Intravenous Immunoglobulin

IVIG is widely accepted as first-line therapy to reduce fever and inflammation, and thus reduce the incidence of CAA in patients with acute KD. When administered in the first 10 days of fever, it reduces CA aneurysms from 25% to less than 5%.[2,3] A single high-dose infusion of IVIG 2 g/kg has been shown to be superior to lower doses and multiple IVIG doses, and is thus the recommended regimen by the AHA guidelines.[16,17] Treatment with IVIG is also recommended for patients who present after 10 days of fever with persistent fever or CA aneurysm with evidence of persistent inflammation.[2] The erythrocyte sedimentation rate (ESR) may be increased following IVIG treatment, so ESR is not a reliable marker of inflammation after IVIG infusion.

Therapy with IVIG is generally well tolerated but there are a few important side effects. Hemolytic anemia is a dose-dependent complication of IVIG administration, and is more frequently encountered in patients with A, B, or AB blood group types and those receiving multiple IVIG doses. Aseptic meningitis can also be encountered, but is usually transient and without sequelae. After IVIG administration, immunization with live viral vaccines including measles, mumps, and varicella should be deferred for 11 months.

Persistent or recrudescent fever greater than or equal to 36 hours after completion of the initial IVIG defines IVIG resistance, occurs in ~15% of patients, and is associated with an increased risk of CAA.[2] There are currently no completed randomized controlled trials to guide choice of therapeutic agent in IVIG-resistant patients. A second dose of IVIG is frequently used in this setting because there is a well-described dose-dependent response to IVIG, although doses greater than 2 g/kg have not been systematically studied.[2,18]

### Corticosteroids

Corticosteroids are widely used in the treatment of other vasculitides, but use in KD has long been controversial (**Table 1**). Corticosteroids were used as the initial therapy before the first report of IVIG efficacy.[19] Early studies were predominantly observational and prone to bias.[19] More recently, convincing evidence for efficacy of corticosteroids in high-risk Japanese children was established in the RAISE (Randomized Controlled Trial to Assess Immunoglobulin Plus Steroid Efficacy for Kawasaki Disease) study.[11] The RAISE study is a multicenter, prospective, randomized, open-label, blinded end points trial to assess the efficacy of IVIG (2 g/kg for 1 day) and aspirin (30 mg/kg/d) plus intravenous prednisolone (2 mg/kg/d) for 5 days followed by an oral steroid taper over ~3 weeks in Japanese patients who are high risk based on clinical scoring criteria (Kobayashi score).[11] The steroid group had a lower incidence of CAA at 4 weeks based on Japanese Ministry of Health criteria (13% vs 3%) and lower treatment resistance rate (40% vs 13%), lower CA z scores, and more rapid resolution of fever and decline in CRP levels. A recent meta-analysis that included the RAISE trial found that a combination of corticosteroid with standard-dose IVIG reduced the rate of CA abnormalities ~3-fold (odds ratio [OR], 0.29 [0.18–0.46]).[19] Two meta-analyses have shown lower rates of CAA in patients with KD who receive IVIG and primary adjunctive corticosteroids compared with IVIG alone.[20,21] The first was a meta-analysis by Wooditch[21] that evaluated 862 patients from 8 randomized trials and found that initial treatment with corticosteroids plus IVIG, compared with IVIG alone, reduced the odds of CAA by ~50% (OR, 0.55 [0.31–0.80]). A more recent meta-analysis evaluated 907 patients with KD in 7 clinical trials of adjunctive corticosteroids and found that patients with KD treated with corticosteroids had reduced CAA (OR, 0.29 [0.18–0.46]), shorter duration of hospital stay, and decreased duration of clinical symptoms compared with patients treated with IVIG alone.[20] Although there is convincing evidence for efficacy of RAISE-dose steroids in high-risk children, there are issues with the ability to generalize to high-risk North American patients because the RAISE study and 3 other Japanese studies in the meta-analyses only included patients at high risk based on the Japanese clinical scoring system and excluded patients with CAA at time of diagnosis.

The only North American prospective study of adjunctive corticosteroids was a phase III, randomized trial of single-dose, intravenous, pulse methylprednisolone (30 mg/kg).[22] There was no difference in CA outcomes at 1 or 5 weeks between

**Table 1**
**Evidence for primary adjunctive therapy and treatment resistance therapy**

| Treatment | Primary Adjunctive | Treatment Resistance |
|---|---|---|
| Corticosteroids | | |
| Japan | RCT: strong benefit on CA and clinical outcomes[11] | Retrospective studies showing benefit[24] |
| North America | RCT: single pulse dose of steroids, no effect on CA or clinical outcomes[22]<br>Retrospective study showing possible benefit[23] | Small case series |
| Meta-analysis | Two meta-analyses showing benefit on CA and clinical outcomes[20,21] | None |
| Infliximab | | |
| Japan/South Korea | None | RCTs: higher rate of defervescence compared with second IVIG in small RCTs[32,33] |
| North America | RCT: reduction on fever days and possible benefit on some CA measures[25] | Phase III trial in United States currently ongoing (infliximab vs second IVIG)[26] |
| Cyclosporine | | |
| Japan | Phase III RCT: no benefit on treatment resistance, no CA benefit when measured by z score[39] | Case series[40] |
| United States | None | — |
| Etanercept | RCT in North America: no effect on treatment resistance, possible benefit on CA in certain subgroups[36] | None |
| Anakinra | Phase I/IIa RCT in United States currently enrolling[34] | Small case series[41,42,44] |
| Cyclophosphamide | None | Case reports[48] |
| Plasmapheresis | None | Case series[45] |

*Abbreviation:* RCT, randomized controlled trial.

patients who received methylprednisolone plus IVIG versus IVIG only. However, in a post hoc subgroup analysis, patients who required repeat treatment due to persistent fever and received methylprednisolone had a lower risk of coronary abnormalities compared with those who received IVIG only. More recently, a North American retrospective multicenter study showed that patients with CA aneurysms at time of diagnosis treated with corticosteroids in addition to IVIG had less progression of CA z score on follow-up compared with patients who received IVIG only.[23]

Corticosteroids are often used as rescue therapy in IVIG-resistant patients with KD, with most reports comprising case series. Kobayashi and colleagues[24] reported on a retrospective cohort of 359 consecutive IVIG-resistant patients and found lower rates of coronary anomalies and lower rate of persistent or recrudescent fever in those retreated with steroids plus IVIG compared with those who received only IVIG or only steroids for rescue therapy.

## Infliximab

Infliximab, a monoclonal antibody to tumor necrosis factor alpha (TNF-α), has also been studied for primary adjunctive treatment (see **Table 1**).[2,25,26] The biological basis of infliximab use in KD is that level of the proinflammatory cytokine TNF-α is increased in the plasma of patients with KD, with highest levels in those who went on to develop CA abnormalities.[27–29] A US randomized, double-blind, placebo controlled trial evaluated the use of infliximab plus IVIG versus infliximab alone for primary adjunctive treatment showed a decrease in the number of days of fever and inflammatory parameters but did not show any difference in IVIG resistance, which was the primary outcome of the study.[25] There was a significant decrease in the left anterior descending coronary z score at 2 weeks but not at later time points, and no statistical difference in the rate of CAA between groups, although the study was not powered for this end point and enrolled both low-risk and high-risk patients. The use of infliximab in high-risk patients was evaluated in a single-center retrospective study. In patients with CAA at diagnosis, treatment with infliximab in addition to IVIG reduced the need for additional therapy, but there was no significant difference in length of stay, CA z scores at 2 to 6 weeks, or decrease in CRP.[30] A recent multicenter, retrospective study comparing adjunctive treatment with either corticosteroids or infliximab in patients with CAA at diagnosis showed that primary treatment intensification with infliximab was associated with less progression of CAA compared with IVIG alone.[23] There was no difference in CAA progression between the patients who received corticosteroids or infliximab in addition to IVIG, and initial treatment resistance varied between groups (21% in IVIG alone, 14% in IVIG plus infliximab, and 0% in IVIG plus RAISE-dose steroids).

Infliximab is frequently used as an alternative to the second dose of IVIG for patients with IVIG resistance.[31] In small Japanese and South Korean randomized trials in IVIG-resistant patients, infliximab was associated with faster resolution of fever but similar CA outcomes compared with a second dose of IVIG.[32,33] A larger Japanese retrospective review comparing infliximab with a second dose of IVIG in IVIG-resistant patients found that infliximab was associated with fewer days of fever and shorter hospital stay but that coronary outcomes were similar.[18] The KIDCARE trial is currently enrolling IVIG-resistant patients in a randomized controlled trial comparing a second dose of IVIG with infliximab and should help to answer the question of optimal rescue therapy in IVIG-resistant patients in the American population.[26,34]

## OTHER THERAPIES

Etanercept is also TNF-α inhibitor that has been used for adjunctive treatment. An open-label prospective trial in North America showed that etanercept was safe, well tolerated, and not associated with recrudescence of fever (see **Table 1**).[35] A phase III, randomized, placebo-controlled trial showed no difference in IVIG resistance in patients who received etanercept plus IVIG compared with IVIG plus placebo.[36] Subanalysis suggested a potential benefit of etanercept in patients more than 1 year of age and African Americans (OR, 0.07; 95% confidence interval, 0.01–0.83), with a lower rate of IVIG resistance in these subgroups. Although there was no significant difference in CAA rate between patients who received etanercept versus placebo, there was less progression of coronary dilation in those with coronary abnormalities after initial therapy in patients who were treated with etanercept.

Cyclosporine is a calcineurin inhibitor that has been used following studies showing that the nuclear factor activated T cells (NFAT) calcineurin pathway was implicated in the susceptibility to KD and CAA formation (see **Table 1**).[37,38]

Cyclosporine inhibits the dephosphorylation of NFAT and the translocation of this transcription factor to the nucleus. The recently published KAICA trial is a randomized, placebo-controlled trial comparing with IVIG plus primary adjunctive cyclosporine with IVIG alone in high-risk Japanese patients based on Kobayashi score.[39] Need for retreatment due to persistent or recrudescent fever was similar between groups. The investigators report a decreased rate of CA abnormalities over the initial 6 weeks based on Japanese Ministry of Health criteria, but, when assessed by z score, the CA abnormality rates were similar between groups. Cyclosporine has also been proposed as a rescue agent for patients with IVIG resistance, but high-quality evidence of efficacy is lacking.[38,40]

Recently, there has been anecdotal evidence of efficacy for anakinra, a recombinant, nonglycosylated form of the human interleukin-1 receptor antagonist, for treatment of IVIG-resistant KD (see **Table 1**).[41–43] In small case series, anakinra led to improvement in clinical and biological inflammation, but no significant change in CA dimensions.[44] A phase I/IIa, open-label, dose-escalation, 2-center trial of anakinra for primary adjunctive therapy in patients with baseline CAA is in progress.[34] In highly treatment-resistant patients, plasmapheresis has been reported to reduce the incidence of CAA, but it is technically complex, requiring placement of large-bore catheters and the commitment of the local blood bank to assist in the exchange.[45,46] In addition, in the most refractory cases of KD where CAAs are enlarging despite multiple other medical therapies, treatment with cytotoxic agents, including cyclophosphamide, has been reported.[47,48]

In conclusion, early diagnosis of KD and treatment with IVIG remains the most critical therapy for prevention of CAA. Increasing evidence suggests that adjunctive, acute antiinflammatory therapy in high-risk patients decreases treatment resistance rates and the progression of CAA. Further research is required to determine the best adjunctive therapy in high-risk patients with KD, IVIG resistance, and patients with CAA at diagnosis.

## DISCLOSURE

No disclosures.

## REFERENCES

1. Newburger JW, Takahashi M, Burns JC. Kawasaki Disease. J Am Coll Cardiol 2016. https://doi.org/10.1016/j.jacc.2015.12.073.
2. McCrindle BW, Rowley AH, Newburger JW, et al. Diagnosis, treatment, and long-term management of Kawasaki disease: A scientific statement for health professionals from the American Heart Association. Circulation 2017. https://doi.org/10.1161/CIR.0000000000000484.
3. Newburger JW, Takahashi M, Burns JC, et al. The Treatment of Kawasaki Syndrome with Intravenous Gamma Globulin. N Engl J Med 2010. https://doi.org/10.1056/nejm198608073150601.
4. Ogata S, Tremoulet AH, Sato Y, et al. Coronary artery outcomes among children with Kawasaki disease in the United States and Japan. Int J Cardiol 2013. https://doi.org/10.1016/j.ijcard.2013.06.027.
5. Salgado AP, Ashouri N, Berry EK, et al. High risk of coronary artery aneurysms in infants younger than 6 months of age with kawasaki disease. J Pediatr 2017. https://doi.org/10.1016/j.jpeds.2017.03.025.
6. Friedman KG, Gauvreau K, Hamaoka-Okamoto A, et al. Coronary artery aneurysms in kawasaki disease: risk factors for progressive disease and adverse

cardiac events in the US population. J Am Heart Assoc 2016. https://doi.org/10.1161/JAHA.116.003289.

7. Friedman KG, Newburger JW. Coronary stenosis after kawasaki disease: size matters. J Pediatr 2018. https://doi.org/10.1016/j.jpeds.2017.11.023.

8. Tsuda E, Tsujii N, Hayama Y. Stenotic lesions and the maximum diameter of coronary artery aneurysms in kawasaki disease. J Pediatr 2018. https://doi.org/10.1016/j.jpeds.2017.09.077.

9. Shulman ST, Rowley AH. Kawasaki disease: Insights into pathogenesis and approaches to treatment. Nat Rev Rheumatol 2015. https://doi.org/10.1038/nrrheum.2015.54.

10. Kobayashi T, Inoue Y, Takeuchi K, et al. Prediction of intravenous immunoglobulin unresponsiveness in patients with Kawasaki disease. Circulation 2006. https://doi.org/10.1161/CIRCULATIONAHA.105.592865.

11. Kobayashi T, Saji T, Otani T, et al. Efficacy of immunoglobulin plus prednisolone for prevention of coronary artery abnormalities in severe Kawasaki disease (RAISE study): A randomised, open-label, blinded-endpoints trial. Lancet 2012. https://doi.org/10.1016/S0140-6736(11)61930-2.

12. Sleeper LA, Minich LL, McCrindle BM, et al. Evaluation of Kawasaki disease risk-scoring systems for intravenous immunoglobulin resistance. J Pediatr 2011. https://doi.org/10.1016/j.jpeds.2010.10.031.

13. Son MBF, Gauvreau K, Kim S, et al. Predicting coronary artery aneurysms in Kawasaki disease at a North American center: An assessment of baseline z scores. J Am Heart Assoc 2017. https://doi.org/10.1161/JAHA.116.005378.

14. Son MBF, Gauvreau K, Tremoulet AH, et al. Risk model development and validation for prediction of coronary artery aneurysms in kawasaki disease in a North American Population. J Am Heart Assoc 2019. https://doi.org/10.1161/JAHA.118.011319.

15. Baumer J, Love S, Gupta A, et al. Salicylate for the treatment of Kawasaki disease in children ( Review ) Salicylate for the treatment of Kawasaki disease in children. Cochrane Database Syst Rev 2009. https://doi.org/10.1002/14651858.CD004175.pub2.Copyright.

16. Newburger JW, Colan SD, Sundel RP, et al. A single intravenous infusion of gamma globulin as compared with four infusions in the treatment of acute kawasaki syndrome. N Engl J Med 1991. https://doi.org/10.1056/NEJM199106063242305.

17. Terai M, Shulman ST. Prevalence of coronary artery abnormalities in Kawasaki disease is highly dependent on gamma globulin dose but independent of salicylate dose. J Pediatr 1997. https://doi.org/10.1016/S0022-3476(97)70038-6.

18. Son MB, Gauvreau K, Burns JC, et al. Infliximab for intravenous immunoglobulin resistance in Kawasaki disease: A retrospective study. J Pediatr 2011. https://doi.org/10.1016/j.jpeds.2010.10.012.

19. Kato H, Koike S, Yokoyama T. Kawasaki disease: Effect of treatment on coronary artery involvement. Pediatrics 1979;63(2):175–9.

20. Wardle AJ, Kiddy HC, Seager MJ, et al. Corticosteroids for the treatment of Kawasaki disease in children. Cochrane Database Syst Rev 2014. https://doi.org/10.1002/14651858.CD011188.

21. Wooditch AC. Effect of initial corticosteroid therapy on coronary artery aneurysm formation in kawasaki disease: a meta-analysis of 862 children. Pediatrics 2005. https://doi.org/10.1542/peds.2005-0504.

22. Newburger JW, Sleeper LA, McCrindle BW, et al. Randomized trial of pulsed corticosteroid therapy for primary treatment of kawasaki disease. N Engl J Med 2007. https://doi.org/10.1056/nejmoa061235.
23. Dionne A, Burns JC, Dahdah N, et al. Treatment intensification in patients with kawasaki disease and coronary aneurysm at diagnosis. Pediatrics 2019. https://doi.org/10.1542/peds.2018-3341.
24. Kobayashi T, Kobayashi T, Morikawa A, et al. Efficacy of intravenous immunoglobulin combined with prednisolone following resistance to initial intravenous immunoglobulin treatment of acute Kawasaki disease. J Pediatr 2013. https://doi.org/10.1016/j.jpeds.2013.01.022.
25. Tremoulet AH, Jain S, Jaggi P, et al. Infliximab for intensification of primary therapy for Kawasaki disease: A phase 3 randomised, double-blind, placebo-controlled trial. Lancet 2014. https://doi.org/10.1016/S0140-6736(13)62298-9.
26. Roberts SC, Jain S, Tremoulet AH, et al. The Kawasaki Disease Comparative Effectiveness (KIDCARE) trial: A phase III, randomized trial of second intravenous immunoglobulin versus infliximab for resistant Kawasaki disease. Contemp Clin Trials 2019. https://doi.org/10.1016/j.cct.2019.02.008.
27. Matsubara T, Furukawa S, Yabuta K. Serum levels of tumor necrosis factor, interleukin 2 receptor, and interferon-γ in Kawasaki disease involved coronary-artery lesions. Clin Immunol Immunopathol 1990. https://doi.org/10.1016/0090-1229(90)90166-N.
28. Hui-Yuen JS, Duong TT, Yeung RSM. TNF-α is necessary for induction of coronary artery inflammation and aneurysm formation in an animal model of kawasaki disease. J Immunol 2006. https://doi.org/10.4049/jimmunol.176.10.6294.
29. Eberhard BA, Andersson U, Laxer RM, et al. Evaluation of the cytokine response in Kawasaki disease. Pediatr Infect Dis J 1995. https://doi.org/10.1097/00006454-199503000-00006.
30. Jone PN, Anderson MS, Mulvahill MJ, et al. Infliximab plus intravenous immunoglobulin (IVIG) versus IVIG alone as initial therapy in children with Kawasaki disease presenting with coronary artery lesions: Is dual therapy more effective? Pediatr Infect Dis J 2018. https://doi.org/10.1097/INF.0000000000001951.
31. Burns JC, Best BM, Mejias A, et al. Infliximab Treatment of Intravenous Immunoglobulin-Resistant Kawasaki Disease. J Pediatr 2008. https://doi.org/10.1016/j.jpeds.2008.06.011.
32. Mori M, Hara T, Kikuchi M, et al. Infliximab versus intravenous immunoglobulin for refractory Kawasaki disease: A phase 3, randomized, open-label, active-controlled, parallel-group, multicenter trial. Sci Rep 2018. https://doi.org/10.1038/s41598-017-18387-7.
33. Youn Y, Kim J, Hong YM, et al. Infliximab as the first retreatment in patients with Kawasaki disease resistant to initial intravenous immunoglobulin. Pediatr Infect Dis J 2016. https://doi.org/10.1097/INF.0000000000001039.
34. Tremoulet AH, Jain S, Kim S, et al. Rationale and study design for a phase I/IIa trial of anakinra in children with Kawasaki disease and early coronary artery abnormalities (the ANAKID trial). Contemp Clin Trials 2016. https://doi.org/10.1016/j.cct.2016.04.002.
35. Choueiter NF, Olson AK, Shen DD, et al. Prospective open-label trial of etanercept as adjunctive therapy for kawasaki disease. J Pediatr 2010. https://doi.org/10.1016/j.jpeds.2010.06.014.
36. Portman MA, Dahdah NS, Slee A, et al. Etanercept with IVIg for acute kawasaki disease: a randomized controlled trial. Pediatrics 2019. https://doi.org/10.1542/peds.2018-3675.

37. Patel RM, Shulman ST. Kawasaki disease: A comprehensive review of treatment options. J Clin Pharm Ther 2015. https://doi.org/10.1111/jcpt.12334.
38. Tremoulet AH, Pancoast P, Franco A, et al. Calcineurin inhibitor treatment of intravenous immunoglobulin-resistant Kawasaki disease. J Pediatr 2012. https://doi.org/10.1016/j.jpeds.2012.02.048.
39. Hamada H, Suzuki H, Onouchi Y, et al. Efficacy of primary treatment with immunoglobulin plus ciclosporin for prevention of coronary artery abnormalities in patients with Kawasaki disease predicted to be at increased risk of non-response to intravenous immunoglobulin (KAICA): a randomised cont. Lancet 2019. https://doi.org/10.1016/S0140-6736(18)32003-8.
40. Izui M, Sano T, Takei A, et al. Two cases of refractory Kawasaki disease successfully treated by cyclosporine. Pediatr Int 2012.
41. Sánchez-Manubens J, Gelman A, Franch N, et al. A child with resistant Kawasaki disease successfully treated with anakinra: A case report. BMC Pediatr 2017. https://doi.org/10.1186/s12887-017-0852-6.
42. Guillaume MP, Reumaux H, Dubos F. Usefulness and safety of anakinra in refractory Kawasaki disease complicated by coronary artery aneurysm. Cardiol Young 2018. https://doi.org/10.1017/S1047951117002864.
43. Gorelik M, Lee Y, Abe M, et al. IL-1 receptor antagonist, anakinra, prevents myocardial dysfunction in a mouse model of Kawasaki disease vasculitis and myocarditis. Clin Exp Immunol 2019. https://doi.org/10.1111/cei.13314.
44. Shafferman A, Birmingham JD, Cron RQ. High dose anakinra for treatment of severe neonatal Kawasaki disease: A case report. Pediatr Rheumatol Online J 2014. https://doi.org/10.1186/1546-0096-12-26.
45. Villain E, Kachaner J, Sidi D, et al. Trial of prevention of coronary aneurysm in Kawasaki's disease using plasma exchange or infusion of immunoglobulins. Arch Fr Pediatr 1987;44(2):79–83.
46. Imagawa T, Mori M, Miyamae T, et al. Plasma exchange for refractory Kawasaki disease. Eur J Pediatr 2004. https://doi.org/10.1007/s00431-003-1267-y.
47. Newburger JW. Kawasaki disease: Medical therapies. Congenit Heart Dis 2017. https://doi.org/10.1111/chd.12502.
48. Wallace CA, French JW, Kahn SJ, et al. Initial intravenous gammaglobulin treatment failure in Kawasaki disease. Pediatrics 2000. https://doi.org/10.1542/peds.105.6.e78.

# Common Left-to-Right Shunts

Dale A. Burkett, MD

## KEYWORDS

- Atrial septal defect (ASD) • Ventricular septal defect (VSD)
- Patent ductus arteriosus (PDA) • Shunt • Left-to-right shunt

## KEY POINTS

- Blood flows to the path of least resistance. The resistance downstream from a shunt varies based on the location of a shunt.
- Atrial septal defects are communications between the atria, volume load the right heart, and are generally asymptomatic in infants and young children.
- Ventricular septal defects are communications between the ventricles, volume load the left heart, and may require intervention early in life.
- A patent ductus arteriosus is a communication between the aorta and pulmonary arteries, volume loads the left heart, and may require intervention in the neonatal period.
- Medical management of left-to-right shunts often involves diuretics to reduce symptoms associated with excessive pulmonary blood flow. Transcatheter or surgical intervention may be necessary.

 Video content accompanies this article at http://www.pediatric.theclinics.com.

Congenital heart disease is often made up of communications between the left and right side of the heart, or the aortic and pulmonary artery, which allow oxygenated blood to shunt into chambers or vessels that normally carry deoxygenated blood, so-called left-to-right shunts. Common shunts include atrial septal defects (ASD), ventricular septal defects (VSD), and a patent ductus arteriosus (PDA). To best understand the shunt physiology in such lesions, it must be emphasized that *blood always flows to the path of least resistance*. The overall resistance that determines shunting differs based on the location of the shunt, but includes the compliance of a chamber (the ability to stretch), downstream stenosis (above, below, or at a valve), and vascular resistance. While the resistance determines the direction of a shunt, the pressure gradient between 2 chambers determines the velocity of the shunt.

Division of Pediatric Cardiology, Heart Institute, Children's Hospital Colorado, University of Colorado, 13123 East 16th Avenue, Aurora, CO, USA
*E-mail address:* Dale.Burkett@ChildrensColorado.org

Pediatr Clin N Am 67 (2020) 821–842
https://doi.org/10.1016/j.pcl.2020.06.007
0031-3955/20/© 2020 Elsevier Inc. All rights reserved.

## ATRIAL SEPTAL DEFECTS

An ASD is a communication between the left and right atria. ASDs comprise about 7% to 8% of congenital heart defects, although up to 50% of children with congenital heart disease have an ASD as a component of their cardiac abnormalities, highlighting how commonly ASDs occur in more complex congenital heart disease.[1,2] ASDs are classified based on their location within the atrial septum and embryologic origin.

A basic knowledge of normal atrial septal anatomy is useful to understand ASD anatomy. Septum primum, the first septum to form, is a thin partition between the atria. It sits on the left atrial (LA) side of a crescentic, thick muscular invagination between the atria, the septum secundum, which forms on the right atrial (RA) side of the partition and forms the limbus of the fossa ovalis; septum primum forms the valve of the fossa ovalis (**Fig. 1**). Superior and inferior endocardial cushions fuse to form the atrioventricular portion of the septum at the crux of the heart. As atrial septation occurs, the left horn of the embryologic sinus venosus becomes the coronary sinus of the heart, draining the venous flow from the heart muscle into the RA.

### Patent Foramen Ovale

A patent foramen ovale (PFO) represents a normal interatrial communication, as the flap between the limbus of the fossa ovalis (septum secundum), and the valve of the fossa ovalis (septum primum) (**Fig. 2**, Video 1). In fetal life, the valve is pushed into the left atrium, with right-to-left atrial shunting allowing oxygenated blood from the ductus venosus to reach the left heart and thus be pumped out to the ascending aorta and brain. However, postnatally, as LA pressure exceeds RA pressure, the fossa ovalis (septum primum) is pressed against the limbus (septum secundum). If these 2 tissues are not fused, blood can pass between the 2 flaps, as a PFO, which is present in nearly all newborns and remains patent in 25% to 30% of adults.[3] The volume of blood that can pass through a PFO is minimal and so there is no hemodynamic compromise: there is insufficient volume to cause right heart dilation, or a flow murmur across the

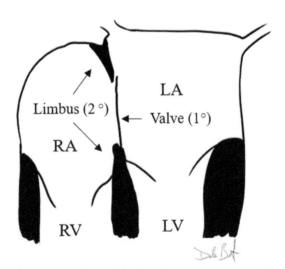

**Fig. 1.** Atrial septal anatomy is formed by the thin septum primum (1°), which forms the valve of the fossa ovalis, and the thicker, crescentic septum secundum (2°), the anteroinferior border of which is known as the limbus.

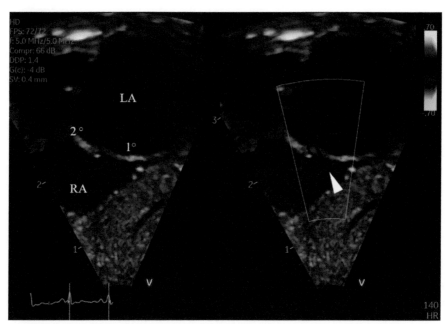

**Fig. 2.** Patent foramen ovale by transthoracic echocardiography, demonstrating flow (*red, arrowhead*) between septum primum and septum secundum. LA, left atrium; RA, right atrium.

pulmonary valve. Although this is thought to be a normal, benign finding, if the rare physiologic conditions are met the interatrial communication does allow possible right-to-left interatrial, thus contributing to paradoxic embolic strokes.

### Atrial Septal Defect Anatomy

ASDs represent a pathologic communication between the LA and RA, although not all communications are truly defects in the septum between the 2 chambers. In fact, some interatrial communications have an entirely normally formed atrial septum. Potential interatrial communications include (**Fig. 3**):

1. *Secundum ASD*—this defect, which accounts for 70% of ASDs and has a female predominance (2:1), is typically the result of a defect in the thin septum primum (single or multiple fenestrations) (**Fig. 4**, Videos 2–6).
2. *Sinus venosus defect*—this defect accounts for 5% to 10% of interatrial communications, and results from a deficiency in the sinus venosus septal tissue between the right pulmonary veins and the superior vena cava (SVC) and RA, most commonly the right upper pulmonary vein and SVC (superior sinus venosus ASD) (**Fig. 5**, Video 7). The interatrial communication is through a pulmonary vein orifice in the LA, allowing LA blood to enter the orifice and drain into the SVC/RA. In addition, pulmonary venous return from the right upper pulmonary vein can directly flow into the SVC/RA. Sinus venosus defects are also associated with anomalous pulmonary venous connections. Rarely, the right lower or middle pulmonary veins communicate with the RA (inferior sinus venosus defect).
3. *Primum ASD*—this interatrial communication is part of the atrioventricular septal defect spectrum, when failure of endocardial cushion fusion results in failure of

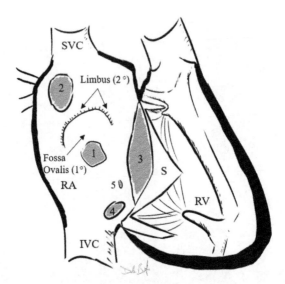

**Fig. 3.** Atrial septal defect (ASD) anatomy, which includes defects in septum primum, known as a secundum ASD (1), superior sinus venosus ASD (2) between the right pulmonary veins and SVC/RA junction, primum ASD (3), coronary sinus ASD (4), and vestibular ASD (5). IVC, inferior vena cava; RV, right ventricle; S, septal leaflet of tricuspid valve; SVC, superior vena cava.

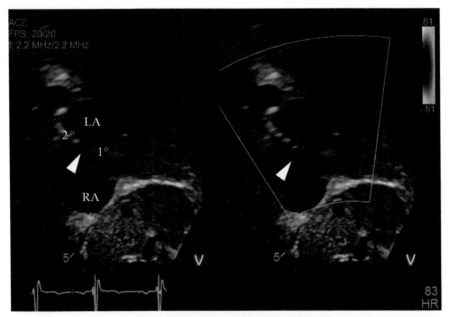

**Fig. 4.** Secundum atrial septal defect (*arrowhead*) by transthoracic echocardiography, demonstrating flow (*red*) from the left atrium (LA) to the right atrium (RA). 1°, septum primum; 2°, septum secundum.

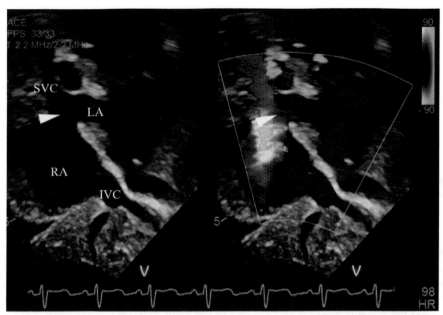

**Fig. 5.** Superior sinus venosus atrial septal defect (*arrowhead*) by transthoracic echocardiography, with flow (*red, arrowhead*) between left atrium (LA) and right atrium (RA). IVC, inferior vena cava; SVC, superior vena cava.

atrioventricular septation (**Figs. 6–8**, Videos 8–11). Some forms of atrioventricular septal defect have only an interatrial shunt, commonly referred to as a "partial" atrioventricular septal defect.

4. *Coronary sinus ASD*—this rare defect results from a deficiency in the septum between with coronary sinus and the LA, allowing LA blood to enter the coronary sinus and drain into the RA. This is usually associated with a persistent left SVC.

5. *Vestibular ASD*—this very rare defect is the result of a deficiency in the atrial septal component derived from the vestibular spine, a muscularized anteroinferior portion of the atrial septum.

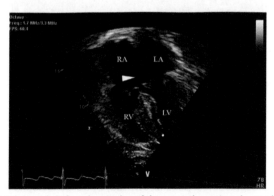

**Fig. 6.** Primum atrial septal defect (*arrowhead*) by transthoracic echocardiography. LA, left atrium; LV, left ventricle; RA, right atrium; RV, right ventricle.

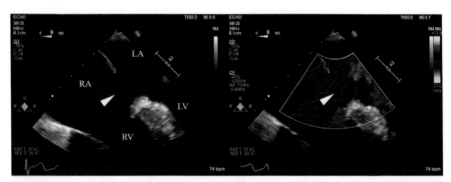

**Fig. 7.** Primum atrial septal defect (*arrowhead*) by transesophageal echocardiography, with flow (blue) from the left (LA) to the right atrium (RA). LV, left ventricle; RV, right ventricle.

## Physiology

As blood flows to the path of least resistance, interatrial shunting is related to atrial compliance, which is, in large part, due to ventricular compliance. The LA is typically less compliant than the right, due to stiffer atrial walls, and the position of the LA between the spine posteriorly and the rest of the heart anteriorly. Importantly, the LA must overcome left ventricular (LV) diastolic pressure, which is typically higher than the right ventricle (RV). The RA is typically more compliant than the left, due to more distensible atrial walls, and the anterior position of the RA with distensible systemic veins. The RA must overcome RV diastolic pressure, which is typically lower than the LV. Mitral and tricuspid valve stenosis can also play important roles in the downstream resistance of each atrium.

Thus, atrial shunting typically flows from a less compliant LA to the more compliant RA. There is typically very little pressure gradient between the atria and so the velocity of the shunt is typically quite low. The shunt results in right heart dilation and increased pulmonary blood flow.

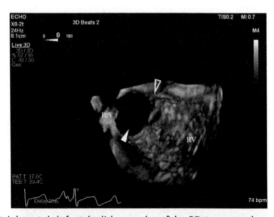

**Fig. 8.** Primum atrial septal defect (*solid arrowhead*) by 3D transesophageal echocardiography, with the defect basal to the atrioventricular valve (*open arrowhead*). RA, right atrium; RV, right ventricle.

### Clinical Features

Increased flow across the pulmonary valve results in turbulence, heard as an ejection murmur, and also delayed closure of the valve, with fixed splitting of S2. A diastolic inflow murmur may be appreciated at the left lower sternal border.

Infants are typically asymptomatic. Even older children with moderate shunts are asymptomatic, whereas those with a large shunt may have fatigue and dyspnea.

### Diagnostic Studies

Radiography may demonstrate cardiomegaly, with engorged pulmonary arteries and distal vasculature. The electrocardiogram often demonstrates RA enlargement, rsR' or RSR' in V1, and possibly prolonged P-R interval.

Echocardiography can visualize the atrial septum, RA and RV dilation, increased flow across the pulmonary valve, pulmonary veins, and the coronary sinus. Transesophageal echocardiography visualizes the atrial septum and pulmonary veins well, although it requires general anesthesia. 3D echocardiography can provide detailed images of interatrial shunts, although it may be limited by imaging windows, limitations in frame rate, or the ability to use an adult-size transesophageal probe.

Contrast-enhanced echocardiography, completed with agitated saline, blood, or albumin, may be able to better define certain ASDs, and importantly can demonstrate right-to-left atrial shunting with visualization of contrast in the left heart.

Cardiac catheterization is typically not necessary for diagnosis of an ASD, although measurement of the effective shunt (pulmonary:systemic blood flow) and identification of anomalous pulmonary venous drainage are possible. It also affords the ability to assess for pulmonary hypertension, a dangerous potential sequela of prolonged increased pulmonary blood flow.

Cardiac MRI can potentially identify interatrial communications, and can also quantify the effective shunt. A computed tomography (CT) scan can identify some interatrial communications, although it involves irradiation and does not quantify the amount of shunting.

### Natural History

ASDs typically have a benign course and are usually asymptomatic in infants and young children. In fact, some do not present for decades. Exercise intolerance, atrial tachyarrhythmias, RV dysfunction, and pulmonary hypertension rates increase with age in those with untreated ASDs. Spontaneous closure or decrease in size of secundum ASDs is common, and more likely if less than 8 mm and younger at the time of diagnosis.[4–7] Spontaneous closure of primum, coronary sinus, and sinus venosus ASDs are unlikely. Pulmonary vascular disease can occur in 5% to 10% of patients with untreated ASDs, with a predominance in women and those over 20 years.[8]

### Treatment

Treatment of secundum ASDs includes both transcatheter and surgical closure, although there is typically little indication for repair in young children. As ASDs are not typically symptomatic in young children, and often decrease in size or even close with increasing age, elective repair is often delayed until at least age 4 to 5 years. In fact, repair in children less than 15 kg rarely improves somatic growth and is associated with complications.[9]

Transcatheter device closure of secundum ASDs is common, with numerous possible devices of various sizes, making closure of a wide range of ASD sizes possible (**Figs. 9** and **10**, Videos 12–15). Complication rates are typically quite low,

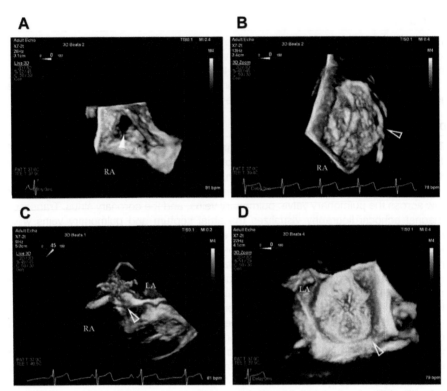

**Fig. 9.** Device closure of a secundum atrial septal defect (*A*) (*solid arrowhead*) by 3D transesophageal echocardiography, with a device (*open arrowhead*) deployed across the atrial septum, viewed from the right atrium (RA) (*B*), above the atrial septum (*C*), and from the left atrium (LA) (*D*). 2°, septum secundum with limbus (*asterisk*); 1°, septum primum.

and success rates very high.[10] Atrial septal rims do limit the candidacy of some patients for transcatheter closure; such patients require surgical closure, which is effective and has a very low rate of death or significant complications in children, although it has a higher rate of complications in adults.[11] In children, compared with transcatheter closure, surgical closure is associated with longer length of stay, higher infection rates, and greater cost.[12]

Surgical closure is usually required for sinus venosus ASDs, which involves patch closure and sometimes rerouting of the SVC (Warden procedure). Surgical closure of coronary sinus ASDs typically involves closure of the coronary sinus ostium, preventing interatrial shunting, but also rerouting of coronary sinus venous return to the left atrium. Surgical closure is also required for vestibular ASDs and primum ASDs, often in conjunction with surgical repair of the left atrioventricular valve.

## VENTRICULAR SEPTAL DEFECTS

A VSD is a communication in the ventricular septum. Behind the bicuspid aortic valve, it is the most common form of congenital heart disease. VSDs are present in ~0.25% of all live births, although they are more commonly identified in studies with screening echocardiography and in premature infants.[13,14] They account for 20% of isolated congenital heart defects.[2]

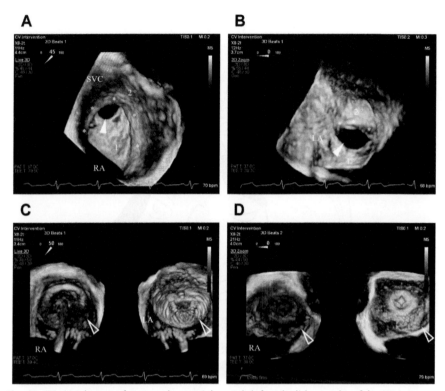

**Fig. 10.** Device closure of a secundum atrial septal defect (*solid arrowhead*) by 3D transeso-phageal echocardiography, as viewed from the right (RA) (*A*) and left (LA) atrium (*B*). A de-vice (*open arrowhead*) is deployed across the atrial septum (*C*), and then released (*D*). 2°, septum secundum with limbus (*asterisk*); 1°, septum primum.

### Ventricular Septal Defect Anatomy

There has been significant historical variability in the description and identification of VSDs, with the same defect having multiple monikers, or a single name applying to a variety of different lesions.[15] However, recent attempts have been made to unify nomenclature (**Fig. 11**):[16]

1. *Perimembranous central VSD*—this defect involves the thin membranous ventricu-lar septum, which lies between the aortic and tricuspid valves (**Figs. 12–14**, Videos 16–18). Once thought to be the most common VSD, the use of echocardiography has demonstrated this defect to be less common than muscular defects in neo-nates, although it is more common in complex congenital heart disease.
2. *Inlet VSD without a common atrioventricular junction* (not associated with an atrio-ventricular septal defect)—such defects open into the RV inlet and extend along the septal leaflet of the tricuspid valve. They can have malalignment between the atrial and ventricular septae, which can result in straddling and/or override of the tricuspid valve.
3. *Trabecular muscular VSD*—these defects are completely bordered by muscle, and are located within the trabecular muscular septum, in the posterior, mid, anterior or apical septum (**Figs. 15** and **16**, Videos 19 and 20). These defects are the most common VSDs, and the most likely to close spontaneously.

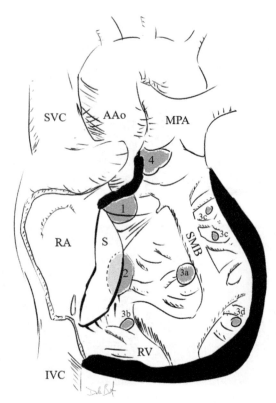

**Fig. 11.** Ventricular septal defect (VSD) anatomy: a perimembranous VSD (1), involving the membranous septum; an inlet VSD without a common atrioventricular junction (2) in the inlet portion of the right ventricle (RV); muscular VSDs in the mid (3a), posterior (3b), and anterior septum (3c), and apical region (3d); outlet VSD (4), cradled between the limbs of the septomarginal trabeculation (SMB). AAo, ascending aorta; IVC, inferior vena cava; MPA, main pulmonary artery; RA, right atrium; S, septal leaflet of the tricuspid valve; SVC, superior vena cava.

4. *Outlet VSD*—these defects lie within the limbs of the septal band (septomarginal trabeculation), just below the RV outlet. They can have no malalignment of the outlet septum, or malalignment of the outlet septum—either anterior or posterior.

Atrioventricular septal defects involve endocardial cushion defects and abnormal atrioventricular septation, frequently with an interventricular shunt present, which is often referred to as an "inlet VSD," although this falls outside of the above nomenclature. With failure of atrioventricular septation, a prominent interventricular shunt may be present.

### Physiology

*Blood flows to the path of least resistance.* For VSDs, downstream resistance is mostly due to pulmonary and systemic vascular resistances, but also includes any arterial stenosis, pulmonary and aortic valve stenosis, and RV and LV outflow tract obstruction. In normal VSD physiology, pulmonary vascular resistance is less than systemic vascular resistance, and so during systole blood flows from LV through the VSD,

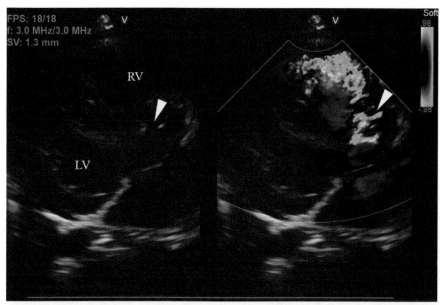

**Fig. 12.** Perimembranous ventricular septal defect (*arrowhead*) by transthoracic echocardiography (parasternal long axis), with a communication and flow (*red*) between the left (LV) and right (RV) ventricles.

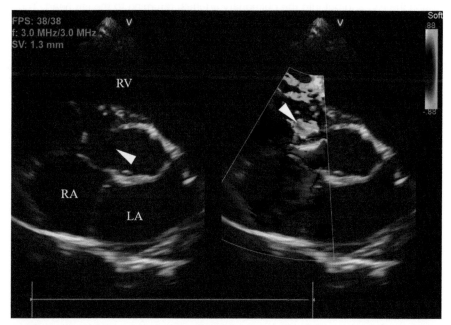

**Fig. 13.** Perimembranous ventricular septal defect (*arrowhead*) by transthoracic echocardiography (parasternal short axis), with a communication and flow (*red*) between the left and right (RV) ventricles. LA, left atrium; RA, right atrium.

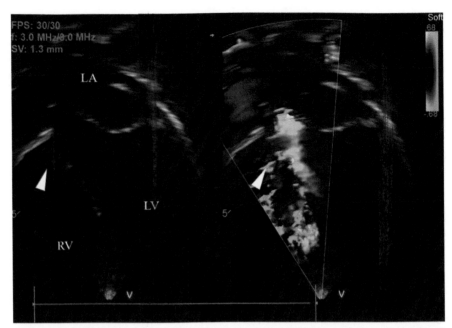

**Fig. 14.** Perimembranous ventricular septal defect (*arrowhead*) by transthoracic echocardi-ography (apical window), with a communication and flow (*red*) between the left (LV) and right (RV) ventricles. LA, left atrium.

through the RV, and out into the pulmonary arteries, returning to the left heart. Thus, VSDs typically lead to left heart dilation. Although resistance determines the direction of blood flow, the interventricular pressure gradient yields the VSD velocity; if the VSD is large, there is minimal pressure gradient between the LV and RV, resulting in low velocity shunting.

At birth, RV pressures are typically increased in the setting of high pulmonary vascular resistance, with minimal interventricular pressure gradient and low velocity

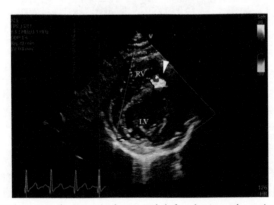

**Fig. 15.** Small anterior muscular ventricular septal defect by transthoracic echocardiography (parasternal short axis) with flow (*red*) through the defect. LV, left ventricle; RV, right ventricle.

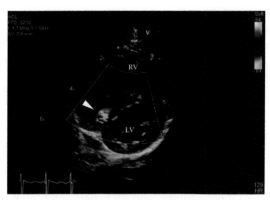

**Fig. 16.** Small posterior muscular ventricular septal defect by transthoracic echocardiography (parasternal short axis) with flow (*red*) through the defect. LV, left ventricle; RV, right ventricle.

VSD flow, which can be difficult to auscultate. Thus, VSDs are commonly not appreciated shortly after birth, but are first heard weeks later, once pulmonary vascular resistance and RV pressures are decreased.

The pressure difference between the LV and RV results in the velocity of the VSD, using the modified Bernoulli equation (pressure difference $= 4 V^2$). With this, we can estimate pulmonary artery systolic pressure. If we know systemic systolic blood pressure, we know the LV systolic pressure (eg, 100 mm Hg), as long as there is no aortic valve stenosis, which would create a discrepancy between the aortic and LV pressures. Using the modified Bernoulli equation, we can calculate the gradient from the LV to the RV (eg, 60 mm Hg), and thus know the RV systolic pressure (eg, 40 mm Hg), which should be similar to the pulmonary artery systolic pressure (in the absence of pulmonary valve stenosis).

VSD location can play an important role for associated findings. Perimembranous and outlet VSDs can be associated with aortic valve prolapse and aortic insufficiency. Perimembranous VSDs can also be associated with both subaortic membranes, which can cause LV outflow tract obstruction and aortic insufficiency, and also a double-chambered RV, where muscle bundles in the RV obstruct outflow. Such findings can be associated with ejection murmurs through the LV outflow and RV outflow, as well as a high-pitched diastolic decrescendo murmur if aortic insufficiency is present. Such findings can persist even if the VSD spontaneously regresses or undergoes repair.

### Clinical Features

At birth, VSDs are often not appreciated on examination. However, over weeks and months, as pulmonary vascular resistance drops, a murmur is often appreciated, with the pitch related to the velocity of the flow through the VSD. As LV pressure quickly exceeds RV pressure during isovolumic contraction, before the aortic valve opens, an S1 coincident holosystolic murmur can be present. Muscular VSDs can squeeze closed during systole as the muscle contracts, resulting in shorter systolic murmurs. The murmur is often harsh (due to multiple frequencies) and best heard at the left lower sternal border. Small defects can allow for a larger interventricular pressure difference, and thus a higher velocity VSD shunt and murmur. Larger defects result in higher RV systolic pressure and thus smaller interventricular pressure gradients, and so shunt murmurs are usually lower pitched.

Children with small VSDs are typically asymptomatic. With moderate and larger VSDs, children can develop tachypnea, increased work of breathing, and sweating, related to increased sympathetic tone and pulmonary edema. Poor feeding can develop, as can poor weight gain despite expected caloric intake, consistent with heart failure in children (caloric intake does not sufficiently meet both the increased cardiovascular metabolic demands and systemic metabolic demands for somatic growth).

### Diagnostic Studies

Radiography is normal in children with small VSDs, although cardiomegaly, pulmonary vascular prominence, and pulmonary edema can be present with large lesions. With small VSDs electrocardiography is typically normal, although left axis deviation, LA abnormality, LV hypertrophy, and RV hypertrophy can be seen with larger lesions.

Echocardiography is able to visualize the ventricular septum well by 2D and 3D imaging. Doppler echocardiography determines the direction and velocity of VSD flow, providing information about RV and pulmonary artery systolic pressures. Echocardiography can also assess associated anomalies, such as aortic valve prolapse, aortic insufficiency, subaortic membranes, double-chamber RV, and straddling mitral or tricuspid valves. Transesophageal echocardiography can demonstrate the anatomy well, perhaps with better visualization than transthoracic echocardiography in older children and adults. 3D echocardiography can detail VSD size and location, as well as pertinent surrounding structures, and has been useful for transcatheter device closure. Cardiac MRI and CT scans can detail VSDs and provide opportunity for 3D modeling, although they are not typically used in those with adequate echocardiography windows.

Cardiac catheterization is not routine for diagnosis of VSDs, but can be useful for quantifying the magnitude of VSD shunting and cardiac output, evaluating pulmonary vascular resistance, and assessing associated lesions.

### Natural History

Although common at birth, VSD spontaneous closure rate is high, with up to 98% of VSDs closing spontaneously by 6 years of life, especially muscular VSDs; even perimembranous VSDs are capable of closing, especially those less than 4 mm.[17,18] Closure of perimembranous VSDs is usually by aneurysmal tricuspid valve septal leaflet tissue growing over the defect, and for muscular VSDs is typically hypertrophy and growth of septal muscle.[19]

Given this trajectory, avoiding surgical intervention, if possible, is warranted, as many VSDs decrease in size enough to preclude intervention. Medical management with diuretics and/or heart failure therapy may allow the VSD time to close.

Untreated moderate and larger VSDs can lead to pulmonary hypertension, and possibly reversal of VSD shunting, with RV-to-LV flow, known as Eisenmenger syndrome. This is associated with cyanosis, polycythemia, iron deficiency, hemoptysis, embolic events, cranial abscesses, and death.

Endocarditis is a recognized potential, though uncommon, complication of untreated VSDs. Although only ~2% of adult patients with untreated VSD develop infective endocarditis, this represents an 11- to 30-fold increased risk for endocarditis over the general population.[20] Currently, subacute bacterial endocarditis prophylaxis risk is not recommended for VSDs, given the substantial number of children with a VSD who undergo spontaneous closure with very low infective endocarditis risk.

## Treatment

Small VSDs do not typically require treatment, given they cannot allow enough blood to flow through them to lead to left heart dilation and heart failure. However, even small VSDs can be complicated by associated defects, such as double-chambered RV, subaortic membrane or aortic valve prolapse, which are often indications in themselves for surgical repair. If such associated lesions are not found, typically small VSDs are monitored intermittently for spontaneous closure.

For larger VSDs, medical management is often attempted. This includes diuretics to treat pulmonary edema and heart failure symptoms. In addition, medications such as digoxin are used, which has been shown to increase ventricular contractility and improve symptoms.[21,22] Medical management can improve symptoms for patients and may allow enough time for VSDs to decrease in size and hemodynamic effect. However, for large defects, medical management is merely a temporizing therapy and does not avoid a definitive repair.

Surgical closure for larger VSDs is often necessary and this remains the most common pediatric cardiovascular surgical repair, with typically very low mortality (<<1%).[11,23,24] Therefore, attention has been turned to reducing morbidity. Factors that lead to increased morbidity, such as prolonged intubation, intensive care stay, or length of admission, include the weight at the time of operation (with smaller infants having a longer length of stay), the presence of a genetic syndrome, and longer cardiopulmonary bypass time.[24,25] Surgical options include primary (suture) and patch closure (**Fig. 17**). Long-term outcomes after surgery include arrhythmias, LV and RV dysfunction, aortic insufficiency, and decreased exercise capacity; risk factors for late events include concomitant cardiac lesions and longer aortic cross-clamp times.[26]

Pulmonary artery banding involves a surgeon placing bands around the pulmonary arteries, increasing the resistance to pulmonary blood flow, and thus reducing excessive pulmonary blood flow. This technique is used when it is thought that, with time, VSDs will eventually close, as is the case for multiple small muscular VSDs that result in a cumulative large interventricular shunt. Once the VSD burden is reduced or resolved, the bands can be removed.

Transcatheter VSD closure has gained popularity in the last 2 decades for closure of muscular VSDs as well as some perimembranous VSDs (Videos 21–25). Risks include residual shunts (16%), arrhythmias (10%), valvular defects (4%), and complete heart block in 1.1%; some studies cite even fewer complications.[27,28] Transcatheter device

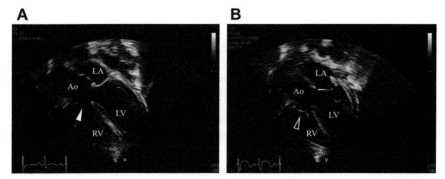

**Fig. 17.** A large anterior malalignment-type ventricular septal defect (*solid arrowhead*) by transthoracic echocardiography (apical window), before (*A*) and after (*B*) surgical patch closure (*open arrowhead*). Ao, aorta; LA, left atrium; LV, left ventricle; RV, right ventricle.

closure is not routinely performed for outlet VSDs or atrioventricular septal defect interventricular communications. Rather, they are typically reserved for muscular VSDs and perimembranous VSD that have a pocket of tissue that can seat the device away from the aortic valve.

## PATENT DUCTUS ARTERIOSUS

The ductus arteriosus, a normal vessel connecting the pulmonary arteries and aorta in fetal life, allows blood entering the RV during fetal life to pass into the aorta. In the fetus, the fluid-filled lungs result in high resistance to flow in the pulmonary arteries, which receive only 16% of the combined ventricular cardiac output. In contrast, the ductus arteriosus sees ~41% of combined cardiac output.[29]

Unlike the walls of other blood vessels, which contain elastic fibers in the medial layer, the ductus arteriosus medial layer contains smooth muscle.[30,31] After birth, the smooth muscle contracts and thickens, and the intimal layer thickens, decreasing the lumen size and resulting in functional closure of the ductus arteriosus, noted in 44% of infants at 24 hours, and 88% at 48 hours. It is during this functional closure that the ductus arteriosus is responsive to therapies to promote patency. Permanent closure is completed in the following days to weeks. It involves necrosis of the subintimal layer and eventual replacement of the muscular layer with fibrosis, forming the ligamentum arteriosum.

Prostaglandins, produced by cyclooxygenase enzymes, relax the ductus arteriosus in fetal life, and administration after birth keeps a ductus arteriosus open in certain forms of congenital heart disease.[32–34] Inhibition of cyclooxygenase enzymes reduces circulating prostaglandin, causing ductus arteriosus constriction both in the fetus and postnatally.[35] At birth, the rise in arterial oxygen tension, and the decrease in circulating prostaglandin levels with removal of the placenta both trigger ductal constriction.

Failure of the ductus arteriosus to close postnatally results in a PDA.[31] The incidence of a PDA at 6 weeks of life among term infants ranges from ~3 to 8/10,000 live births, with a 2:1 female predominance. Prematurity is the most substantial risk factor for a PDA, with an overall greater than 10-fold increase risk of PDA in premature infants.[36,37] The more premature an infant, the greater the risk of a PDA: more than 80% of those less than 1250 g have a PDA. The rate increases with altitude, with a slight increase in those greater than 3000 m (9842 feet), and a substantial increase in those above 4000 m (13,123 feet); infants greater than 4500 m (14,763 feet) have a 30-fold increased risk of a PDA.[38,39]

### Patent Ductus Arteriosus Anatomy

Although both right and left PDAs are possible, by far the most common is a left-sided PDA, between the main pulmonary artery and the proximal descending aorta (**Fig. 18**, Videos 26–29). The vessel usually tapers from aortic to pulmonary arterial end. Even with closure of the PDA, the ductal ampulla is often still present and visible, giving some clue as to the location of the ductus arteriosus ligament. This can prove helpful in the evaluation for a vascular ring when the PDA is closed. In premature infants and those with ductal-dependent cardiovascular lesions, the PDA can be quite large, even similar in size to the aorta.

### Physiology

Pulmonary and systemic vascular resistance are the primary determinants of PDA shunting; arterial obstruction may also play a role. The length and diameter contribute

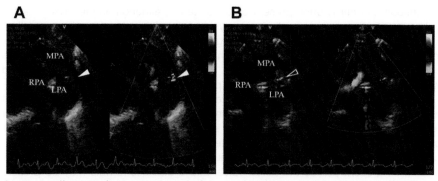

**Fig. 18.** Small patent ductus arteriosus (*solid arrowhead*) by transthoracic echocardiography, with flow (*red*) through the ductus from the aorta into pulmonary arteries (*A*). After device (*open arrowhead*) closure of the ductus arteriosus (*B*) there is no residual shunt. LPA, left pulmonary artery; MPA, main pulmonary artery; RPA, right pulmonary artery.

to the resistance to shunting through a PDA. Immediately after birth, when pulmonary vascular resistance is still high, flow through a PDA is often bidirectional, with right-to-left flow in systole. As pulmonary vascular resistance drops, the shunt becomes all left-to-right.

Left-to-right shunting through the PDA results in increased pulmonary blood flow and thus pulmonary venous return to the left heart, and increased flow through the aortic valve and ascending aorta. A large shunt will thus cause pulmonary edema, left heart dilation, and increased flow through the mitral and aortic valves. This physiology results in increased sympathetic tone, leading to tachypnea, tachycardia, and sweating. Although compensatory mechanisms are more fully developed in older children and adults, they are not well developed in newborns, and even less-so in premature infants. Premature infants also have fewer contractile elements within the myocardium, and lower calcium levels than term infants.[40] Thus, premature infants can develop heart failure earlier than term infants with the same size PDA.

The size of the PDA can play a role in pulmonary artery pressures, as a large PDA will essentially cause equalization of pulmonary and aortic pressures. A small PDA can provide enough restriction to flow to allow a gradient to form between the 2 vessels. The presence of such a gradient can be helpful when trying to estimate pulmonary artery systolic pressure, as the aortic pressure is obtained from the systemic blood pressure.

### Clinical Features

Clinical features vary based on the size of the PDA shunt. For small PDAs, with less than 1.5:1 pulmonary:systemic blood flow ratio, there is enough restriction to prevent any significant amount of increased pulmonary blood flow, and thus left heart dilation. The restriction to flow may allow a pressure gradient between the aorta and pulmonary artery, which can yield a murmur as turbulent flow enters the pulmonary artery; this will be continuous ("machine-like") if the pressure difference between the vessels is always increased, as is seen when pulmonary vascular resistance has dropped. The respiratory examination is usually normal, and pulses are normal.

With a moderate PDA (pulmonary:systemic blood flow ratio of 1.5–2.2:1), the volume load to the left heart is large enough to cause dilation. In addition, pulmonary edema is common, and may cause respiratory distress in premature infants. A continuous murmur is often present on auscultation, although as the PDA is larger, pulmonary pressures are usually higher with a lower interarterial gradient and thus lower pitched murmur. A flow murmur might also be heard across the aortic valve. With diastolic run-off from the aorta into the PDA, diastolic systemic blood pressure can be low, with a wide pulse pressure. This pulse pressure is what is palpated when pulses are felt, and so the palpated pulses are typically increased.

Infants with a large PDA (pulmonary:systemic blood flow ratio of >2.2:1) will present with left heart dilation, pulmonary edema, and heart failure, with poor weight gain, poor feeding, increased work of breathing, and sweating. Tachycardia and tachypnea are common, as are rales. Given the large defect, a significant pressure gradient is typically absent, and so a continuous murmur may not be present. However, a flow murmur is present across the aortic valve, and a diastolic rumble may be present across the mitral valve. P2 may be loud given increased pulmonary artery pressures. Diastolic blood pressure is lower, and the pulse pressure is wide, resulting in bounding pulses.

### Diagnostic Studies

Radiography is typically normal with a small PDA. However, with moderate and larger PDAs, there is evidence of left heart dilation and cardiomegaly, as well as increased pulmonary vascular markings proximally and distally. The electrocardiogram is typically normal in small PDAs, although with moderate and large PDAs, left axis deviation, LA abnormality, and LV hypertrophy are often present.

Echocardiography can visualize the PDA and the shunt direction and velocity using Doppler imaging. Estimations of the interarterial pressure gradient can be calculated from the PDA velocity, although long tubular PDAs are a poor use of the Bernoulli equation.

Cardiac catheterization is rarely used for diagnosis of a PDA, although it is regularly used to close the PDA. In such situations, angiography can detail the duct, and the surrounding aorta and pulmonary arteries. Assessment of the hemodynamic impact of the shunt is feasible, as is evaluation for pulmonary hypertension.

Cardiac MRI and CT scans are able to demonstrate the PDA well, and can provide 3D reconstructions of the vessel and surrounding anatomy. Cardiac MRI is also capable of quantifying the shunt.

### Natural History

In the current era, most PDAs are detected in infancy and treated. However, before widespread diagnosis and treatment, infant mortality, infective endarteritis/endocarditis, heart failure, and pulmonary vascular obstructive disease were frequently encountered, and the mortality rate was as high as 60% by age 60 years, although closure was documented in a wide range of adults.[41] In premature infants with a significant PDA, mortality may be as high as 20% at 1 year, although this is not attributable entirely to the PDA alone, and it is difficult to isolate the role of the PDA in the development of intracranial bleeds, necrotizing enterocolitis, sepsis, and respiratory failure.[42] Bacterial endocarditis/endarteritis is extremely uncommon in developed countries, but is associated with PDAs in underdeveloped countries, although the risk is lower than that for VSDs. Currently, subacute bacterial endocarditis prophylaxis is not recommended for PDAs.

### Treatment

Treatment is recommended for moderate or larger PDAs associated with left heart volume overload or reversible pulmonary hypertension; in those with severe, suprasystemic pulmonary hypertension, a PDA may prove advantageous to allow a "pop-off" for the pulmonary circulation and can help preserve RV function.

Therapeutic options for PDA closure include pharmacotherapy, transcatheter closure, and surgical ligation. As cyclooxygenase produces prostaglandins, which maintain a PDA, the use of medications that inhibit cyclooxygenase have been successfully used to induce PDA closure. This includes indomethacin and ibuprofen, though indomethacin is typically ineffective for term infants and older patients. Interestingly, acetaminophen has also proven effective at closure of PDAs.[43] In a recent meta-analysis of the use of indomethacin, ibuprofen, and acetaminophen, high-dose oral ibuprofen was shown to have the best odds for closure of hemodynamically significant PDA in premature infants.[44] There have been clinician concerns for necrotizing enterocolitis with the use of oral ibuprofen, although high-dose oral ibuprofen was actually shown to have the best cumulative probability for preventing necrotizing enterocolitis, suggesting the risk of necrotizing enterocolitis is likely related to the presence of the PDA rather than the treatment.[44] Interestingly, no statistical difference in mortality was noted for treatment of PDA versus placebo, suggesting that closure of a hemodynamically significant PDA may not actually reduce mortality in preterm infants.[44] Similarly, others have found that as much as 85% of very-low-birth-weight infants will have spontaneous closure of their PDA.[45]

Transcatheter closure of PDAs has been gaining popularity in the previous decades over surgical ligation (see **Fig. 18**, Video 30). Recent devices can be very successful at PDA closure, reaching as high as 100% efficacy.[46–49] Complications include device embolization, infection, femoral vessel damage or thrombosis, and vascular or valvar damage, although rates of complications are low.

Surgical ligation was once the predominant method for closure of a PDA. It is typically approached from a lateral thoracotomy, although video-assisted thoracopic surgery has also been undertaken. Although success rate is high, complication rates include recurrent laryngeal nerve paralysis, infection, respiratory compromise, scoliosis, pleural effusions, and pneumothorax. Compared with transcatheter closure in a meta-analysis, surgery was shown to be more successful at PDA closure, and length of stay was shorter for the transcatheter approach.[50] This study did not use the more recent and successful devices.

## DISCLOSURE

The author has no relationships to disclose.

## SUPPLEMENTARY DATA

Supplementary data related to this article can be found online at https://doi.org/10.1016/j.pcl.2020.06.007.

## REFERENCES

1. Hoffman JI, Kaplan S. The incidence of congenital heart disease. J Am Coll Cardiol 2002;39:1890–900.

2. Botto LD, Correa A, Erickson JD. Racial and temporal variations in the prevalence of heart defects. Pediatrics 2001;107:E32.

3. Hagen PT, Scholz DG, Edwards WD. Incidence and size of patent foramen ovale during the first 10 decades of life: an autopsy study of 965 normal hearts. Mayo Clin Proc 1984;59:17–20.

4. Radzik D, Davignon A, van Doesburg N, et al. Predictive factors for spontaneous closure of atrial septal defects diagnosed in the first 3 months of life. J Am Coll Cardiol 1993;22:851–3.

5. Hanslik A, Pospisil U, Salzer-Muhar U, et al. Predictors of spontaneous closure of isolated secundum atrial septal defect in children: a longitudinal study. Pediatrics 2006;118:1560–5.

6. Helgason H, Jonsdottir G. Spontaneous closure of atrial septal defects. Pediatr Cardiol 1999;20:195–9.

7. Brassard M, Fouron JC, van Doesburg NH, et al. Outcome of children with atrial septal defect considered too small for surgical closure. Am J Cardiol 1999;83: 1552–5.

8. Steele PM, Fuster V, Cohen M, et al. Isolated atrial septal defect with pulmonary vascular obstructive disease—long-term follow-up and prediction of outcome after surgical correction. Circulation 1987;76:1037–42.

9. Bartakian S, Fagan TE, Schaffer MS, et al. Device closure of secundum atrial septal defects in children <15 kg: complication rates and indications for referral. JACC Cardiovasc Interv 2012;5:1178–84.

10. Jalal Z, Hascoet S, Gronier C, et al. Long-term outcomes after percutaneous closure of ostium secundum atrial septal defect in the young: a nationwide cohort study. JACC Cardiovasc Interv 2018;11:795–804.

11. Goldberg JF. Long-term follow-up of "simple" lesions—atrial septal defect, ventricular septal defect, and coarctation of the aorta. Congenit Heart Dis 2015;10: 466–74.

12. Ooi YK, Kelleman M, Ehrlich A, et al. Transcatheter versus surgical closure of atrial septal defects in children: a value comparison. JACC Cardiovasc Interv 2016;9:79–86.

13. Roguin N, Du ZD, Barak M, et al. High prevalence of muscular ventricular septal defect in neonates. J Am Coll Cardiol 1995;26:1545–8.

14. Ooshima A, Fukushige J, Ueda K. Incidence of structural cardiac disorders in neonates: an evaluation by color Doppler echocardiography and the results of a 1-year follow-up. Cardiology 1995;86:402–6.

15. Jacobs JP, Burke RP, Quintessenza JA, et al. Congenital Heart Surgery Nomenclature and Database Project: ventricular septal defect. Ann Thorac Surg 2000; 69:S25–35.

16. Lopez L, Houyel L, Colan SD, et al. Classification of ventricular septal defects for the eleventh iteration of the international classification of diseases-striving for consensus: a report from the International Society for Nomenclature of Paediatric and Congenital Heart Disease. Ann Thorac Surg 2018;106:1578–89.

17. Cresti A, Giordano R, Koestenberger M, et al. Incidence and natural history of neonatal isolated ventricular septal defects: Do we know everything? A 6-year single-center Italian experience follow-up. Congenit Heart Dis 2018;13:105–12.

18. Zhao QM, Niu C, Liu F, et al. Spontaneous closure rates of ventricular septal defects (6,750 consecutive neonates). Am J Cardiol 2019;124:613–7.

19. Eroglu AG, Oztunc F, Saltik L, et al. Evolution of ventricular septal defect with special reference to spontaneous closure rate, subaortic ridge and aortic valve prolapse. Pediatr Cardiol 2003;24:31–5.

20. Berglund E, Johansson B, Dellborg M, et al. High incidence of infective endocarditis in adults with congenital ventricular septal defect. Heart 2016;102:1835–9.

21. Kimball TR, Daniels SR, Meyer RA, et al. Effect of digoxin on contractility and symptoms in infants with a large ventricular septal defect. Am J Cardiol 1991; 68:1377–82.

22. Stewart JM, Hintze TH, Woolf PK, et al. Nature of heart failure in patients with ventricular septal defect. Am J Physiol 1995;269:H1473–80.

23. Bol-Raap G, Weerheim J, Kappetein AP, et al. Follow-up after surgical closure of congenital ventricular septal defect. Eur J Cardiothorac Surg 2003;24:511–5.

24. Schipper M, Slieker MG, Schoof PH, et al. Surgical repair of ventricular septal defect; contemporary results and risk factors for a complicated course. Pediatr Cardiol 2017;38:264–70.

25. Anderson BR, Stevens KN, Nicolson SC, et al. Contemporary outcomes of surgical ventricular septal defect closure. J Thorac Cardiovasc Surg 2013;145:641–7.

26. Menting ME, Cuypers JA, Opic P, et al. The unnatural history of the ventricular septal defect: outcome up to 40 years after surgical closure. J Am Coll Cardiol 2015;65:1941–51.

27. Santhanam H, Yang L, Chen Z, et al. A meta-analysis of transcatheter device closure of perimembranous ventricular septal defect. Int J Cardiol 2018;254: 75–83.

28. Mandal KD, Su D, Pang Y. Long-term outcome of transcatheter device closure of perimembranous ventricular septal defects. Front Pediatr 2018;6:128.

29. Prsa M, Sun L, van Amerom J, et al. Reference ranges of blood flow in the major vessels of the normal human fetal circulation at term by phase-contrast magnetic resonance imaging. Circ Cardiovasc Imaging 2014;7:663–70.

30. Gittenberger-de Groot AC, van Ertbruggen I, Moulaert AJ, et al. The ductus arteriosus in the preterm infant: histologic and clinical observations. J Pediatr 1980; 96:88–93.

31. Fay FS, Cooke PH. Guinea pig ductus arteriosus. II. Irreversible closure after birth. Am J Physiol 1972;222:841–9.

32. Clyman RI. Ontogeny of the ductus arteriosus response to prostaglandins and inhibitors of their synthesis. Semin Perinatol 1980;4:115–24.

33. Clyman RI. Ductus arteriosus: current theories of prenatal and postnatal regulation. Semin Perinatol 1987;11:64–71.

34. Coceani F, Olley PM. Role of prostaglandins, prostacyclin, and thromboxanes in the control of prenatal patency and postnatal closure of the ductus arteriosus. Semin Perinatol 1980;4:109–13.

35. Takahashi Y, Roman C, Chemtob S, et al. Cyclooxygenase-2 inhibitors constrict the fetal lamb ductus arteriosus both in vitro and in vivo. Am J Physiol Regul Integr Comp Physiol 2000;278:R1496–505.

36. Danilowicz D, Rudolph AM, Hoffman JI. Delayed closure of the ductus arteriosus in premature infants. Pediatrics 1966;37:74–8.

37. Kitterman JA, Edmunds LH Jr, Gregory GA, et al. Patent ducts arteriosus in premature infants. Incidence, relation to pulmonary disease and management. N Engl J Med 1972;287:473–7.

38. Alzamora-Castro V, Battilana G, Abugattas R, et al. Patent ductus arteriosus and high altitude. Am J Cardiol 1960;5:761–3.

39. Penaloza D, Arias-Stella J, Sime F, et al. The heart and pulmonary circulation in children at high altitudes: physiological, anatomical, and clinical observations. Pediatrics 1964;34:568–82.

40. Friedman WF. The intrinsic physiologic properties of the developing heart. Prog Cardiovasc Dis 1972;15:87–111.

41. Campbell M. Natural history of persistent ductus arteriosus. Br Heart J 1968; 30:4–13.

42. Gersony WM, Peckham GJ, Ellison RC, et al. Effects of indomethacin in premature infants with patent ductus arteriosus: results of a national collaborative study. J Pediatr 1983;102:895–906.

43. Hammerman C, Bin-Nun A, Markovitch E, et al. Ductal closure with paracetamol: a surprising new approach to patent ductus arteriosus treatment. Pediatrics 2011;128:e1618–21.

44. Mitra S, Florez ID, Tamayo ME, et al. Association of placebo, indomethacin, ibuprofen, and acetaminophen with closure of hemodynamically significant patent ductus arteriosus in preterm infants: a systematic review and meta-analysis. JAMA 2018;319:1221–38.

45. Semberova J, Sirc J, Miletin J, et al. Spontaneous closure of patent ductus arteriosus in infants ≤1500 g. Pediatrics 2017;140.

46. Pass RH, Hijazi Z, Hsu DT, et al. Multicenter USA Amplatzer patent ductus arteriosus occlusion device trial: initial and one-year results. J Am Coll Cardiol 2004;44: 513–9.

47. Gruenstein DH, Ebeid M, Radtke W, et al. Transcatheter closure of patent ductus arteriosus using the Amplatzer duct occluder II (ADO II). Catheter Cardiovasc Interv 2017;89:1118–28.

48. Moore JW, Greene J, Palomares S, et al. Results of the combined U.S. Multicenter Pivotal Study and the Continuing Access Study of the Nit-Occlud PDA device for percutaneous closure of patent ductus arteriosus. JACC Cardiovasc Interv 2014; 7:1430–6.

49. Delaney JW, Fletcher SE. Patent ductus arteriosus closure using the Amplatzer(R) vascular plug II for all anatomic variants. Catheter Cardiovasc Interv 2013;81:820–4.

50. Lam JY, Lopushinsky SR, Ma IWY, et al. Treatment options for pediatric patent ductus arteriosus: systematic review and meta-analysis. Chest 2015;148: 784–93.

# Update on Prevention and Management of Rheumatic Heart Disease

Craig Sable, MD

## KEYWORDS

- Rheumatic heart disease • Acute rheumatic fever • Primary prophylaxis
- Secondary prophylaxis • Echocardiography screening • Cardiac surgery

## KEY POINTS

- Rheumatic heart disease remains the most common cause of cardiovascular morbidity and mortality globally in children and young adults.
- Primary prevention is designed to prevent group A streptococci from causing acute rheumatic fever.
- Secondary prophylaxis is designed to prevent recurrent episodes of rheumatic fever and end-stage valvular disease.
- Echocardiography screening holds promise for detecting rheumatic heart disease in a large number of children at a stage when secondary prophylaxis may have a greater chance of success.
- Definitive catheter and surgical interventions are the only treatments that can improve outcomes of patients with moderate or severe rheumatic heart disease. Access to intervention remains very limited in endemic regions.

Rheumatic heart disease (RHD) remains the most common cause of cardiovascular morbidity and mortality globally in children and young adults, with a worldwide prevalence of more than 39 million people affected (http://ghdx.healthdata.org/gbd-results-tool). Nearly 300,000 deaths and 10 million disability-adjusted life years (DALYs) are attributable to RHD each year.[1] Although the prevalence and mortality of RHD have declined significantly in high-income countries, the disease persists in low-income countries and in marginalized populations within middle-income and high-income countries.[1] A recent analysis found that RHD received the least funding relative to disease burden (based on DALYs) across a range of 16 tropical diseases,

Dr. Sable has funding (Center Director) for research on rheumatic heart disease from the American Heart Association (Award ID 17SFRN33630027) Strategically Focused Research Children's Network.
Cardiology, Children's National Hospital, 111 Michigan Avenue, Northwest, Washington, DC 20010, USA
E-mail address: csable@childrensnational.org

including human immunodeficiency virus (HIV)/acquired immunodeficiency syndrome (AIDS), tuberculosis, and malaria (RHD funding/DALYs 100-fold less than HIV/AIDS).[2] Limited data on disease burden, poverty and inequality, ineffective advocacy, and health systems that are incapable and/or have not prioritized RHD control all contribute to the large disease burden that has persisted for 75 years after the original Jones Criteria for acute rheumatic fever (ARF) were published.[3] This article focuses on prevention and management of RHD, highlighting critical gaps that need to be addressed to effectively reduce the burden of RHD.

## PREVENTION OF RHEUMATIC HEART DISEASE

Understanding of the pathophysiology of ARF and RHD informs opportunities for primordial, primary, and secondary prevention of RHD and the most serious sequelae, end-stage valve disease. A detailed discussion of prevention as well as treatment of initial episodes of ARF is beyond the scope of this article, but a brief overview is helpful to put prevention in context with management of RHD. The association between ARF and group A β-hemolytic streptococcal (GAS) infection is well described. It is postulated that a complex interaction between a susceptible host, virulent strains of GAS, and environmental risk factors results in the autoimmune reaction that causes ARF.[4] Primordial prevention involves strategies to avoid GAS infection and is focused on environmental conditions. Interestingly, the decline of ARF in the United States and Western Europe predated the widespread introduction of penicillin by more than decade, suggesting an important role of overcrowding (and frequent untreated GAS infections) in the pathogenesis of ARF and RHD.[5]

### Primary Prevention

Primary prevention is designed to prevent GAS infection from causing ARF and most commonly involves treating the GAS pharyngitis with antibiotics.[4] GAS pharyngitis is asymptomatic or causes only a mild sore throat in many cases, and, as result, children and parents do not seek treatment; this is especially common in low-resource settings where ARF and RHD are endemic. Development of an effective GAS vaccine could revolutionize primary prevention and is one of the cornerstones of global RHD control advocacy. Research has entered phase I clinical trials[6]; however, the complex nature of GAS and its variability around the globe add to the challenge of developing a vaccine that would be effective in the most endemic regions.[7]

### Secondary Prevention

Secondary prophylaxis consists of the continuous delivery of antibiotics to prevent recurrent episodes of ARF, usually with monthly benzathine penicillin G (BPG) injections or daily oral penicillin. Up to 80% of patients with a primary episode of ARF have carditis. The overall risk of developing long-term RHD following the first episode of ARF is approximately 60% to 65%.[8] Risk of progression to chronic severe RHD depends on the severity of initial carditis and the number of ARF recurrences.[4] Recurrence of ARF is most common in the first 5 years after the initial episode and may occur in up to 75% of patients who do not receive regular secondary prophylaxis. The benefits of secondary prophylaxis have been recognized since the 1950s.[9] Continuous adherence to secondary prophylaxis leads to a reduction in recurrent episodes of ARF, improvement in the severity of RHD (including complete regression of mild valvulitis within 5–10 years in up to 70% of cases), and reduced mortality.

Current American Heart Association guidelines recommend intramuscular BPG for secondary prophylaxis with an every-4-week schedule for most individuals, although a

3-week schedule can be considered for those at high risk or those who experience recurrent ARF despite high adherence to a 4-week schedule. The duration of secondary antibiotic prophylaxis is based on echocardiographic findings: (1) individuals with ARF and no carditis remain on prophylaxis for 5 years, or until 21 years of age (whichever is longer); (2) individuals with ARF with carditis but no residual heart disease remain on prophylaxis for 10 years or until 21 years of age (whichever is longer); and (3) individuals with ARF with carditis and residual heart disease remain on prophylaxis for 10 years or until 40 years of age (whichever is longer), and sometimes require lifelong treatment.[10] Extension of prophylaxis is then based on severity of underlying residual disease. Maintaining appropriate BPG adherence remains a global challenge and more research is needed into improved delivery, update, and adherence to BPG.[11] Registry-based care may improve uptake and is currently recommended for optimal delivery of secondary prophylaxis.[11]

Adverse reactions to BPG limit compliance and can have a negative impact on regional control programs. Until recently, deaths after BPG injection have been presumed to be anaphylactic. However, a growing number of anecdotal reports of immediate or nearly immediate BPG-related deaths do not seem to be from classic anaphylaxis. In a recent case review of 10 deaths from 5 countries, the common presentation was that of children with severe valvular RHD who lost consciousness shortly after BPG injection and could not be resuscitated.[12] These deaths seem predominantly hemodynamic, with a BPG injection leading to hypotension (presumably vagal), decreased coronary perfusion, ventricular arrhythmias, and death in high-risk patients with tenuous underlying cardiovascular physiology. These reactions are likely exacerbated by conditions common in low-income and middle-income countries (LMICs): dehydrated and hungry patients who have traveled long distances and waited hours for injections. Additional research is needed, but these cases have led to a growing global dialogue questioning whether the benefits of BPG compared with oral penicillin outweigh the risks in all settings, and whether specific guidelines for administration of penicillin can be developed in those at highest risk.

### Echocardiography Screening

Up to one-third of patients with ARF report no history of a sore throat.[13] Similarly, the REMEDY study, an international registry, reports that up to three-quarters of people living with RHD have no previous history of ARF.[14] The diagnosis of ARF using the Jones Criteria remains challenging in LMIC, where the differential diagnosis for a febrile illness with joint pain is wide, public awareness of GAS/ARF is poor, and advanced diagnostic testing is not routinely available.[3] In these settings, where millions of children may already have established but undiagnosed RHD, echocardiographic screening for early disease may hold hope for detecting RHD at a stage when secondary prophylaxis may have a greater chance of success.[15]

The 2012 World Health Federation echocardiographic guidelines were developed to facilitate echocardiographic screening, and, for individuals less than 20 years of age, it divides RHD into 2 major categories: borderline or definite RHD.[16] RHD found on echocardiography screening that was not detected by auscultation or other clinical tools is known as latent or subclinical RHD. The pooled prevalence of subclinical RHD (21.1 per 1000 people; 95% confidence interval [CI], 14.1–31.4) is about 7 times higher than that of clinical disease (2.7 per 1000 people; 95% CI, 1.6–4.4).[17,18] Studies have also shown that borderline RHD progresses to more severe forms of RHD at a greater rate (relative risk of 8.2), compared with matched controls.[19] Before recommending population-based screening for RHD on the global stage, several issues must be addressed. These issues include achieving a better understanding of the natural history of subclinical disease, consideration of the cost-effectiveness of such programs, the worldwide gap in access to echocardiography, and a lack of infrastructure and providers to care for an increased number of patients. Ongoing research efforts, including a randomized controlled trial to determine the impact of BPG on the progression of latent RHD (https://clinicaltrials.gov/ct2/show/NCT03346525), are helping to answer some of these critical questions.

## RHEUMATIC HEART DISEASE MEDICAL MANAGEMENT
### Medical Management of Heart Failure

Management principles for RHD in children are derived from valvular heart disease guidelines for adult patients. These principles primarily focus on surgical and catheter-based intervention for severe or symptomatic valvular heart disease.[20] In contrast, there is little evidence-based support for pharmacologic management of severe valvular heart disease to alter outcomes. Most of the global burden of symptomatic RHD exists in locations where surgical or catheter-based treatment is not available or only available for a minority of those in need.[1,21] For such patients, pharmacologic management is often the only option to achieve any symptomatic improvement.[22]

Symptomatic medical management of moderate to severe rheumatic mitral regurgitation (MR) includes afterload reduction with vasodilator therapy, most often angiotensin-converting enzyme inhibition (ACEI), angiotensin II receptor blockers, and diuretics (loop diuretics and spironolactone). In addition, digoxin and beta-blockade may also be considered. There are a few studies worth noting. Enalapril resulted in a significant reduction in left ventricular diameter and volume relative to placebo in 47 patients with MR, 26 with RHD.[23] A Turkish study reported that addition of ACEI reduced left ventricular end-diastolic volume and atrial natriuretic peptide levels after 20 days of treatment.[24] Both enalapril and nicorandil resulted in decreased left ventricular systolic volume and increased ejection fraction in 87 patients with RHD with severe RHD over 6 months.[25] Other causes of MR in patients suspected of having RHD must also be considered, including ischemia and dilated cardiomyopathy.

The only long-lasting effective treatment of mitral stenosis (MS) is catheter or surgical intervention; children with moderate to severe MS have a rapidly worsening course if they do not undergo definitive intervention. Loop diuretics are useful in acute pulmonary edema and for chronic management. However, overdiuresis can reduce preload and compromise cardiac output. Other diuretics, such as aldosterone blockers (spironolactone and eplerenone) and thiazide diuretics (metolazone and chlorthalidone) can also be used. β-Blockers may provide some symptomatic relief by reducing the heart rate, allowing greater diastolic filling and decreasing left atrial pressure.

No medical therapy has been shown to reduce progression of aortic regurgitation (AR) in RHD; treatment is predominantly targeted at symptom relief and treatment of underlying left ventricle (LV) dysfunction and heart failure (HF). Treatment with ACEI, angiotensin-receptor blockers, and β-blockers has been shown to be beneficial in large population cohort studies in patients with AR and in particular those with LV dysfunction.[26] Treatment of other associated comorbidities, such as hypertension, should also be considered. In patients with mixed MR and AR, medical therapy with afterload reduction, diuretics, and possibly beta-blockade may be complementary. In patients with MR and MS, diuretics may be the only medical therapy available.

### Atrial Fibrillation

Atrial fibrillation is a common complication of RHD and is associated with a poor prognosis.[27,28] Factors associated with atrial fibrillation include number of valves involved, age, left ventricular ejection fraction, left atrial size, left atrial strain, and right atrial pressure.[29] Complications of atrial fibrillation include HF, stroke, peripheral thromboembolism, and premature death.[27] Small single-center randomized trials have shown that nondihydropyridine calcium channel blockers or β-blockers can provide rhythm control of symptomatic atrial fibrillation. Maintenance of sinus rhythm has been shown after electrical and pharmacologic (usually amiodarone) cardioversion or catheter ablation,[30] but these strategies are not readily generalizable to all patients.

Anticoagulation with vitamin K oral antagonists (eg, warfarin) or direct thrombin or factor Xa inhibitors (direct oral anticoagulants [DOACs]) is recommended for prevention of stroke in patients with RHD with atrial fibrillation.[31] However, patients with moderate/severe rheumatic mitral valve stenosis were excluded from the DOAC randomized clinical trials; warfarin remains the primary anticoagulation agent in these patients.[31] Warfarin compliance and International Normalized Ratio monitoring remain a significant challenge in patients with RHD in LMIC. The Investigation of rheumatic Atrial Fibrillation Treatment Using Vitamin K Antagonists, Rivaroxaban or Aspirin Studies, Noninferiority (INVICTUS-VKA noninferiority trial) is currently enrolling to evaluate DOAC (rivaroxaban) versus standard vitamin K antagonist therapy in patients with RHD and atrial fibrillation/flutter (https://clinicaltrials.gov/ct2/show/NCT02832531). Atrial fibrillation can occur even after successful catheter or surgical treatment of MR and/or MS; therefore, monitoring of rhythm during follow-up is important, and anticoagulation is indicated for patients with intermittent or persistent atrial fibrillation.

### Endocarditis

Infective endocarditis (IE) still carries high mortalities, approaching 30% at 1 year. The role of RHD as a risk factor for both acquiring IE and having complications from IE is significant in regions of the world endemic for RHD.[32] RHD was found to be the underlying valve disease in 5.4% to 77% of cases of IE in LMIC.[33] In New Caledonia, a French Pacific island, Oceanic Islanders had a significantly higher incidence of IE compared with non-Oceanic (mainly European) populations. RHD was the most common underlying valve condition among Oceanic islanders, with a proportion of approximately one-third being viridians group streptococci (VGS) IE.[34] Guidelines, including those published in 2007 by the American Heart Association, have limited the role of antibiotic prophylaxis before dental procedures.[35] Several publications from high-income countries have supported these guidelines; showing no increase in rates of VGS IE.[36] However, there are no data specifically addressing whether this practice should be applied to LMICs where dental hygiene is much poorer and RHD is endemic. Access to oral health services in patients with RHD in LMICs is an important part of the care of this population and should be prioritized at the public policy level as well.

### Pregnancy

RHD is more common in women than in men and fertility rates often track with rates of RHD. Women with unrepaired RHD have an increased risk of poor maternal and fetal outcome, which is exacerbated by ventricular dysfunction, pulmonary hypertension, atrial fibrillation, and any signs of HF. Stenotic lesions are less well tolerated than regurgitant lesions and occasionally require catheter or surgical interventions or termination of pregnancy.[37] Undiagnosed RHD can be unmasked during pregnancy when cardiac output increases and systemic vascular resistance decreases.[37,38] A recent study of 3506 pregnant women who underwent echocardiography screening in Uganda showed that 1.7% had cardiac disease, 88% of which was RHD.[39] Less than 5% of women were aware of their diagnosis, and 50% required medical intervention and/or change in delivery planning. The attributable risk of heart disease on maternal mortality was 11%. Maternal and infant mortality was higher in women with heart disease.

Management of women before, during, and after pregnancy with unoperated and operated RHD requires a multidisciplinary team of cardiologists, obstetricians, nurses, community health workers, and sometimes cardiothoracic surgeons. Appropriate preconception counseling including advice on contraception should be the goal but only happens infrequently. The REMEDY study found that only 5% of women with prosthetic heart valves and 2% of those with severe MS were on contraception.[14] Women with mechanical valve replacement require anticoagulation throughout the pregnancy, which can include warfarin, unfractionated heparin, or low-molecular-weight heparin.[40] In women needing warfarin less than or equal to 5 mg/d, the medication can be continued until the end of the pregnancy, whereas in others a more complex treatment regimen is required.[40]

## INTERVENTIONAL TREATMENT OF RHEUMATIC HEART DISEASE

The Ugandan RHD registry includes more than 2000 patients that have been followed for almost a decade. Recent analysis of 612 children with clinical RHD enrolled between 2011 and 2018 highlights the severity of RHD and critical need for interventional treatment.[41] The overall mortality in the pediatric population was 31% with a median time to death of 7.8 months (interquartile range, 18 months) from time of enrollment. Kaplan-Meier curves showed a striking difference in the 8-year survival between the 73 children who received surgical or catheter-based intervention (97% survival) versus the 535 children who only received medical management (58% survival, *P*<.001). These data highlight not only the critical impact of intervention but also the significant gap in access that exists in LMIC. The REMEDY study also highlights this critical gap; only 1% and 11% of children and adults, respectively, in LMIC in need of catherization and surgery received it.[14]

### Percutaneous Interventions

Catheter-based intervention for RHD is primarily focused on balloon mitral valvuloplasty (BMV) for MS. Low cost, less invasiveness, and rapid turnaround time associated with BMV compared with open heart surgery make it the preferable treatment of moderate to severe MS (with mild or less MR). Patients with isolated MS make up about 5% to 15% of the RHD population who require intervention,[14,22] and MS is most prevalent in countries that are highly endemic for RHD. Long-term outcomes for BMV are comparable with open mitral commissurotomy.[42] The echocardiographic Wilkins score[43] provides guidance regarding the suitability of the mitral valve morphology for percutaneous balloon mitral valvotomy. It considers the degree of (1) valve calcification, (2) leaflet mobility, (3) leaflet thickening, and (4) disease of the subvalvular apparatus. Each item is graded on increasing severity from 0 to 4, with 0 being normal and 4 being the most abnormal. Almost 80% of symptomatic patients with severe rheumatic MS are candidates for BMV (Wilkins score of 8 or less).[44] For pregnant women with severe MS, BMV can be lifesaving and can be accomplished with minimal complication and low fluoroscopy times.

The infrastructure for BMV includes access to cardiac catheterization as well as surgical backup for immediate catastrophic complications. Complications occur in 2% to 5% of procedures and include cardiac tamponade, stroke, and acute MR. A ruptured valve leaflet requires urgent surgery. Developing a sustainable, low-cost model for BMV in environments that need them most is a high priority for RHD. This goal includes training skilled personnel; installing and maintaining equipment; and having reliable access to disposable supplies, most importantly mitral balloons (most commonly the Inoue balloon). The procedure can often be done with conscious sedation and transthoracic echocardiography guidance, and the possibility of resterilization and reuse of the balloon makes it relatively affordable. Low-cost options are available as alternatives to the Inoue balloon. Percutaneous valve implantation holds promise,[45] especially if this work can be expanded to the mitral valve. However, the application of these technologies in young rheumatic patients seems less probable in the foreseeable future; current techniques and devices are less appropriate for rheumatic disorders with very large annulus sizes.

### Surgery

Indications for surgery for RHD are similar to those for nonrheumatic valvular disease for the mitral and the aortic valves.[20] When there is severe valvular dysfunction, especially if the patient is symptomatic, surgery is recommended. Accompanying tricuspid regurgitation is often present alongside chronic rheumatic mitral valve disease and requires simultaneous surgery. The question of repair versus replacement is always paramount, and is very relevant in young patients and women of reproductive age, especially in LMIC. The challenges of compliance and the requirement of monitoring long-term oral anticoagulation after mitral valve replacement drives mitral valve repair as the ideal care for RHD.[46,47] Experienced surgeons have reported feasibility of repair in 75% to 80% of these patients.[46] Patient survival and survival free from prosthetic valve complications are lower after valve replacement with either mechanical or biological prostheses than repair, because of higher rates of thromboembolism in the former and of faster degenerative process in the latter. The lower incidence of these complications with aortic prostheses and the greater difficulty with aortic valve repair makes aortic valve replacement more acceptable.

However, the durability of repair of the rheumatic mitral valve is generally poorer than in nonrheumatic valves[48] and is, in part, determined by compliance with secondary penicillin prophylaxis. In RHD endemic regions, reoperation may not be an option and the surgical team may be more expert in valve replacement than repair. These considerations are significant in most low-resource environments and often influence the decision at the time of initial operation.

Access to surgery remains one of the most important problems in LMICs where RHD is endemic. A 2014 study found that there is only 1 cardiac surgeon per 3.3 million people in sub-Saharan Africa.[49] Only a small number of countries in sub-Saharan Africa have cardiac surgical facilities, and access to surgery abroad is limited and often prohibitively expensive. It is estimated that there is a need of 250 RHD operations per million population in countries with endemic RHD, creating a huge gap in need for cardiac surgery with less than 10% of patients in need of surgery receiving it. The population of sub-Saharan Africa is approximately 1 billion people, resulting in a need for 250,000 RHD surgeries per year (in addition to 100,000 congenital heart operations).[50]

## SUMMARY

The 71st World Health Organization (WHO) Assembly adopted a resolution on RHD in June 2018. Twenty-six member states and 6 nongovernmental organizations spoke in support of the resolution, recognizing that RHD remains a significant public health concern in many countries. Prevention and management strategies for RHD described in this article highlight many of the gaps that need to be addressed to operationalize the WHO resolution. Vaccine development; increased awareness of GAS, ARF, and RHD; along with early diagnosis, including echocardiography screening, hold promise for developing prevention strategies that can decrease the need for intervention.

The recently published, "Cape Town Declaration on Access to Cardiac Surgery in the Developing World," which was jointly published in 10 journals, highlights the critical need for expanded surgical and interventional services.[50] The aims are (1) to establish an international working group (coalition) of individuals from cardiac surgery societies and representatives from industry, cardiology, and government to evaluate and endorse the development of cardiac care in LMICs; and (2) to advocate for the training of cardiac surgeons and other key specialized caregivers at identified and endorsed centers in LMICs. Given the minimal benefits of medical management, increased access to intervention is the only hope for the current generation of people with RHD and who are beyond benefitting from prevention strategies.

## REFERENCES

1. Watkins DA, Johnson CO, Colquhoun SM, et al. Global, regional, and national burden of rheumatic heart disease, 1990-2015. N Engl J Med 2017;377(8): 713–22.
2. Macleod CK, Bright P, Steer AC, et al. Neglecting the neglected: the objective evidence of underfunding in rheumatic heart disease. Trans R Soc Trop Med Hyg 2019;113(5):287–90.
3. Gewitz MH, Baltimore RS, Tani LY, et al. Revision of the Jones criteria for the diagnosis of acute rheumatic fever in the era of Doppler echocardiography: a scientific statement from the American Heart Association. Circulation 2015;131(20): 1806–18.
4. Carapetis JR, Beaton A, Cunningham MW, et al. Acute rheumatic fever and rheumatic heart disease. Nat Rev Dis Primers 2016;2:15084.
5. Kaplan EL. T. Duckett Jones Memorial Lecture. Global assessment of rheumatic fever and rheumatic heart disease at the close of the century. Influences and dynamics of populations and pathogens: a failure to realize prevention? Circulation 1993;88(4 Pt 1):1964–72.
6. Pastural E, McNeil SA, MacKinnon-Cameron D, et al. Safety and immunogenicity of a 30-valent M protein-based group a streptococcal vaccine in healthy adult volunteers: a randomized, controlled phase I study. Vaccine 2020;38(6):1384–92.
7. Woldu B, Bloomfield GS. Rheumatic heart disease in the twenty-first century. Curr Cardiol Rep 2016;18(10):96.
8. Bland EF, Jones TD. The natural history of rheumatic fever: a 20 year perspective. Ann Intern Med 1952;37(5):1006–26.
9. Stollerman GH, Rusoff JH, Hirschfeld I. Prophylaxis against group A streptococci in rheumatic fever; the use of single monthly injections of benzathine penicillin G. N Engl J Med 1955;252(19):787–92.
10. Gerber MA, Baltimore RS, Eaton CB, et al. Prevention of rheumatic fever and diagnosis and treatment of acute Streptococcal pharyngitis: a scientific statement from the American Heart Association Rheumatic Fever, Endocarditis, and Kawasaki Disease Committee of the Council on Cardiovascular Disease in the Young, the Interdisciplinary Council on Functional Genomics and Translational Biology, and the Interdisciplinary Council on Quality of Care and Outcomes Research: endorsed by the American Academy of Pediatrics. Circulation 2009; 119(11):1541–51.

11. Palafox B, Mocumbi AO, Kumar RK, et al. The WHF roadmap for reducing CV morbidity and mortality through prevention and control of RHD. Glob Heart 2017;12(1):47–62.
12. Marantelli S, Robert H, Carapetis J, et al. Severe adverse events following benzathine penicillin G injection for rheumatic heart disease prophylaxis: cardiac compromise more likely than anaphylaxis. Heart Asia 2019;11:e011191.
13. Carapetis JR, Steer AC, Mulholland EK, et al. The global burden of group A streptococcal diseases. Lancet Infect Dis 2005;5(11):685–94.
14. Zuhlke L, Engel ME, Karthikeyan G, et al. Characteristics, complications, and gaps in evidence-based interventions in rheumatic heart disease: the Global Rheumatic Heart Disease Registry (the REMEDY study). Eur Heart J 2015; 36(18):1115–1122a.
15. Tompkins DG, Boxerbaum B, Liebman J. Long-term prognosis of rheumatic fever patients receiving regular intramuscular benzathine penicillin. Circulation 1972; 45(3):543–51.
16. Remenyi B, Wilson N, Steer A, et al. World Heart Federation criteria for echocardiographic diagnosis of rheumatic heart disease–an evidence-based guideline. Nat Rev Cardiol 2012;9(5):297–309.
17. Rothenbuhler M, O'Sullivan CJ, Stortecky S, et al. Active surveillance for rheumatic heart disease in endemic regions: a systematic review and meta-analysis of prevalence among children and adolescents. Lancet Glob Health 2014; 2(12):e717–26.
18. Mirabel M, Tafflet M, Noel B, et al. Prevalence of rheumatic heart disease in the pacific: from subclinical to symptomatic heart valve disease. J Am Coll Cardiol 2016;67(12):1500–2.
19. Remond M, Atkinson D, White A, et al. Are minor echocardiographic changes associated with an increased risk of acute rheumatic fever or progression to rheumatic heart disease? Int J Cardiol 2015;198:117–22.
20. Nishimura RA, Otto CM, Bonow RO, et al. 2017 AHA/ACC focused update of the 2014 AHA/ACC guideline for the management of patients with valvular heart disease: a report of the American College of Cardiology/American Heart Association Task Force on Clinical Practice Guidelines. J Am Coll Cardiol 2017;70(2):252–89.
21. Watkins D, Zuhlke L, Engel M, et al. Seven key actions to eradicate rheumatic heart disease in Africa: the Addis Ababa communique. Cardiovasc J Afr 2016; 27(3):184–7.
22. Zhang W, Okello E, Nyakoojo W, et al. Proportion of patients in the Uganda rheumatic heart disease registry with advanced disease requiring urgent surgical interventions. Afr Health Sci 2015;15(4):1182–8.
23. Sampaio RO, Grinberg M, Leite JJ, et al. Effect of enalapril on left ventricular diameters and exercise capacity in asymptomatic or mildly symptomatic patients with regurgitation secondary to mitral valve prolapse or rheumatic heart disease. Am J Cardiol 2005;96(1):117–21.
24. Kula S, Tunaoglu FS, Olgunturk R, et al. Atrial natriuretic peptide levels in rheumatic mitral regurgitation and response to angiotensin-converting enzyme inhibitors. Can J Cardiol 2003;19(4):405–8.
25. Gupta DK, Kapoor A, Garg N, et al. Beneficial effects of nicorandil versus enalapril in chronic rheumatic severe mitral regurgitation: six months follow up echocardiographic study. J Heart Valve Dis 2001;10(2):158–65.
26. Elder DH, Wei L, Szwejkowski BR, et al. The impact of renin-angiotensin-aldosterone system blockade on heart failure outcomes and mortality in patients

identified to have aortic regurgitation: a large population cohort study. J Am Coll Cardiol 2011;58(20):2084–91.

27. Zuhlke L, Karthikeyan G, Engel ME, et al. Clinical outcomes in 3343 children and adults with rheumatic heart disease from 14 low- and middle-income countries: two-year follow-up of the global rheumatic heart disease registry (the REMEDY study). Circulation 2016;134(19):1456–66.

28. Wang B, Xu ZY, Han L, et al. Impact of preoperative atrial fibrillation on mortality and cardiovascular outcomes of mechanical mitral valve replacement for rheumatic mitral valve disease. Eur J Cardiothorac Surg 2013;43(3):513–9.

29. Negi PC, Sondhi S, Rana V, et al. Prevalence, risk determinants and consequences of atrial fibrillation in rheumatic heart disease: 6 years hospital based-Himachal Pradesh- Rheumatic Fever/Rheumatic Heart Disease (HP-RF/RHD) registry. Indian Heart J 2018;70(Suppl 3):S68–73.

30. Nair M, Shah P, Batra R, et al. Chronic atrial fibrillation in patients with rheumatic heart disease: mapping and radiofrequency ablation of flutter circuits seen at initiation after cardioversion. Circulation 2001;104(7):802–9.

31. January CT, Wann LS, Calkins H, et al. 2019 AHA/ACC/HRS focused update of the 2014 AHA/ACC/HRS guideline for the management of patients with atrial fibrillation: a report of the American College of Cardiology/American Heart Association Task Force on Clinical Practice Guidelines and the Heart Rhythm Society. J Am Coll Cardiol 2019;74(1):104–32.

32. Cabell CH, Jollis JG, Peterson GE, et al. Changing patient characteristics and the effect on mortality in endocarditis. Arch Intern Med 2002;162(1):90–4.

33. Mirabel M, Rattanavong S, Frichitthavong K, et al. Infective endocarditis in the Lao PDR: clinical characteristics and outcomes in a developing country. Int J Cardiol 2015;180:270–3.

34. Mirabel M, Andre R, Barsoum P, et al. Ethnic disparities in the incidence of infective endocarditis in the Pacific. Int J Cardiol 2015;186:43–4.

35. Wilson W, Taubert KA, Gewitz M, et al. Prevention of infective endocarditis: guidelines from the American Heart Association: a guideline from the American Heart Association Rheumatic Fever, Endocarditis, and Kawasaki Disease Committee, Council on Cardiovascular Disease in the Young, and the Council on Clinical Cardiology, Council on Cardiovascular Surgery and Anesthesia, and the Quality of Care and Outcomes Research Interdisciplinary Working Group. Circulation 2007;116(15):1736–54.

36. Duval X, Delahaye F, Alla F, et al. Temporal trends in infective endocarditis in the context of prophylaxis guideline modifications: three successive population-based surveys. J Am Coll Cardiol 2012;59(22):1968–76.

37. Sliwa K, Johnson MR, Zilla P, et al. Management of valvular disease in pregnancy: a global perspective. Eur Heart J 2015;36(18):1078–89.

38. Sliwa K, Anthony J. Late maternal deaths: a neglected responsibility. Lancet 2016;387(10033):2072–3.

39. Beaton A, Okello E, Scheel A, et al. Impact of heart disease on maternal, fetal and neonatal outcomes in a low-resource setting. Heart 2019;105(10):755–60.

40. Regitz-Zagrosek V, Roos-Hesselink JW, Bauersachs J, et al. 2018 ESC guidelines for the management of cardiovascular diseases during pregnancy. Eur Heart J 2018;39(34):3165–241.

41. Zimmerman M, Kitooleko S, Okello E, et al. Clinical outcomes of children with rheumatic heart disease: a retrospective registry-based study in Uganda. Circulation 2019;140(Suppl_1):A13933.

42. Song JK, Kim MJ, Yun SC, et al. Long-term outcomes of percutaneous mitral balloon valvuloplasty versus open cardiac surgery. J Thorac Cardiovasc Surg 2010;139(1):103–10.

43. Wilkins GT, Weyman AE, Abascal VM, et al. Percutaneous balloon dilatation of the mitral valve: an analysis of echocardiographic variables related to outcome and the mechanism of dilatation. Br Heart J 1988;60(4):299–308.

44. Meneguz-Moreno RA, Costa JR Jr, Gomes NL, et al. Very long term follow-up after percutaneous balloon mitral valvuloplasty. JACC Cardiovasc Interv 2018; 11(19):1945–52.

45. Ntsekhe M, Scherman J. TAVI for rheumatic aortic stenosis - The next frontier? Int J Cardiol 2019;280:51–2.

46. Krishna Moorthy PS, Sivalingam S, Dillon J, et al. Is it worth repairing rheumatic mitral valve disease in children? Long-term outcomes of an aggressive approach to rheumatic mitral valve repair compared to replacement in young patients. Interact Cardiovasc Thorac Surg 2019;28(2):191–8.

47. Remenyi B, Webb R, Gentles T, et al. Improved long-term survival for rheumatic mitral valve repair compared to replacement in the young. World J Pediatr Congenit Heart Surg 2013;4(2):155–64.

48. Antunes MJ. Repair for rheumatic mitral valve disease. The controversy goes on! Heart 2018;104(10):796–7.

49. Yankah C, Fynn-Thompson F, Antunes M, et al. Cardiac surgery capacity in subsaharan Africa: quo vadis? Thorac Cardiovasc Surg 2014;62(5):393–401.

50. Zilla P, Bolman RM, Yacoub MH, et al. The Cape Town declaration on access to cardiac surgery in the developing world. Eur J Cardiothorac Surg 2018;54(3): 407–10.

# Diagnosis, Evaluation, and Treatment of Myocarditis in Children

Adam Putschoegl, DO[a],*, Scott Auerbach, MD[b]

## KEYWORDS

- Myocarditis • Pediatrics • Etiology • Diagnosis • Treatment

## KEY POINTS

- Myocarditis is a ubiquitous disease that can present in myriad ways requiring a high index of suspicion.
- Diagnosis requires a full armamentarium of diagnostic tools including various laboratory values and imaging modalities.
- The best treatment course remains controversial with many practitioners using immune modulators such as intravenous immunoglobulin and steroids.

## INTRODUCTION

Myocarditis is defined as an inflammatory myocardial disease diagnosed by a combination of histologic, immunologic, and immunohistochemical criteria.[1] More simply, it is known as inflammation of the myocardium or heart muscle. Myocarditis is caused by a wide range of infections, inflammatory diseases, and toxins. Clinical severity of myocarditis ranges to mild chest discomfort without other symptoms to cardiogenic shock. Fulminant myocarditis was recently defined as sudden and severe inflammation of the myocardium resulting in myocyte necrosis, edema, and cardiogenic shock.[2] However, the diagnosis is challenging due to a wide variety of symptoms that overlap with a myriad of other disease processes. Varying results in studies of treatment of myocarditis have resulted in varied and inconsistent approaches to management.

## EPIDEMIOLOGY

The incidence and prevalence of myocarditis in children is likely underestimated because many will have only mild symptoms without need for medical attention. The annual incidence in children ranges from 0.26 to 2 cases per 100,000 children.[3–8] Multiple studies have shown a bimodal peak in incidence. Most cases occur in infancy

[a] Department of Pediatrics, Children's Hospital & Medical Center/University of Nebraska Medical Center, 8200 Dodge Street, Omaha, NE 68114, USA; [b] Department of Pediatrics, Children's Hospital Colorado, 13123 East 16th Avenue, Aurora, CO 80045, USA
* Corresponding author.
*E-mail address:* aputschoegl@childrensomaha.org

Pediatr Clin N Am 67 (2020) 855–874
https://doi.org/10.1016/j.pcl.2020.06.013
0031-3955/20/© 2020 Elsevier Inc. All rights reserved.

and adolescents, with those in infancy having worse outcomes.[3,9-12] There may be a higher prevalence among men.[5,11]

Myocarditis is also known to be a cause of sudden cardiac death, with some reports showing a rate of 1.8% of all deaths and 3% to 7% of cardiac deaths.[13-16] Myocarditis has been associated with 16% to 20% of cases of sudden infant death syndrome.[17-19]

## CAUSE

Myocarditis is most commonly caused by viral infection, but other causes must be considered and include bacterial, fungal, and parasitic infections; autoimmune diseases; hypersensitivity reactions; toxins; and other possible exposures (**Table 1**).[20] Viral infection is thought to be the most common cause. Trends in viral causes of myocarditis change longitudinally, so investigations into the causative agent will need to cast a wide net (**Fig. 1**).[20,21] In a multicenter registry in Germany (MYKKE), 44% of 226 biopsies were positive for cardiotropic viruses. The most common virus detected was parvovirus B19 (59%) followed by human herpesvirus 6 (HHV-6) (12%), enterovirus (3%), cytomegalovirus (2%), and Epstein-Barr virus (1%).[22] In another study by Gagliardi and colleagues,[23] they evaluated biopsies on 63 children admitted for heart failure and found a cardiotropic virus in 35%, with, again, parvovirus B19 being the most common at 41%. Interestingly, enterovirus and adenovirus were not detected in any of the samples, despite findings of previous studies.[24] Parvovirus B19 or HHV-6 can persist in endomyocardial biopsy (EMB) specimens in up to 80% of patients after 7 months.[25] This has also been seen in asymptomatic adults and suggests a lifelong asymptomatic persistent of these viruses in the myocardium after a primary infection.[26] In areas with low vaccination rates, consideration should be given to diphtheria (especially in patients with heart block) and mumps. Rarer causes of myocarditis have included clozapine, exposure to penicillin, Tylenol, and cannabis.[27-30]

## PATHOPHYSIOLOGY

Much of our understanding of the pathogenesis of myocarditis has come from murine models and can be broken down into 3 separate phases (**Figs. 2** and **3**). Phase 1 (1–7 days) is characterized by myocellular invasion of a virus via endocytosis and rapid viral replication, myocellular necrosis and apoptosis, and innate immune responses. Phase 2 (1–4 weeks) involves transition from innate immune response to adaptive immunity, infiltration of T cells, and presence of cardiac autoantibodies. Phase 3 (months to years) is associated with clearance of virus and recovery or disease progression. Myocardial damage may persist in phase 3, possibly leading to fibrosis, increased cardiac mass, and a dilated cardiomyopathy.[31-33]

## CLINICAL PRESENTATION

Symptoms of myocarditis at presentation are often nonspecific. Therefore, it is important to have a high index of suspicion to avoid a delay in diagnosis. Gastrointestinal (GI) symptoms, such as abdominal pain, nausea, poor appetite, and vomiting, have been some of the most common clinical manifestations.[12,34,35] Other common presenting symptoms include decrease exercise capacity, upper respiratory infection symptoms, fever, angina, dyspnea, arrhythmia, and syncope.[35-41] Durani and colleagues[35] found that 85% of patients required at least a second visit with a provider before they were diagnosed with myocarditis. Of those patients, just more than half required another visit within 14 days before myocarditis was diagnosed. In addition,

**Table 1**
**Causes of myocarditis**

| | |
|---|---|
| Viral agents and disorders | Rickettsial diseases |
|   Adenovirus |   Q fever |
|   Arbovirus |   Rocky mountain spotted |
|   Coxsackievirus B |   Fever |
|   Cytomegalovirus |   Typhus |
|   Dengue virus | Protozoal diseases |
|   Echovirus |   African sleeping sickness |
|   Epstein-Barr virus |   Amebiasis |
|   Hepatitis C |   Chagas disease |
|   Herpesvirus |   Leishmaniasis |
|   Human immunodeficiency virus |   Malaria |
|   Influenza virus |   Toxoplasmosis |
|   Mumps | Helminthic agents and diseases |
|   Parvovirus B19 |   Ascariasis |
|   Poliomyelitis |   Echinococcosis |
|   Rabies |   Filariasis |
|   Rubella |   Paragonimiasis |
|   Rubeola |   Schistosomiasis |
|   Varicella |   *Strongyloides* |
|   Variola |   Trichinosis |
|   Yellow fever | |
| Bacterial agents and disorders | Cardiotoxins |
|   Brucella |   Alcohol |
|   Chlamydia |   Anthracyclines |
|   Cholera |   Arsenic |
|   Clostridia |   Carbon monoxide |
|   Diphtheria |   Catecholamines |
|   Hemophilus |   Cocaine |
|   Legionella |   Heavy metals |
|   Meningococcus | Causes of hypersensitivity reactions |
|   Mycoplasma |   Antibiotics |
|   Neisseria gonorrhoeae |   Clozapine |
|   Psittacosis |   Diuretics |
|   Salmonella |   Insect bites |
|   Staphylococcus |   Lithium |
|   Streptococcus |   Snake bites |
|   Tetanus |   Tetanus toxoid |
|   Tuberculosis |   Mesalamine |
|   Tularemia | |
| Spirochetal disorders | Systemic disorders |
|   Leptospirosis |   Celiac disease |
|   Lyme disease |   Connective tissue disorders |
|   Relapsing fever |   Hypereosinophilia |
|   Syphilis |   Kawasaki disease |
| Mycotic agents and disorders |   Sarcoidosis |
|   *Actinomyces* |   Thyrotoxicosis |
|   *Aspergillus* |   Wegener granulomatosis |
|   *Blastomyces* | |
|   Candida | |
|   Coccidioidomycosis | |
|   Cryptococcosis | |
|   *Histoplasma* | |
|   Mucormycosis | |
|   *Nocardia* | |
|   Sporotrichosis | |

*From* Schultz J, Hilliard A, Cooper Jr L, Rihal C. Diagnosis and Treatment of Viral Myocarditis. *Mayo Clin Proc.* 2009;84(11):1001-1009; with permission.

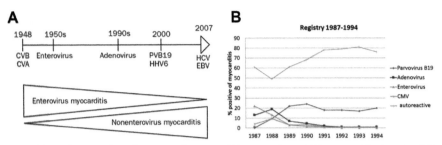

**Fig. 1.** (A) Evolution of viral causes of myocarditis over time. CVA, coxsackievirus A; CVB, coxsackievirus B; EBV, Epstein-Barr virus; HCV, hepatitis C virus; HHV6, human herpesvirus 6; PV-B19, parvovirus B19. (B) Epidemiologic shift in the Myocarditis Registry from entero- (*green line*) and adenoviruses (*brown line*) to Parvovirus B 19 (*dark blue line*) in the late 1980s. The number of patients with nonviral myocarditis (*light blue line*) varied from 50% to 80% in the same time span. (*From* [A] Schultz J, Hilliard A, Cooper Jr L, Rihal C. Diagnosis and Treatment of Viral Myocarditis. *Mayo Clin Proc.* 2009;84(11):1001-1009; with permission (Figure 5 in original); and [B] Maisch B. Cardio-Immunology of Myocarditis: Focus on Immune Mechanisms and Treatment Options. *Front Cardiovasc Med.* 2019;6; with permission (Figure 6A in original).)

62% of patients admitted to a single pediatric intensive care unit were diagnosed with a respiratory illness before a diagnosis of myocarditis.[42]

When symptoms at presentation were compared based on the degree of ventricular dysfunction, the most common symptoms in those with moderate to severely depressed function were a viral prodrome, GI symptoms, malaise/fatigue, dyspnea, chest pain, and respiratory distress. Those with mildly depressed to normal function

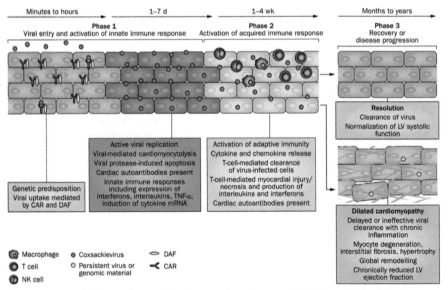

**Fig. 2.** Temporal phases of coxsackievirus-mediated myocarditis. (*From* Pollack A, Kontorovich AR, Fuster V, Dec GW. Viral myocarditis-diagnosis, treatment options, and current controversies. *Nat Rev Cardiol.* 2015;12(11):670-680; with permission (Figure 2 in original).)

# Pathogenesis Viral and Inflammatory Cardiomyopathy

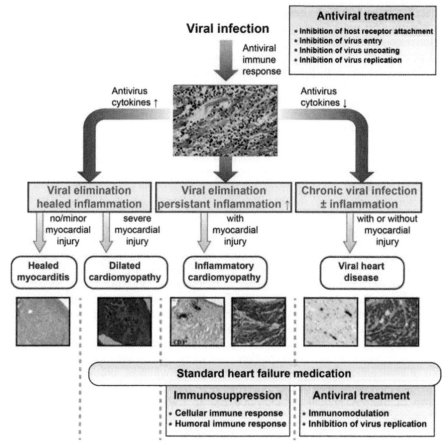

**Fig. 3.** Infection of cardiac endothelial cells or cardiac myocytes by virus causes direct cellular damage and subsequently an innate and adaptive immune response, all of which contribute to cardiomyopathy. (*From* Schultheiss H-P, Kü Hl U, Cooper LT. The management of myocarditis. https://doi.org/10.1093/eurheartj/ehr165 with permission (Figure 2 in original).)

were most likely to have chest pain followed by respiratory distress, viral prodrome, dyspnea, GI symptoms, and malaise/fatigue.[12]

Neonates may be especially difficult to diagnose with myocarditis, given their inability to express symptoms with providers relying on physical examination findings and laboratory evaluation.[43,44] Early recognition in this population is critical, as neonatal myocarditis has been associated with lower likelihood of recovery and high mortality. The initial presentation is often mistaken for, or associated with clinical sepsis, so a high index of suspicion is critical.[45]

## DIAGNOSIS

Multiple data sources are required to make a diagnosis of myocarditis. Clinical signs and symptoms at presentation can range from mild chest pain with a normal physical examination to cardiogenic shock. Laboratory findings consistent with myocarditis include elevated levels of inflammatory markers, cardiac troponin levels, and natri-uretic peptides.

Laboratory testing for an infectious or noninfectious cause must be performed in a manner specific to each cause (**Table 2**).[46]

Noninvasive testing should include an electrocardiogram (ECG), echocardiogram, and possibly an MRI. The gold standard for diagnosis has been and remains the use of EMB despite one study that suggested 17 EMB specimens would be required for 79% diagnostic sensitivity.[47] However, the use of EMB has been decreasing with increasing use of MRI.[11] The classification for diagnostic certainty of myocarditis can be a helpful tool for incorporating the clinical signs and symptoms with the diagnostic studies obtained (**Table 3**).[48]

Cardiac troponin levels can be used to aid in the diagnosis of myocarditis but cannot be relied on as a single marker for definitive diagnosis. Studies have shown that a negative troponin is helpful for ruling out myocarditis but has low specificity.[38,40,42] Therefore, it is important to interpret the troponin value in the context of the entire clinical picture and diagnostic results when considering a diagnosis of myocarditis.

## ELECTROCARDIOGRAM

Multiple studies of children with myocarditis have shown that ECG abnormalities are detected in nearly all patients.[34,38,49,50] The most common ECG abnormalities in a study of 24 pediatric myocarditis cases were abnormal Q waves (67%), negative T waves (63%), wide QRS (58%), and abnormalities of ST segments (46%).[34] It has been reported that an abnormal ECG finding was 100% sensitive; however, a normal ECG does not exclude a diagnosis of myocarditis.[24,50]

It is clear that an abnormal ECG is nearly universal in patients with myocarditis; however, certain patients will have more significant arrhythmias necessitating a higher degree of intervention. Patients may develop tachyarrhythmias, bradyarrhythmias, or advanced atrioventricular block.[10,51] When an arrhythmia is present in myocarditis, choice of therapy should be individualized to the patient and their presenting arrhythmia.[52]

## ECHOCARDIOGRAM

Echocardiogram is a mainstay in the evaluation of suspected myocarditis and can determine if there is ventricular dysfunction, atrioventricular valve regurgitation, pericardial or pleural effusions, or atrial or ventricular thrombosis. Findings can be completely normal in mild cases. Often, there will be left ventricular (LV) dysfunction without associated dilation. When LV enlargement is present, it is often less severe when compared with those with idiopathic dilated cardiomyopathy.[40] Myocarditis was also associated with more frequent wall motion abnormalities, less mitral valve regurgitation, and less severely depressed systolic function. Patients with fulminant myocarditis are more likely to have increased ventricular septal thickness, markedly decreased systolic function, and normal dimensions of the LV when compared with patients with acute myocarditis.[53]

## MRI

MRI use for the diagnosis of myocarditis has been increasing since the advent of the Lake Louise Criteria (LLC) and our increasing understanding of the limitations of the Dallas Criteria for EMB.[11] The strength of MRI comes from its ability to evaluate for edema, hyperemia, fibrosis, and scarring of the myocardium, all of which help

**Table 2**
**Specific diagnostic testing for myocarditis**

| | Infections Agent | % pos. In MMR | Comments Diagnosis Made via: |
|---|---|---|---|
| **1. Infectious myocarditis** | | | |
| Bacteria | Chlamydia pneumoniae | 0.03 | Serodiagnosis |
| | Mycobacterium tuberculosis | 0.02 | IGRA (QuantiFERON) or microscopy from sputum, pericardial fluid, in Africa more frequent |
| | Haemophilus influenzae | 0.002 | Serodiagnosis |
| | Staphylococci | 0.03 | Blood culture, in sepsis or endocarditis |
| | Streptococci | 0.02 | In rheumatic fever, in cooperation with Chandigarh |
| Spirochete | Syphilis | 0.001 | Serodiagnosis |
| | Borrelia burgdorferi | 0.7 | ELISA and western blot or PCR from EMB |
| Rickettsia | Coxiella bumeti | 0.005 | Serodiagnosis, predominant pericarditis |
| Fungi | Candida | 0.002 | In immunocompromised patients, diagnosed by culture |
| Protozoa | Plasmodium falciparum (malaria) | 0.002 | Microscopy (thick blood film) |
| | Toxoplasma gondii | 0.002 | Serodiagnosis |
| Helminthic infections | - | 0 | None in MMR |
| **Viruses (RNA subtype)** | | | |
| Picornaviruses | Coxsackie A + B | 0.019 | All by PCR, epidemiologic shift in late 1990s, none since 2002 |
| | Echo | 0.005 | PCR |
| | Hepatitis B and C | 0.002 | Serodiagnosis or PCR |
| Orthomyxoviruses | Influenza A or B | 0.002 | Serodiagnosis |
| | H1N1 | 0.001 | Serodiagnosis |
| Paramyxoviruses | Mumps | 0.001 | Serodiagnosis |
| | Measles | 0.002 | Serodiagnosis |
| Toga-/Rubivirus | Rubella | 0.001 | Serodiagnosis |
| Flavi-/Arbovirus | Dengue | 0.001 | Serodiagnosis |
| **Viruses (DNA subtype)** | | | |

(continued on next page)

**Table 2**
*(continued)*

| | Infections Agent | % pos. In MMR | Comments Diagnosis Made via: |
|---|---|---|---|
| Adenoviruses | A1, 2,3,5 | 0.011 | PCR |
| Erythroviruses | Parvovirus B19 types 1–3 | 28 | PCR |
| | Herpesviruses: human herpesvirus 6 | 0.03 | PCR; sometimes together with PVB 19 virus |
| | Cytomegalovirus | 0.02 | PCR or ISH |
| | Epstein-Barr virus | 0.012 | PCR |
| | Varicella zoster | 0.001 | Serodiagnosis |
| | Retrovirus: HIV | 0.005 | PCR or by serodiagnosis |
| | Rhabdovirus | 0.001 | – |
| 2. Noninfectious myocarditis | Autoreactive myocarditis | 53 | Exclusion of microbial agents |
| Systemic autoimmune diseases | Giant cell myocarditis | 0.03 | Histology |
| | Wegener granulomatosis | 0.01 | Histology |
| | Sarcoid heart disease | 0.015 | Histology |
| | Rheumatoid arthritis | 0.03 | Histology and serology |
| | Sjögren syndrome | 0.02 | Serology |
| | Systemic lupus | 0.05 | Serodiagnosis |
| | Crohn disease | 0.02 | Serodiagnosis |
| | Dermatomyositis | 0.02 | Serodiagnosis |
| | Kawasaki syndrome | 0.015 | – |
| Rejection | After heart transplantation | 1 | In cooperation with Hannover Medical School |
| | After stem cell transplantation | 0.002 | – |
| Hypereosinophilic Syndrome (HES) | Löffler endomyocarditis | 0.01 | Biopsy and histology |
| | Churg-Strauss syndrome | 0.01 | Biopsy and histology |
| 3. Toxicity | | | |
| Alcohol | Alcoholic cardiomyopathy | 0.2 | History, negative PCR on microorganisms |

| | | |
|---|---|---|
| Drug toxicity | Aminophylline, amphetamine, anthracycline, chloramphenicol, cocaine, cyclophosphamide, d5-fluorouracil, mesylate, methylsergide, Phenytoin, trastuzumab, zidovudine, ipilimumab, and nivolumab antibodies | 0.02 | Only anthracycline induced CMP in the MMR |
| Hypersensitivity reaction (drugs) | Azithromycin, benzodiazepine, clozapine, cephalosporin, dobutamine, lithium, diuretics, methyldopa, mexiletine, streptomycin, sulfonamides, NSAIDs, tetracycline, tricyclic antidepressants | 0.001 | Only one patient with lithium intoxication in MMR |
| Hypersensitivity reactions (venoms) | Bees, wasps, scorpions, snakes, spider | 0 | |
| Radiation injury | - | 0.015 | History + biopsy + imaging |
| Metabolic disorder | Diabetic cardiomyopathy | 0.02 | History + biopsy + imaging in diabetes patients |
| 4. Other patients with DCM | - | 16.62 | - |

*From* Maisch B, Alter P. Treatment options in myocarditis and inflammatory cardiomyopathy: Focus on i.v. immunoglobulins. *Herz.* 2018;43(5):423-430: with permission.

**Table 3**
**A 3-tiered clinical classification for the diagnosis of myocarditis based on the level of diagnostic certainty**

|  | Criteria | Histologic Confirmation | Biomarker, ECG, or Imaging Abnormalities Consistent with Myocarditis | Treatment |
|---|---|---|---|---|
| Possible subclinical acute myocarditis | In the clinical context of possible myocardial injury without cardiovascular symptoms but with at least one of the following: 1. Biomarkers of cardiac injury raised 2. ECG findings that suggest cardiac injury 3. Abnormal cardiac function on echocardiogram or cardiac MRI | Absent | Needed | Not known |
| Probable acute myocarditis | In the clinical context of possible myocardial injury with cardiovascular symptoms and at least one of the following: 1. Biomarkers of cardiac injury raised 2. ECG findings that suggest cardiac injury 3. Abnormal cardiac function on echocardiogram or cardiac MRI | Absent | Needed | Per clinical syndrome |
| Definite myocarditis | Histologic or immunohistologic evidence of myocarditis | Needed | Not needed | Tailored to specific cause |

*From* Sagar S, Liu PP, Cooper Jr LT. Myocarditis. Reprinted with permission from Elsevier (The Lancet, Sagar S, Liu PP, Cooper Jr LT. Myocarditis, March 2012, 379, 738-747).

delineate the diagnosis of myocarditis. The entire myocardium can be assessed, rather than just the right ventricular septal wall (which is biopsied on EMB). According to the LLC, at least 2 of the 3 following findings would fulfill the diagnosis of myocarditis: regional or global myocardial S1 increase in T2-weighted images, increased global myocardial early gadolinium enhancement (EGE) ratio between myocardium and skeletal muscle in gadolinium-enhanced T1-weighted images, and at least 1 focal lesion with nonischemic regional distribution in inversion recovery–prepared gadolinium-enhanced T1-weighted images.[54] In one of the largest pediatric MRI myocarditis studies, late gadolinium enhancement was present in 81% of 141 patients, with the most common pattern being subepicardial. T2-weighted imaging was abnormal in 74% and EGE in 60%.[55]

Since the release of the LLC, T1 and T2 mapping, which allow for comparison of quantified myocardial parameters with normal reference values, have improved the diagnostic accuracy of MRI for myocarditis.[56] Mean global T1 and T2 mapping values have been shown to be significantly elevated in patients with clinically suspected myocarditis compared with healthy controls with a sensitivity of 91% for both T1 and T2 mapping.[57] Combining T1 and T2 mapping with LLC led to a greater sensitivity than the LLC alone.

Timing of performing an MRI will most likely depend on the patient's clinical condition and index of suspicion of a diagnosis of myocarditis. Risk of sedation and endotracheal intubation causing clinical deterioration must be considered before use of MRI. Sensitivity of MRI was better when done in the acute phase versus the recovery phase, as myocardial edema began to resolve 14 days after onset of symptoms.[58]

MRI has become a potential alternative imaging modality if there is suspicion for myocarditis in a patient presenting with acute myocardial infarction symptoms. In one study, up to 21% of adolescents presenting with myocarditis were thought to have an acute myocardial infarction with cardiac MRI being able to distinguish between myocarditis and coronary ischemia.[59]

## ENDOMYOCARDIAL BIOPSY

Biopsy has been considered the gold standard in diagnosis of myocarditis since the proposal of the Dallas criteria in 1986.[60] These criteria require an inflammatory infiltrate and associated myocyte necrosis or damage not characteristic of an ischemic event. Borderline myocarditis requires a less intense inflammatory infiltrate and no light microscopic evidence of myocyte destruction.[61] Obtaining a biopsy is also an opportunity to detect a cardiotropic virus, which may increase confidence in the diagnosis of myocarditis. Reported performance of EMB has varied from 56% to 100% and is based on center preference and expertise.[62,63] Up to 72% of biopsies may show inflammation with cardiotropic viruses detected in 24% to 41% of patients.[22,64] Risk of obtaining EMB and lack of sensitivity should be incorporated into clinical decision-making. EMB should only be obtained if it will change clinical management.

Despite EMB being considered the gold standard for diagnosis of myocarditis, its use has decreased over time and its utility has been questioned.[60] Reasons for this include low sensitivity due to sampling error, variability in pathologic interpretation, and potential complications such as myocardial perforation and tamponade.[65–69]

## TREATMENT

Treatment efficacy continues to be controversial in pediatric patients with myocarditis. Assessing options depend on presenting symptoms, clinical stability, phase of illness, and long-term prognosis. Initial treatment may require use of inotropes or mechanical circulatory support (MCS) if the patient presents with fulminant myocarditis and hemo-dynamic instability. Some patients may present with minimal symptoms and normal hemodynamics that may require acute treatment without the need for long-term ther-apy. If patients with more severe presenting symptoms do not recover, proceeding to heart transplantation may be their best option for a good long-term outcome.

For years, the mainstay of therapy has been immune modulation. Opinions vary on which form to use. Nonsteroidal antiinflammatory drugs (NSAIDS), intravenous immu-noglobulin (IVIG), and corticosteroids have been most commonly used. NSAIDS can be used in patients with no more than mild ventricular dysfunction until inflammatory markers have normalized. Corticosteroids or IVIG tend to be used in more severe cases. Plasmapheresis may be used when antimyocyte antibodies are thought to be contributing to fulminant myocarditis. Side effects must be considered when formulating a treatment plan, including decrease in glomerular filtration rate (GFR) with NSAIDs; volume overload and decrease in GFR from IVIG; infection risk, hyper-tension, hyperglycemia, and psychological changes with steroids; and infection risk and need for vascular access with plasmapheresis.

Studies of immune modulation in humans have been limited by the use of historical controls, inclusion of patients with dilated cardiomyopathy rather than myocarditis, and administrative databases that rely on implantable cardioverter defibrillator codes for diagnosis.[12,70,71] Despite this, multiple studies of IVIG have been performed with conflicting outcomes.[70,72,73] Steroids and immunosuppressive agents have also been considered in addition to IVIG with mixed results.[74–78]

Until there is better evidence, treatment modalities should target the suspected in-fectious agent (if possible) and suspected immunologic mechanism at the estimated phase of the disease (**Fig. 4**). It has even been suggested that children with DCM

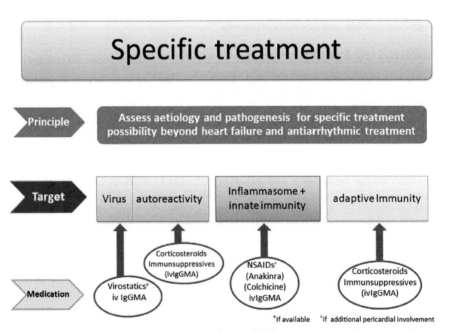

**Fig. 4.** Etiology-driven treatment in myocarditis and inflammatory cardiomyopathy. (*From* Maisch B. Management of pericarditis and pericardial effusion, constrictive and effusive-constrictive pericarditis. *Herz.* 2018:663-678; with permission (Figure 7 in original).)

should be evaluated for inflammatory cardiomyopathy in hopes of using immune modulating therapy as treatment.[79,80]

## MECHANICAL SUPPORT

MCS may be necessary in patients with severe to fulminant forms of myocarditis (11%–55%) and can provide time for myocardial recovery.[36,81,82] MCS may also act as a bridge to transplantation in the absence of recovery. Risk factors for the need

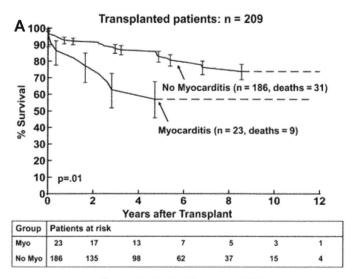

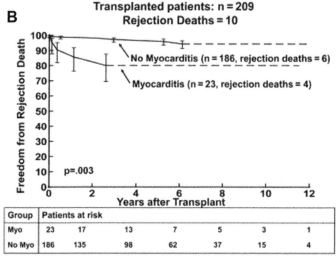

**Fig. 5.** (*A*) Kaplan-Meier posttransplantation survival curve for children with the diagnosis of myocarditis versus no myocarditis (at presentation). (*B*) Kaplan-Meier curves comparing freedom from rejection death posttransplantation for children with the diagnosis of myocarditis versus no myocarditis. The error bars represent 70% confidence limits. (*From* Pietra BA, Kantor PF, Bartlett HL, et al. Early Predictors of Survival to and After Heart Transplantation in Children with Dilated Cardiomyopathy; with permission.)

for MCS include female sex, vomiting, weakness, seizure, arrhythmia, and lower ejection fraction (EF).[41] Survival to hospital discharge following mechanical support has been reported to be anywhere from 70% to 92%.[81,83,84] ECMO is a rapidly deployable form of MCS and is used as a bridge to recovery when recovery is expected within 1 to 2 weeks. If recovery requires more time and lung function is intact, temporary or durable VAD placement can be used as a bridge to either recovery or decision for transplantation.

## TRANSPLANT

Myocarditis can lead to end-stage heart failure with only transplantation as an option for long-term survival. Nearly 5% of children listed for heart transplant had a diagnosis of myocarditis.[85] Children listed for transplant due to myocarditis are often sicker than those with other causes and more likely to have risk factors for poor posttransplant outcomes, such as mechanical ventilation, MCS, or renal dysfunction at the time of listing.[85–90] Studies are conflicting about the impact of myocarditis on survival posttransplant. A linked analysis of the Pediatric Cardiomyopathy Registry and Pediatric Heart Transplant Society database found that myocarditis was a risk factor for posttransplant mortality and cause of death was associated with acute rejection (**Fig. 5**).[91] A subsequent analysis of the Organ Procurement and Transportation Network suggested that an association between myocarditis was no longer seen after controlling for other risk factors (**Table 4**).[85,90,91] Individual centers need to determine how to incorporate these mixed results into their posttransplant treatment protocols.

## PREDICTING FACTORS AND OUTCOMES

The outcomes for patients diagnosed with myocarditis likely depend on multiple factors including severity of presentation, location, expertise of care, and timing of potential treatment. It is estimated that rate of survival after a diagnosis of myocarditis is anywhere from 75.6% to 98.6%.[3,5,11,12,34,92–94] Factors associated with poor

| Table 4 Multivariable predictors of waitlist mortality | | |
|---|---|---|
| Variable | Hazard Ratio (95% CI) | P Value |
| Myocarditis | 1.3 [0.9, 2.0] | .11 |
| Age <1 y | 2.3 [1.7, 3.3] | <.001 |
| Assisted ventilation at listing | 2.2 [1.5, 3.1] | <.001 |
| MCS at listing | | .02 |
| ECMO | 1.7 [1.1,2.7] | |
| BiVAD | 2.4 [1.2, 4.7] | |
| LVAD | 1.4 [0.8, 2.3] | |
| Renal dysfunction | | <.001 |
| Moderate | 2.3 [1.6, 3.2] | |
| Severe | 2.9 [1.7, 5.0] | |

Includes patients who became too sick to transplant.

*Abbreviations:* BiVAD, biventricular assist device; CI, confidence interval; ECMO, extracorporeal membrane oxygenation; LVAD, left ventricular assist device.

*From* Garbern JC, Gauvreau K, Blume ED, Singh TP. Is Myocarditis an Independent Risk Factor for Post-Transplant Mortality in Pediatric Heart Transplant Recipients? *Circ Hear Fail.* 2016;9(1); with permission.

outcomes include New York Heart Association class IV dyspnea, elevated brain natriuretic peptide, troponin, tachyarrhythmias, and a reduced rejection fraction.[10,12,92,95]

Historically, those presenting with fulminant myocarditis were thought to be more likely to survive. However, recent research has started to question this teaching.[96,97] Earlier studies had a low number of fulminant myocarditis cases, leading to low statistical power, longer time frame between symptom onset and study entry leading to a selection bias (omitting more aggressive courses), and different entry criteria compared with more recent studies. Overall, more recent studies suggest worse outcomes with fulminant myocarditis.[3] Persistence of a cardiotropic virus in the myocardium of patients with reduced LV function was associated with ongoing impairment of the LV EF.[98] This has potential to guide longer term treatment against specific viruses in an effort to preserve ventricular function.[23]

## SUMMARY

Myocarditis presents challenges for providers in determining appropriate diagnosis and treatment options. One must use a full armamentarium of clinical findings, laboratory testing, and imaging modalities to make the diagnosis. As technology improves and further study continues, diagnostic criteria may become clearer and treatment options more specific. Although overall outcomes are acceptable, there is room for improvement in our ability to specifically target infectious and immune mechanisms that lead to the sequelae of myocarditis. Such improvements have the potential to reduce mortality and improve the chances for recovery in children diagnosed with myocarditis.

## DISCLOSURE

The authors have nothing to disclose.

## REFERENCES

1. Richardson P, McKenna RW, Bristow M, et al. Report of the 1995 World Health Organization/International Society and Federation of Cardiology Task Force on the definition and classification of cardiomyopathies. Circulation 1996;93(5): 841–2.
2. Kociol RD, Cooper LT, Fang JC, et al. Recognition and initial management of fulminant myocarditis. Circulation 2020;141(6). https://doi.org/10.1161/cir. 0000000000000745.
3. Matsuura H, Ichida F, Saji T, et al. Clinical features of acute and fulminant myocarditis in children. Circ J 2016;80:2362–8.
4. Nugent AW, Daubeney PE, Chondros P, et al. The epidemiology of childhood cardiomyopathy in Australia. Vol 17. 2003. Available at: www.nejm.org. Accessed January 14, 2020.
5. Arola A, Pikkarainen E, Sipilä JOT, et al. Occurrence and features of childhood myocarditis: a nationwide study in Finland. J Am Heart Assoc 2017;6(11). https://doi.org/10.1161/JAHA.116.005306.
6. Lipshultz SE, Sleeper LA, Towbin JA, et al. The incidence of pediatric cardiomyopathy in two regions of the United States. Vol 17. 2003. Available at: www.nejm. org. Accessed January 14, 2020.
7. Wu MH, Wu ET, Wang CC, et al. Contemporary postnatal incidence of acquiring acute myocarditis by age 15 years and the outcomes from a Nationwide Birth Cohort. Pediatr Crit Care Med 2017;18(12):1153–8.

8. Friedman RA, Schowengerdt KO. The science and practice of pediatric cardiology. 2nd edition. Baltimore (MD): Williams & Wilkins; 1998. p. 1777.

9. Messroghli DR, Pickardt T, Fischer M, et al. Toward evidence-based diagnosis of myocarditis in children and adolescents: Rationale, design, and first baseline data of MYKKE, a multicenter registry and study platform From the Trial Design. Am Hear J 2017;187:133–77.

10. Anderson BR, Silver ES, Richmond ME, et al. Usefulness of arrhythmias as predictors of death and resource utilization in children with myocarditis. Am J Cardiol 2014. https://doi.org/10.1016/j.amjcard.2014.07.074.

11. Ghelani SJ, Spaeder MC, Pastor W, et al. Demographics, trends, and outcomes in pediatric acute myocarditis in the United States, 2006 to 2011. Circ Cardiovasc Qual Outcomes 2012;5(5):622–7.

12. Butts RJ, Boyle GJ, Deshpande SR, et al. Characteristics of clinically diagnosed pediatric myocarditis in a contemporary multi-center cohort. Pediatr Cardiol 2017;38(6):1175–82.

13. Weber MA, Ashworth MT, Risdon RA, et al. Clinicopathological features of paediatric deaths due to myocarditis: an autopsy series. Arch Dis Child 2008. https://doi.org/10.1136/adc.2007.128686.

14. Bagnall RD, Weintraub RG, Ingles J, et al. A prospective study of sudden cardiac death among children and young adults. N Engl J Med 2016;374(25):2441–52.

15. Meyer L, Stubbs B, Fahrenbruch C, et al. Incidence, causes, and survival trends from cardiovascular-related sudden cardiac arrest in children and young adults 0 to 35 years of age: a 30-year review. Circulation 2012;126(11):1363–72.

16. Gajewski KK, Saul JP. Sudden cardiac death in children and adolescents (excluding Sudden Infant Death Syndrome). Ann Pediatr Cardiol 2010;3(2):107–12.

17. Shatz A, Hiss J, Arensburg B. Myocarditis misdiagnosed as sudden infant death syndrome (SIDS). Med Sci Law 1997;37(1):16–8.

18. Rajs J, Hammarquist F. Sudden infant death in Stockholm. A forensic pathology study covering ten years. Acta Paediatr Scand 1988;77(6):812–20.

19. Rasten-Almqvist P, Eksborg S, Rajs J. Myocarditis and sudden infant death syndrome. APMIS 2002;110(6):469–80.

20. Schultz J, Hilliard A, Cooper L Jr, et al. Diagnosis and treatment of viral myocarditis. Mayo Clin Proc 2009;84(11):1001–9. Available at: www.mayoclinicproceedings.com. Accessed March 3, 2020.

21. Maisch B. Cardio-immunology of myocarditis: focus on immune mechanisms and treatment options. Front Cardiovasc Med 2019;6. https://doi.org/10.3389/fcvm.2019.00048.

22. Degener F, Opgen-Rhein B, Wagner R, et al. Virus detection within endomyocardial biopsy in pediatric myocarditis: results from the German Multi-Center Registry "MYKKE." Cardiol Young 2019;29:S8-S9 (Abstract).

23. Gagliardi MG, Fierabracci A, Pilati M, et al. The impact of specific viruses on clinical outcome in children presenting with acute heart failure. Int J Mol Sci 2016;17(4):1–10.

24. Bowles NE, Ni J, Kearney DL, et al. Detection of viruses in myocardial tissues by polymerase chain reaction: Evidence of adenovirus as a common cause of myocarditis in children and adults. J Am Coll Cardiol 2003;42(3):466–72.

25. den Boer SL, Meijer RPJ, van Iperen GG, et al. Evaluation of the diagnostic workup in children with myocarditis and idiopathic dilated cardiomyopathy. Pediatr Cardiol 2015;36(2):409–16.

26. Schenk T, Enders M, Pollak S, et al. High prevalence of human parvovirus B19 DNA in myocardial autopsy samples from subjects without myocarditis or dilative cardiomyopathy. J Clin Microbiol 2009;47(1):106–10.
27. Aykac K, Ozsurekci Y, Kahyaoglu P, et al. Myocarditis associated with influenza infection in five children. J Infect Public Health 2018;11(5):698–701.
28. Ben Khelil M, Chkirbene Y, Mlika M, et al. Penicillin-Induced Fulminant Myocarditis: A Case Report and Review of the Literature. Am J Forensic Med Pathol 2017;38(1):29–31.
29. Nappe T, Hoyte C. Pediatric Death Due to Myocarditis After Exposure to Cannabis. Clin Pract Cases Emerg Med 2017;1(3):166–70.
30. Gosselin M, Dazé Y, Mireault P, et al. Toxic Myocarditis Caused by Acetaminophen in a Multidrug Overdose. Am J Forensic Med Pathol 2017;38(4):349–52.
31. Kawai C. From myocarditis to cardiomyopathy: Mechanisms of inflammation and cell death: Learning from the past for the future. Circulation 1999;99(8):1091–100.
32. Pollack A, Kontorovich AR, Fuster V, et al. Viral myocarditis-diagnosis, treatment options, and current controversies. Nat Rev Cardiol 2015;12(11):670–80.
33. Schultheiss H-P, Kü Hl U, Cooper LT. The management of myocarditis. Eur Heart J 2011. https://doi.org/10.1093/eurheartj/ehr165.
34. Abe T, Tsuda E, Miyazaki A, et al. Clinical characteristics and long-term outcome of acute myocarditis in children. Heart Vessels 2013;28(5):632–8.
35. Durani Y, Egan M, Baffa J, et al. Pediatric myocarditis: presenting clinical characteristics. Am J Emerg Med 2009;27:942–7.
36. Degener F, Opgen-Rhein B, Böhne M, et al. Four-Year Experience of the German Multicenter Registry for Pediatric Patients with Suspected Myocarditis: MYKKE. In: 50th Annual Meeting of the German Society for Pediatric Cardiology (DGPK). Vol 66. Georg Thieme Verlag KG; 2018. doi:10.1055/s-0038-1628324.
37. Niu L, An X-J, Tian J, et al. 124 cases of clinical analysis of children with viral myocarditis. Eur Rev Med Pharmacol Sci 2015;19:2856–9.
38. Price S, Bodys A, Celińska A, et al. Interlibrary Loan The value of chosen diagnostic tools in evaluating myocarditis in children and adolescents. Pediatr Pol J Paediatr 2018;93(5):389–95.
39. Rodriguez-Gonzalez M, Sanchez-Codez MI, Lubian-Gutierrez M, et al. Clinical presentation and early predictors for poor outcomes in pediatric myocarditis: A retrospective study. World J Clin Cases 2019;7(5):548–61.
40. Suthar D, Dodd DA, Godown J. Identifying Non-invasive Tools to Distinguish Acute Myocarditis from Dilated Cardiomyopathy in Children. Pediatr Cardiol 2018;39(6):1134–8.
41. Wu HP, Lin MJ, Yang WC, et al. Predictors of Extracorporeal Membrane Oxygenation Support for Children with Acute Myocarditis. Biomed Res Int 2017;2017. https://doi.org/10.1155/2017/2510695.
42. Rady HI, Zekri H. Prevalence of myocarditis in pediatric intensive care unit cases presenting with other system involvement. J Pediatr (Rio J) 2015;91(1):93–7.
43. De Vetten L, Bergman KA, Elzenga NJ, et al. Neonatal myocardial infarction or myocarditis? Pediatr Cardiol 2011;32(4):492–7.
44. Jedidi M, Tilouche S, Masmoudi T, et al. Infant acute myocarditis mimicking acute myocardial infarction. Autops Case Rep 2016. https://doi.org/10.4322/acr.2016.052.
45. Freund MW, Kleinveld G, Krediet TG, et al. Prognosis for neonates with enterovirus myocarditis. Arch Dis Child Fetal Neonatal Ed 2010;95(3):F206–12.
46. Maisch B, Alter P. Treatment options in myocarditis and inflammatory cardiomyopathy: Focus on i. v. immunoglobulins. Herz 2018;43(5):423–30.

47. Chow LH, Radio SJ, Sears TD, et al. Insensitivity of right ventricular endomyocardial biopsy in the diagnosis of myocarditis. J Am Coll Cardiol 1989;14;915-20.

48. Sagar S, Liu PP, Cooper Jr LT. Myocarditis. Lancet. 2012;379(9817):738-47.

49. Eisenberg MA, Green-Hopkins I, Alexander ME, et al. Cardiac troponin t as a screening test for myocarditis in children. Pediatr Emerg Care 2012;28(11): 1173–8.

50. Chong S-L, Bautista D, Ang A-Y. Diagnosing paediatric myocarditis: what really matters. Emerg Med J 2015;32:138–43.

51. Batra AS, Epstein D, Silka MJ. The clinical course of acquired complete heart block in children with acute myocarditis. Pediatr Cardiol 2003;24:495–7.

52. Loevets TS, Boldina NM, Vershinina TL, et al. The approach to drug therapy of arrythmias in children with suspected myocarditis. Cardiol. Young 2019;29:S76(Abstract).

53. Felker GM, Boehmer JP, Hruban RH, et al. Echocardiographic findings in fulminant and acute myocarditis. J Am Coll Cardiol 2000;36(1):227–32.

54. Friedrich MG, Sechtem U, Schulz-Menger J, et al. Cardiovascular Magnetic Resonance in Myocarditis: A JACC White Paper. J Am Coll Cardiol 2009; 53(17):1475–87.

55. Banka P, Robinson JD, Uppu SC, et al. Cardiovascular magnetic resonance techniques and findings in children with myocarditis: a multicenter retrospective study. J Cardiovasc Magn Reson 2015;17(1). https://doi.org/10.1186/s12968-015-0201-6.

56. Kim PK, Hong YJ, Im DJ, et al. Myocardial T1 and T2 mapping: Techniques and clinical applications. Korean J Radiol 2017;18(1):113–31.

57. Cornicelli MD, Rigsby CK, Rychlik K, et al. Diagnostic performance of cardiovascular magnetic resonance native T1 and T2 mapping in pediatric patients with acute myocarditis. J Cardiovasc Magn Reson 2019;21(1). https://doi.org/10.1186/s12968-019-0550-7.

58. Lv J, Han B, Wang C, et al. The Clinical Features of Children With Acute Fulminant Myocarditis and the Diagnostic and Follow-Up Value of Cardiovascular Magnetic Resonance. Front Pediatr 2019;7. https://doi.org/10.3389/fped.2019.00388.

59. Martinez-Villar M, Gran F, Sabaté-Rotés A, et al. Interlibrary Loan Acute Myocarditis with Infarct-like Presentation in a Pediatric Population: Role of Cardiovascular Magnetic Resonance. Pediatr Cardiol 2018. https://doi.org/10.1007/s00246-017-1726-2.

60. Baughman KL. Diagnosis of myocarditis: death of Dallas criteria. Circulation 2006;113(4):593–5.

61. Aretz HT, Billingham ME, Edwards WD, et al. Myocarditis. A histopathologic definition and classification. Am J Cardiovasc Pathol 1987;1(1):3–14.

62. Degener F, Opgen-Rhein B, Wagner R, et al. Impact of endomyocardial biopsy on treatment and outcome in pediatric myocarditis: results from the german multicenter registry for pediatric myocarditis "MYKKE." In: 51st Annual Meeting German Society for Pediatric Cardiology. Vol 67. Georg Thieme Verlag KG; 2019. doi:10.1055/s-0039-1679088.

63. Giulia Gagliardi M, Bevilacqua M, Bassano C, et al. Long term follow up of children with myocarditis treated by immunosuppression and of children with dilated cardiomyopathy. Heart 2004;90(10):1167–71.

64. Brighenti M, Donti A, Giulia Gagliardi M, et al. Endomyocardial biopsy safety and clinical yield in pediatric myocarditis: An Italian perspective. Catheter Cardiovasc Interv 2016;87(4):762–7.

65. Daly KP, Marshall AC, Vincent JA, et al. Endomyocardial biopsy and selective coronary angiography are low-risk procedures in pediatric heart transplant recipients: Results of a multicenter experience. J Heart Lung Transplant 2012;31(4): 398–409.

66. Pophal SG, Sigfusson G, Booth KL, et al. Complications of endomyocardial biopsy in children. J Am Coll Cardiol 1999;34(7):2105–10.

67. Mahrholdt H, Goedecke C, Wagner A, et al. Cardiovascular Magnetic Resonance Assessment of Human Myocarditis: A Comparison to Histology and Molecular Pathology. Circulation 2004;109(10):1250–8.

68. Shanes JG, Ghali J, Billingham ME, et al. Interobserver variability in the pathologic interpretation of endomyocardial biopsy results. Circulation 1987;75(2): 401–5.

69. Martin AB, Webber S, Fricker FJ, et al. Acute myocarditis: Rapid diagnosis by PCR in children. Circulation 1994;90(1):330–9.

70. Drucker NA, Colan SD, Lewis AB, et al. $\gamma$-Globulin treatment of acute myocarditis in the pediatric population. Circulation 1994;89(1):252–7.

71. McNamara DM, Holubkov R, Starling RC, et al. Controlled trial of intravenous immune globulin in recent-onset dilated cardiomyopathy. Circulation 2001;103(18): 2254–9.

72. Robinson J, Hartling L, Vandermeer B, et al. Intravenous immunoglobulin for presumed viral myocarditis in children and adults (Review) Summary of findings for the main comparison. Cochrane Database Syst Rev 2015;(5). https://doi.org/10.1002/14651858.CD004370.pub3. Available at: www.cochranelibrary.com.

73. Yen CY, Hung MC, Wong YC, et al. Role of intravenous immunoglobulin therapy in the survival rate of pediatric patients with acute myocarditis: A systematic review and meta-analysis. Sci Rep 2019;9(1). https://doi.org/10.1038/s41598-019-46888-0.

74. Kim HJ, Yoo GH, Kil HR. Clinical outcome of acute myocarditis in children according to treatment modalities. Korean J Pediatr 2010;53(7):745–52.

75. English RF, Janosky JE, Ettedgui JA, et al. Outcomes for children with acute myocarditis. Cardiol Young 2004;14(5):488–93.

76. Huang X, Sun Y, Su G, et al. Intravenous immunoglobulin therapy for acute myocarditis in children and adults a meta-analysis. Int Heart J 2019. https://doi.org/10.1536/ihj.18-299.

77. Limongelli G, Merlo M, He B, et al. Immunosuppressive treatment for myocarditis in the pediatric population: a meta-analysis. Front Pediatr 2019;7:430. Available at: www.frontiersin.org.

78. Lin MS, Tseng YH, Chen MY, et al. In-hospital and post-discharge outcomes of pediatric acute myocarditis underwent after high-dose steroid or intravenous immunoglobulin therapy. BMC Cardiovasc Disord 2019;19(1). https://doi.org/10.1186/s12872-018-0981-3.

79. Canter CE, Simpson KP. Diagnosis and treatment of myocarditis in children in the current era. Circulation 2014;129(1):115–28.

80. Maisch B. Management of pericarditis and pericardial effusion, constrictive and effusive-constrictive pericarditis. Herz 2018;663–78.

81. Nosaka N, Muguruma T, Fujiwara T, et al. Effects of the elective introduction of extracorporeal membrane oxygenation on outcomes in pediatric myocarditis cases. Acute Med Surg 2015;2(2):92–7.

82. Saji T, Matsuura H, Hasegawa K, et al. Comparison of the clinical presentation, treatment, and outcome of fulminant and acute myocarditis in cshildren. Circ J 2012;76:1222–8.

83. Jung Y, Shin HJ, Jung JW, et al. Extracorporeal life support can be a first-line treatment in children with acute fulminant myocarditis. Interact Cardiovasc Thorac Surg 2016. https://doi.org/10.1093/icvts/ivw114.
84. Xiong H, Xia B, Zhu J, et al. Clinical outcomes in pediatric patients hospitalized with fulminant myocarditis requiring extracorporeal membrane oxygenation: a meta-analysis. Pediatr Cardiol 2017;38(2):209–14.
85. Garbern JC, Gauvreau K, Blume ED, et al. Is Myocarditis an Independent Risk Factor for Post-Transplant Mortality in Pediatric Heart Transplant Recipients? Circ Hear Fail 2016;9(1). https://doi.org/10.1161/CIRCHEARTFAILURE.115.002328.
86. Davies RR, Russo MJ, Mital S, et al. Predicting survival among high-risk pediatric cardiac transplant recipients: An analysis of the United Network for Organ Sharing database. J Thorac Cardiovasc Surg 2008;135(1). https://doi.org/10.1016/j.jtcvs.2007.09.019.
87. Almond CS, Gauvreau K, Canter CE, et al. A risk-prediction model for in-hospital mortality after heart transplantation in US children. Am J Transplant 2012;12(5):1240–8.
88. Dipchand AI, Kirk R, Edwards LB, et al. The registry of the international society for heart and lung transplantation: Sixteenth official pediatric heart transplantation report - 2013; Focus theme: Age. J Heart Lung Transplant 2013;32(10):979–88.
89. Gandhi R, Almond C, Singh TP, et al. Factors associated with in-hospital mortality in infants undergoing heart transplantation in the United States. J Thorac Cardiovasc Surg 2011;141(2):531–6.e1.
90. Kirk R, Naftel D, Hoffman TM, et al. Outcome of pediatric patients with dilated cardiomyopathy listed for transplant: a multi-institutional study. J Heart Lung Transpl 2009. https://doi.org/10.1016/j.healun.2009.05.027.
91. Pietra BA, Kantor PF, Bartlett HL, et al. Early predictors of survival to and after heart transplantation in children with dilated cardiomyopathy. Circulation 2012. https://doi.org/10.1161/CIRCULATIONAHA.110.011999.
92. Abrar S, Ansari MJ, Mittal M, et al. Predictors of mortality in paediatric myocarditis. J Clin Diagn Res 2016;10(6):SC12–6. https://doi.org/10.7860/JCDR/2016/19856.7967.
93. Degener F, Opgen-Rhein B, Boehne M, et al. Survival and outcome in pediatric myocarditis-3 year data from the german multicenter prospective myocarditis registry: "MYKKE."
94. Towbin JA, Lowe AM, Colan SD, et al. Incidence, causes, and outcomes of dilated cardiomyopathy in children. J Am Med Assoc 2006;296(15):1867–76.
95. Al-Biltagi M, Issa M, Hagar HA, et al. Circulating cardiac troponins levels and cardiac dysfunction in children with acute and fulminant viral myocarditis. Acta Paediatr Int J Paediatr 2010;99(10):1510–6.
96. McCarthy RE, Boehmer JP, Hruban RH, et al. Long-term outcome of fulminant myocarditis as compared with acute (nonfulminant) myocarditis. N Engl J Med 2000;342(10):690–5.
97. Ammirati E, Lilliu M, Cipriani M, et al. Mid-term outcome of acute fulminant myocarditis presenting with cardiogenic shock: a single centre experience does time on ventricular assist device compromise post-transplant outcome? J Heart Lung Transplant 2015;34(4): S178.
98. Kühl U, Pauschinger M, Seeberg B, et al. Viral persistence in the myocardium is associated with progressive cardiac dysfunction. Circulation 2005. https://doi.org/10.1161/CIRCULATIONAHA.105.548156.

# Pediatric Infective Endocarditis: A Clinical Update

Daniel A. Cox, DO*, Lloyd Y. Tani, MD

## KEYWORDS

• Antibiotic • Echocardiography • Endocarditis • Infection • Pediatric • Valve

## KEY POINTS

• Infective or bacterial endocarditis is an infectious process that involves the heart valves or cardiovascular structures.
• Endocarditis prophylaxis recommendations are more selective for when and for which patients should receive prophylactic antibiotics.
• Transthoracic and transesophageal echocardiography remains the main imaging modalities that assist in diagnosis of infective endocarditis in pediatrics.
• Bioprosthetic valve endocarditis is becoming a more common source of endocarditis, even in the pediatric population.

## INTRODUCTION

Infective endocarditis (IE) is an infection of the endocardium of the heart and vascular endothelium. This process can include the native endocardium of the heart chambers or the endothelium associated with the cardiac valves or prosthetic hardware or material (prosthetic valves, conduits, grafts, patches, or pacemaker generator or leads). IE development is a complex process that involves the susceptibility of a valve or tissue to bacterial adherence, survival of the bacteria on the tissue or associated structure, and propagation of the infected vegetation.[1] Most commonly, IE involves a bacterial infection, but can also include a fungal infection. In the pediatric population of developed countries, a shift away from rheumatic heart disease predisposition has occurred. Prior studies estimated that 30% to 50% of children in the United States who eventually developed IE had prior rheumatic heart disease.[2]

With the decrease in the prevalence of rheumatic heart disease in developed countries, nonrheumatic predisposing conditions such as congenital heart disease are more common. It should be noted that endocarditis complicating rheumatic heart

University of Utah School of Medicine, 81 North Mario Capecchi Drive, Salt Lake City, UT 84113, USA
* Corresponding author.
*E-mail address:* d.cox@hsc.utah.edu

Pediatr Clin N Am 67 (2020) 875–888
https://doi.org/10.1016/j.pcl.2020.06.011
0031-3955/20/© 2020 Elsevier Inc. All rights reserved.

disease continues to occur in many patients in parts of the world where rheumatic heart disease continues to be prevalent. With this said, 8% to 10% of pediatric IE cases develop in structurally normal hearts, most commonly being associated with *Staphylococcus aureus*.[3] Between the 1960s and 1980s, it has been estimated that endocarditis was responsible for an estimated 1 in 500 to 1 in 1000 pediatric hospitalizations.[4] More recent studies have estimated there to be 0.43 cases per 100,000 children.[5] This finding differs significantly from the reported incidence in an adult population of 15 cases per 100,000 adults.[6] The infectious process involving the endocardium, and the inflammatory process associated with the infection, carries significant risk of morbidity and mortality if not identified early with implementation of effective treatment. Updates published over the past several years take into account the change in pathogenic variance as well as patient-related changes.[7] Although guidelines have been written for pediatric IE, the majority of recommendations are extrapolated from adult studies and guidelines. Diagnostic criteria have been proposed and modified over the past several decades, including the Beth Israel criteria and the Duke criteria.[8,9] More recently, a set of modified Duke criteria has been more readily used to aid in diagnosis: **Box 1**.[10] These criteria help to define definitive IE, possible IE, or rejection of a diagnosis of IE.[10] Certain bacteria or infectious processes, such as that seen with *Staphylococcus*, have become more commonly associated with IE, and have also affected outcomes. However, there has been an increase in streptococcal IE seen in pediatric populations, more commonly with underlying cardiac conditions.[5] Unfortunately, despite medical and surgical advances, outcomes have not been greatly affected over the past few decades.[4]

## SOURCE OF INFECTION

Variable sources of IE have been identified, as have the potential cardiovascular structures involved. Commonly involved structures include native cardiac valves, prosthetic valves (bioprosthetic or mechanical), nonvalvar cardiovascular structures (unrepaired ventricular septal defects, patent ductus arteriosus), prosthetic materials (patches, shunts, conduits, stents), implanted devices (pacemaker, leads, ventricular assist devices). Treatment strategies differ based on the structures involved. In adult populations, intravenous drug use remains a common source of IE with the incidence continuing to increase nationally.[11] Although less common in the pediatric population, intravenous drug use should not be excluded as a potential source of infection, especially when right-sided IE is identified. Central lines, implanted devices, synthetic shunts or grafts, increasing numbers of children with cyanotic heart disease, and general immunodeficiencies also contribute to the shifting etiologies associated with IE. In children with an underlying congenital heart condition, the incidence of IE has been estimated at 6.1 per 1000 children with 34% occurring in cyanotic cardiac conditions. In addition, children who had undergone cardiac surgery in the prior 6 months are more than 5 times more likely to develop IE compared with those who had not undergone a cardiac surgery or intervention.[12] The most common associated bacteria include gram-positive organisms (staphylococci, streptococci, enterococci) and less commonly gram-negative bacteria such as the HACEK organisms (*Haemophilus aphrophilus* [more recently identified as *Aggregatibacter aphrophilus* and *Aggregatibacter paraphrophilus*], *Actinobaccillus actinomycetemcomitans* [more recently identified as *Aggregatibacter actinomycetemcomitans*], *Cardiobacterium hominis*, *Eikenella corrodens*, and *Kingella kingae*). Culture-negative endocarditis can also occur (discussed in the section on Diagnostic Modalities). Fungal IE most commonly occurs with candida or *Aspergillus* species.

**Box 1**
**The modified Duke criteria for the diagnosis of IE**

Definitive IE
  Pathologic criteria
  • Micro-organisms demonstrated by culture or histologic examination of vegetation, vegetation that has embolized, or an intracardiac abscess specimen; or
  • Pathologic lesions; vegetation or intro cardiac abscess confirmed by histologic examination showing active endocarditis.
  Clinical criteria
  • Two major and 0 minor criteria; or
  • One major and 3 minor criteria; or
  • No major and 5 minor criteria.
  Major criteria
  • Positive blood culture positive for IE
    ○ Typical endocarditis organism from 2 separate blood cultures
      ■ Viridans streptococci or *Streptococcus bovis*
      ■ HACEK organisms
      ■ *Staphylococcus aureus*
      ■ Community-acquired enterococcus in absence of primary focus
    ○ Micro-organisms consistent with IE from persistently positive blood cultures:
      ■ Two separate blood cultures from samples drawn greater than 12 hours apart
      ■ Three, or a majority of 4 or more, separate blood cultures (first and last sample drawn 1 hour apart)
      ■ Single positive blood culture for *Coxiella burnetii* or an antiphase I IgG antibody titer of greater than 1:800
  • Evidence of endocardial involvement
  • Echocardiogram positive for IE
    ○ Oscillating intracardiac mass on valve or supporting structures, in the path of regurgitant jets, or on implanted material in the absence of an alternative anatomic explanation; or
    ○ Abscess; or
    ○ New partial dehiscence of prosthetic valve or new valvular regurgitation.
  • New valvular regurgitation (worsening or changing of preexisting murmur not sufficient)
  Minor criteria
  • Predisposing heart condition or intravenous drug use
  • Fever, temperature greater than 38° C (100.4° F)
  • Vascular phenomena: major arterial emboli, septic pulmonary infarcts, mycotic aneurysm, intracranial bleed, conjunctival hemorrhages, Janeway lesions
  • Immunologic phenomena: glomerulonephritis, Osler nodes, Roth spots, rheumatoid factor
  • Microbiological evidence: positive blood culture, but does not meet a major criterion as noted or serologic evidence of an active infection with organism consistent with IE (excluding single positive culture for coagulase-negative staphylococci and other common contaminants)

Possible IE
  Clinical criteria
  • One major criterion and one minor criterion; or
  • Three minor criteria

Rejected diagnosis
  • Firm alternative diagnosis explaining evidence of IE; or
  • Resolution of IE syndrome with antibiotic therapy for less than or equal to 4 days; or
  • No pathologic evidence of IE at surgery or autopsy, with antibiotic therapy for less than or equal to 4 days; or
  • Does not meet criteria for possible IE, as described

*Adapted from* Li JS, Sexton DJ, Mick N, et al. Proposed modifications to the Duke criteria for the diagnosis of infective endocarditis. *Clin Infect Dis.* 2000;30(4):633-638; with permission.

## RISK FACTORS FOR ENDOCARDITIS

For IE to occur, 2 factors are required: bacteremia (or less commonly fungemia) and disruption of the endocardium or endothelial lining. With an increasing number of children with complex congenital heart disease surviving past infancy, the number of IE cases is shifting from pediatric patients with no structural heart conditions to those with structural heart conditions.

IE commonly develops on areas exposed to blood flow from a high-pressure system through a narrow orifice with the site of infection being in the low-pressure area distal to the narrowing. It is theorized that this area of lower pressure may predispose the tissue to hypoxia and poor metabolic perfusion, and in turn lead to deformation of the valve or vessel wall leading to a propensity to develop IE. In turn, tricuspid and mitral valve vegetations are commonly identified on the atrial surface adjacent to the line of closure. Aortic and pulmonary valve vegetations more commonly occur on the ventricular surface, with aortic insufficiency-related IE also potentially involving the anterior leaflet of the mitral chordae and muscular attachments. IE associated with a ventricular septal defect commonly occurs on the right ventricle side (**Fig. 1**).[13]

There seems to be a bimodal distribution of IE cases with a peak during infancy and another during late adolescence. IE in neonates has increased over the past decades and is often associated with indwelling lines and right-sided vegetations.[14]

Additionally, prosthetic valves are becoming a more common source of infection in the pediatric population. There seems to be a propensity to IE with bovine jugular vein valves, including the Contegra surgical valve and the Melody transcatheter valve (Medtronic Inc, Minneapolis, MN), when compared with other valve types. The transcatheter valves are used more frequently in the pediatric and adolescent populations as experience with the valves and number of implanted valves increase. One systematic review of IE in bioprosthetic valves in the pulmonic position reported a 5.4% incidence in the bovine jugular vein valves regardless of mode of implantation, compared with 1.2% in other valve types.[15] Additional studies have indicated that IE associated with the transcatheter Melody valve implanted in the pulmonary position may also be higher with an incidence of 3.2% to 25% with an annualized incidence rate of 1.3% to 9.1% per patient-year.[16]

## CLINICAL FINDINGS AND SYMPTOMS OF INFECTIVE ENDOCARDITIS

In pediatrics, higher risk symptoms and physical examination findings should raise suspicion for IE. Unexplained and persistent fevers without a potential source in a patient who carries a high risk for IE should be evaluated thoroughly. Nonspecific findings commonly include new-onset fatigue, night sweats or chills, generalized malaise, and weight loss. With IE associated with a cardiac valve, a murmur will likely become evident. It can be challenging to differentiate a new pathologic murmur from an innocent murmur in times of illness, but can be potentially differentiated by a skilled provider with good auscultation. A new diastolic murmur or an abnormal systolic murmur (often regurgitant or holosystolic) should raise suspicion in a patient without a history of structural heart disease. In patients with bioprosthetic valves, a new diastolic murmur or a rapidly changing or progressive systolic ejection murmur should also raise high suspicion.

As the infectious process proceeds, progressive heart failure symptoms related to valve insufficiency or stenosis may become more evident, as may embolic events. In addition to the infectious process that occurs in relation to IE, the inflammatory and immune response will often contribute to the associated clinical findings and symptoms. This response may include myalgias, neurologic changes, dermatologic

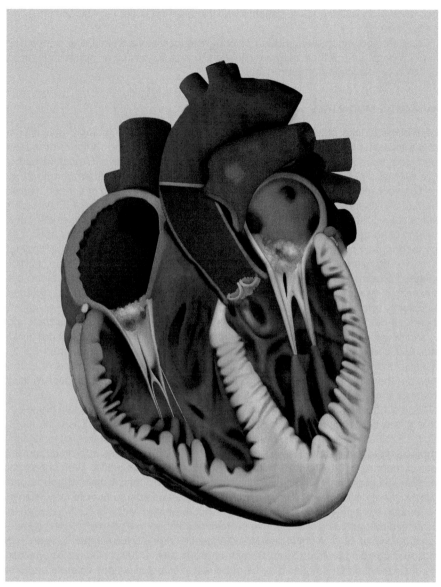

**Fig. 1.** Representation of common areas of endocarditis, including the atrial side of the tricuspid and mitral valve, ventricular side of the aortic valve.

findings such as splinter hemorrhages, Roth spots (retinal hemorrhagic lesions), Janeway lesions (painless hemorrhagic lesions of the distal extremities), or Osler nodes (painful nodules of the distal extremities). The skin manifestations, if present, are associated with an increased risk of complications. Servy and colleagues[17] noted in a population-based study in 2008 that 11.9% of patients with definite IE had skin manifestations consisting of purpura in 8.0%, Osler nodes in 2.7%, and Janeway lesions in 1.6%. These patients carried a 32.8% risk of cerebral emboli, compared with 18.4% of those without skin manifestations, with Janeway lesions correlating with a 75.0% risk of cerebral emboli. In addition, patients with purpura had larger vegetations (18.1 mm vs 13.7 mm).[17]

Visual changes such as a sudden or complete loss of vision in 1 eye or eye pain should prompt an ophthalmologic evaluation to look for retinal or ophthalmic artery occlusion or associated endophthalmitis.

## DIAGNOSTIC MODALITIES

The modified Duke criteria for diagnosis of IE incorporate pathologic and clinical criteria to assist in the diagnosis of IE (see **Box 1**)[10] Major and minor criteria have been recommended to stratify patients into 3 categories: definitive IE (positive pathologic criteria, 2 major and no minor criteria, 1 major and 3 minor criteria, or no major and 5 minor criteria), possible IE (1 major and 1 minor criteria, or no major and 3 minor criteria), and rejected diagnosis of IE (alternative diagnosis, resolution of IE syndrome with antibiotic therapy for less than or equal to 4 days, no pathologic evidence of IE at the time of surgery or autopsy and having received less than 4 days of antibiotic therapy, or not meeting the other criteria for IE). Major criteria include pathologic findings of micro-organisms demonstrated by culture or histologic examination from a collected specimen showing active infection. They also include a positive blood culture with a typical endocarditis micro-organism from 2 separate blood cultures, persistently positive blood cultures with micro-organisms consistent with IE, evidence of endocardial involvement, an echocardiogram positive for findings consistent with IE, and new valve regurgitation. Minor criteria include a predisposing heart condition, intravenous drug use, a febrile illness with a temperature of greater than 38° C, vascular phenomena, immunologic phenomena, microbiological evidence of IE that does not meet a major criterion, or serologic evidence of an active infection with an organism that is consistent with IE.[10]

Blood cultures are the mainstay of diagnosis. It is not necessary to obtain blood cultures at the time of fever because the bacteremia associated with IE is continuous. Ideally, 3 cultures drawn from separate sites should be obtained before administering empiric antibiotic therapy. Even in the setting where blood culture sampling occurs in a correct manner, 5% to 10% of cases of IE remain culture negative. With suspected endocarditis in patients who have been treated for fewer than 4 days without a prior blood culture, cessation of antibiotic therapy can be considered to potentially identify a pathogen if the patient is clinically stable.[4] Acute phase reactants such as an erythrocyte sedimentation rate, C-reactive protein, or an abnormal platelet count may support a diagnosis, but are not included in diagnostic criteria because they are generally nonspecific findings related to inflammatory processes. Other molecular or polymerase chain reaction techniques may be of benefit in select situations where a bacterial source has not been detected.

Although echocardiographic imaging plays an important role, the initiation of treatment after obtaining blood cultures in highly suspicious cases should not be delayed before obtaining echocardiographic imaging.

Echocardiographic imaging should be performed on any patient with suspected endocarditis to assist in diagnosis. Echocardiographic imaging of intracardiac masses, noninfectious thrombus, and vegetations associated with IE may be indistinguishable (**Fig. 2**). Without additional clinical findings, echocardiographic imaging alone is insufficient to diagnose IE and is inappropriate to use as a screening test. In the pediatric population, transesophageal echocardiographic imaging has not been shown to increase the diagnostic potential. In a majority of cases, transthoracic imaging is sufficient for the initial evaluation of suspected IE. In cases where

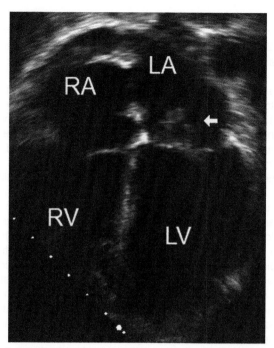

**Fig. 2.** Transthoracic echocardiogram 4-chamber view with large vegetation (*arrow*) associated with the anterior leaflet of the mitral valve. LA, left atrium; LV, left ventricle; RA, right atrium; RV, right ventricle.

transthoracic windows for imaging are poor with incomplete visualization of higher risk structures, transesophageal imaging should be considered. These factors may include patients with a prominent lung artifact, a larger body habitus, or a prosthetic valve or material that is positioned behind the sternum or other location not well-visualized by transthoracic imaging. In addition, persistent bacteremia or a high clinical suspicion for IE with normal transthoracic imaging should prompt consideration of transesophageal echocardiographic imaging. In the younger pediatric patient, transesophageal imaging can be challenging to perform without general anesthesia. In a controlled setting with older children, transesophageal echocardiography can be performed with conscious sedation. A negative echocardiogram does not mean that the patient does not have endocarditis. In some cases, repeat imaging may be indicated. Serial imaging studies can also provide valuable information in regard to therapy success or progressive disease.

Other imaging modalities such as computed tomography scans, MRI, and cardiac PET may be used in select situations. The use of these modalities are increasing in utility in the setting of concern for prosthetic valve IE or abscess formation not identified by echocardiographic imaging. An electrocardiogram, in general, is not helpful in the diagnosis of IE, but a new conduction abnormality or bundle branch block should raise concern for abscess formation affecting the conduction system.

## MANAGEMENT OF INFECTIOUS ENDOCARDITIS

Treatment of IE requires a multidisciplinary approach. The subspecialty teams involved commonly include cardiology, infectious disease, and cardiothoracic surgery, with other providers involved on an as-needed basis. An infectious disease consultation is strongly recommended to assist in guidance of appropriate antibiotic therapy early in the workup and treatment of IE. Successful management includes the diagnosis, early initiation of appropriate antibiotic therapy, and surveillance for, identification of, and management of complications, along with determining the need for and potential timing of surgery. Antibiotic therapy is the mainstay of treatment with an attempt to clear the associated bacteremia and sterilize the infected source. The course of antibiotic therapy varies based on the pathogen and the site(s) involved in the primary infectious process and any potential embolic sites. Owing to the complexity of potential antibiotic therapies, this topic will not be addressed in detail in this article. A common duration of antibiotic therapy consists of 4 to 6 weeks of treatment, depending on the organism identified, antibiotic susceptibility, and native versus prosthetic valve IE.[4] Transitioning from inpatient to outpatient therapy can be considered for part of the antibiotic course in lower risk patients with close outpatient monitoring. Because a higher risk of complications generally exists during the first 2 weeks of antibiotic therapy, outpatient therapy during this time is generally discouraged. Outpatient therapy may be considered for lower risk patients after the initial 2 weeks of antibiotic therapy. This includes patients who are medically stable, free of systemic symptoms, have negative blood culture results, have a stable electrocardiogram, have a stable home environment, have an appropriate monitoring plan in place, and have acute care access readily available.[18] Outpatient antibiotic treatment is not recommended in high-risk patients with unstable hemodynamics or symptoms, sepsis or ongoing bacteremia, perivalvar abscess, new conduction abnormalities, vegetations greater than 10 mm in diameter, or other serious complications.[18]

When a valve is directly involved, progressive stenosis or insufficiency may ensue. Depending on the rate of progression and the ability to clear the potential infectious process, heart failure management may be required in an acute or chronic setting, and surgery is often indicated in these cases.

Blood culture–negative IE is a complicated situation when a micro-organism cannot be identified by blood culture, but there is clinical or imaging concerns for IE, or pathologic examination of a valve or tissue after surgery. This situation may occur for several reasons that include antibiotic therapy before blood cultures are obtained, improper sampling or laboratory evaluation of samples, IE associated with a fastidious bacteria or nonbacterial micro-organism, or right-sided IE. With the administration of antibiotic therapy before blood cultures, the recovery rate of bacteria may be decreased by up to 40%.[19] This scenario emphasizes the importance of cultures being obtained before antibiotic administration, unless the clinical context warrants immediate administration of antibiotics in patients at risk.

Fungal IE presents a challenging situation because the complications may be compounded, with larger vegetations often being present, an increased risk of embolic events, and a high risk of perivalvar abscess formation. Antifungal therapies, including amphotericin B, have a poor ability to penetrate infected material and surgery is commonly required if complications arise. Antifungal therapy using oral fluconazole, because a long-term suppressive therapy has been reported for uncomplicated IE related to fungal infection, with the mortality rate no worse than those receiving combined medical and surgical therapy.[20]

The timing of potential surgical intervention relies on many associated factors that may occur in isolation or in combination. The decision about surgical intervention should be individualized in the pediatric patient. These determinants include the tolerance of associated symptoms such as heart failure symptoms necessitating surgery in 60% of patients with IE, the size and location of a vegetation in 48%, inability to clear the infection or refractory sepsis in 40%, or embolic episodes in 18%.[21] Surgical intervention, including debridement or extraction of any involved tissue, valve repair, or valve replacement, often becomes a necessity in the setting of IE. Surgery may be required in up to 25% of acute infections and 40% of subacute or chronic cases.[22]

Perioperative risks remain high with the complexity of intervention and potential for multiorgan involvement with reports of a 6% to 25% risk of perioperative mortality with long-term survival of approximately 70% in adult studies.[22] Note that these studies include many older patients with additional comorbidities.

The potential need for, or timing of, any intervention can be challenging. Determining factors include left-sided IE versus right-sided IE, vegetations that are progressively increasing in size while on appropriate antibiotics, or significant mobility of the vegetation. Prior studies have attempted to recommend indications for surgical removal of a vegetation based on its size. Although these recommendations should be considered, they should not be used as definitive indications to intervene because they do not carry good confirmatory evidence and these indications remain controversial, even more so in the pediatric patient. Echocardiographic features that have been described in the adult literature in regard to the timing of potential surgical intervention include persistent vegetation after systemic embolization, anterior mitral valve leaflet vegetation size of greater than 10 mm, 1 or more embolic events during the first 2 weeks of antimicrobial therapy, 2 or more embolic events during or after antimicrobial therapy, or an increase in vegetation size after 4 weeks of antimicrobial therapy. Surgery should be considered with valvular dysfunction contributing to signs of ventricular decompensation associated with aortic or mitral valve insufficiency with heart failure that is unresponsive to medical therapy. Finally, perivalvar extension that includes valve perforation, dehiscence, rupture, or fistula creation as well as new heart block, or a large abscess with extension despite antimicrobial therapy, are indications for surgical intervention in select patients (**Box 2**). Although indicated for other reasons (eg, mechanical prosthetic valve), anticoagulation is not indicated in IE. In some situations, such as IE associated with mycotic aneurysms or other high-risk intracranial complications, anticoagulation may be contraindicated.[19]

## MORBIDITY AND MORTALITY ASSOCIATED WITH INFECTIVE ENDOCARDITIS

Complications related to IE are variable with an emphasis placed on early diagnosis and initiation of antibiotic therapy before clinical decompensation. There are many factors that may predispose pediatric patients to cardiac and noncardiac complications that may require intervention. Complication risks are higher in patients with prosthetic valves, left-sided IE, IE owing to S aureus or fungi, prior IE, prolonged clinical symptoms lasting months, cyanotic congenital heart disease, systemic to pulmonary artery shunts, and those with poor clinical response to antimicrobial therapy.[19]

Sepsis can be a late complication after the infectious process has spread, leading to multiorgan failure and shock. Early recognition and standard shock protocols should be used. Embolic events may involve many organ systems, including the brain, lungs, peripheral vasculature, kidneys, and other organs depending on the primary locations of IE. Attempts to predict the risk of embolic events have been difficult, including identification of higher risk groups for which surgery would be recommended to avoid risk of an embolic event. IE associated with staphylococcal or fungal infections, as well as those involving the anterior leaflet of the mitral valve, may carry a higher risk of embolization.[19]

Stroke, meningitis, intracranial abscess, and other neurologic manifestations complicate the course in roughly 30% of patients, with roughly 60% of patients having

---

**Box 2**
**Criteria to consider in determining surgical indications for IE**

Echocardiographic features suggesting potential need for surgical intervention
Vegetation
- Persistent vegetation after systemic embolization
- Anterior mitral valve leaflet vegetation size of greater than 10 mm
- One or more embolic events during the first 2 weeks of antimicrobial therapy
- Two or more embolic events during or after antimicrobial therapy
- Increase in vegetation size after 4 weeks of antimicrobial therapy
Valvular dysfunction
- Acute aortic or mitral insufficiency with sings of ventricular failure
- Heart failure unresponsive to medical therapy
- Valve perforation or rupture
Perivalvular extension
- Valvular dehiscence, rupture, or fistula
- New heart block
- Large abscess or extension of abscess despite appropriate antimicrobial therapy

*From* Bayer AS, Bolger AF, Taubert KA, et al. Diagnosis and management of infective endocarditis and its complications. *Circulation.* 1998;98(25):2936-2948. Reprinted with permission, Circulation. 1998.98;2936-2948 © 1998 American Heart Association, Inc. All requests to use this information must come through the AHA.

---

a neurologic finding as their chief complaint or one of the major presenting symptoms.[23] Congestive heart failure is often related to associated valve pathology and can have a great impact on overall prognosis. Heart failure symptoms may develop early in the process of IE owing to rapid degeneration of an infected valve. These symptoms may occur owing to a progressive obstructive or regurgitant process, as well as potential dehiscence of a valve or development of a new intracardiac shunt. Surgical intervention should be strongly considered in these cases complicated by heart failure.

Overall in-hospital mortality related to IE has been estimated to occur in between 1.1% and 5.0% of patients, with staphylococcal IE being associated with increased mortality. Patients with certain congenital heart conditions have an increased risk of mortality, with death occurring in 48% of patients with tetralogy of Fallot and pulmonary atresia and 8% in patients with prosthetic valve IE.[5,14,24] A high risk of mortality also exists in premature infants, occurring in 31% of patients in 1 study.[14]

## INFECTIVE ENDOCARDITIS PREVENTION AND PROPHYLACTIC RECOMMENDATIONS

Prevention of IE is of utmost importance. Patients and their families should be made aware of potential risk factors and ways to minimize the risk of acquiring IE. Some procedural risks cannot be avoided, but sterile technique and other infection reduction protocols should be used.

In 2007, the American Heart Association and American College of Cardiology revised the antibiotic prophylactic guidelines to restrict preprocedural antibiotics to a few cardiac conditions that remain at higher risk for adverse outcomes related to IE.[25] The historical rational for, or against, the prophylactic use of antibiotics before certain invasive procedures included the association between bacteremia and IE. It should be noted that bacteremia can occur with daily activities such as teeth brushing, flossing, and chewing. Although certain higher risk procedures may contribute to transient bacteremia, justification for the recommendation to continue to use preprocedural prophylactic antibiotics in select situations has included the following:

Streptococci and Enterococci are a part of the normal flora and carry a higher suscep- tibility to antibiotics recommended for prophylaxis, previously published cases of IE have had a potential temporal relationship with IE and certain procedures, the risk of antibiotic prophylaxis is overall low, and the potential for complications associated with IE are high.[6] These updated guidelines note that, although these factors remained valid, they did not compensate for the lack of published data to support the use of pro- phylactic antibiotics. No prospective, randomized, placebo-controlled studies having been published in regard to the efficacy of antibiotic prophylaxis to prevent IE when undergoing dental procedures.

This updated guideline acknowledges that the effectiveness is unknown, but that it is reasonable to use prophylactic antibiotic therapy only in select situations.[25] Anti- biotic prophylaxis is reasonable for dental procedures that may perforate the oral mu- cosa or involve the gingiva or periapical tooth manipulation, for respiratory tract procedures, and for procedures that involve skin infections, skin structures, or muscu- loskeletal tissue for those at risk (**Box 3**). Recommendations for antibiotic prophylaxis include a single antibiotic dose 30 to 60 minutes before a procedure (**Table 1**). In the event a dose is not administered before the procedure, it can be administered up to 2 hours after the procedure. If patients are already receiving an antibiotic, a drug from a different class should be considered. Antibiotic prophylaxis is not required for patients undergoing gastrointestinal or genitourinary procedures. With limited data to fully support the use and benefit of antibiotic prophylaxis, emphasis should still be placed on good oral and skin hygiene.

## CONTROVERSIES IN MANAGEMENT

In the pediatric population, clear guidelines remain limited and many treatment strate- gies are inferred from adult guidelines. It is unlikely that large randomized controlled trials will be performed, but population-based or case-control studies could prove useful toward improving recommendations for prophylaxis and infection prevention. The authors of the Modified Duke Criteria have encouraged others to assist in

---

**Box 3**
**Indications for endocarditis prophylaxis**

Prosthetic cardiac valve or prosthetic material used for cardiac valve repair

Previous IE

Congenital heart disease
- Unrepaired cyanotic congenital heart disease, including palliative shunts and conduits
- Completely repaired congenital heart defect with prosthetic material or device, whether placed by surgery or catheter intervention, during the first 6 months after the procedure
- Repaired congenital heart disease with residual defects at the site or adjacent to the site of a prosthetic patch or prosthetic device (which inhibit endothelialization)

Cardiac transplant recipients who develop cardiac valvulopathy

*From* Wilson W, Taubert KA, Gewitz M, et al. Prevention of infective endocarditis: guidelines from the American Heart Association: a guideline from the American Heart Association Rheu- matic Fever, Endocarditis, and Kawasaki Disease Committee, Council on Cardiovascular Disease in the Young, and the Council on Clinical Cardiology, Council on Cardiovascular Surgery and Anesthesia, and the Quality of Care and Outcomes Research Interdisciplinary Working Group. *Circulation.* 2007;116(15):1736-1754. Reprinted with permission, Circulation.2007;116:1736- 1754 ©2007 American Heart Association, Inc. All requests to use this information must come through the AHA.

**Table 1**
**Antibiotic dosing for prophylaxis before procedures carrying increased IE risk**

| Regimens for a Dental Procedure | | | | |
|---|---|---|---|---|
| | Antibiotic | Route | Children | Adult |
| Usual therapy | Amoxicillin | Oral | 50 mg/kg | 2 g |
| Unable to take oral medication | Ampicillin | IV or IM | 50 mg/kg | 2 g |
| | Cephazolin or ceftriaxone | IV or IM | 50 mg/kg | 1 g |
| Allergic to penicillins or ampicillin | Clindamycin or | Oral | 20 mg/kg | 600 mg |
| | Cephalexin[a,b] or | Oral | 50 mg/kg | 2 g |
| | Azithromycin or clarithromycin | Oral | 15 mg/kg | 500 mg |
| Allergic to penicillins or ampicillin and unable to take oral medication | Clindamycin | IV | 20 mg/kg | 600 mg |
| | Cefazolin/ceftriaxone | IV or IM | 50 mg/kg | 1 g |

Regimen: single dose 30 to 60 minutes before procedure.
*Abbreviations*: IM, intramuscularly; IV, intravenous.
[a] Or other first- or second-generation oral cephalosporins in equivalent adult or pediatric dosage.
[b] Cephalosporins should not be used in an individual with a history of anaphylaxis, angioedema, or urticaria with penicillins or ampicillin.
*From* Wilson W, Taubert KA, Gewitz M, et al. Prevention of infective endocarditis: guidelines from the American Heart Association: a guideline from the American Heart Association Rheumatic Fever, Endocarditis, and Kawasaki Disease Committee, Council on Cardiovascular Disease in the Young, and the Council on Clinical Cardiology, Council on Cardiovascular Surgery and Anesthesia, and the Quality of Care and Outcomes Research Interdisciplinary Working Group. *Circulation.* 2007;116(15):1736-1754. Reprinted with permission, Circulation.2007;116:1736-1754 ©2007 American Heart Association, Inc. All requests to use this information must come through the AHA.

evaluating additional modifications to these criteria to further improve the diagnostic capability.[10]

More recent studies from adult populations have shown that a change from intravenous antibiotic therapy to early oral antibiotic therapy was not associated with delayed treatment failure for patients whose conditions have stabilized with left-sided endocarditis.[26,27] These results have not been reproduced in pediatrics to date.

## DISCLOSURE

The authors have nothing to disclose.

## REFERENCES

1. Sullam PM, Drake TA, Sande MA. Pathogenesis of endocarditis. Am J Med 1985; 78(6B):110-5.

2. Stull TL, LiPuma JJ. Endocarditis in children. In: D K, editor. Infective endocarditis. 2nd edition. New York: Raven Press, Ltd; 1992. p. 313-27.

3. Valente AM, Jain R, Scheurer M, et al. Frequency of infective endocarditis among infants and children with Staphylococcus aureus bacteremia. Pediatrics 2005; 115(1):e15-9.

4. Baltimore RS, Gewitz M, Baddour LM, et al. Infective endocarditis in childhood: 2015 update: a scientific statement from the American Heart Association. Circulation 2015;132(15):1487-515.

5. Gupta S, Sakhuja A, McGrath E, et al. Trends, microbiology, and outcomes of infective endocarditis in children during 2000-2010 in the United States. Congenit Heart Dis 2017;12(2):196–201.

6. Pant S, Patel NJ, Deshmukh A, et al. Trends in infective endocarditis incidence, microbiology, and valve replacement in the United States from 2000 to 2011. J Am Coll Cardiol 2015;65(19):2070–6.

7. Baddour LM, Wilson WR, Bayer AS, et al. Infective endocarditis in adults: diagnosis, antimicrobial therapy, and management of complications: a scientific statement for healthcare professionals from the American Heart Association. Circulation 2015;132(15):1435–86.

8. Von Reyn CF, Levy BS, Arbeit RD, et al. Infective endocarditis: an analysis based on strict case definitions. Ann Intern Med 1981;94(4 pt 1):505–18.

9. Durack DT, Lukes AS, Bright DK. New criteria for diagnosis of infective endocarditis: utilization of specific echocardiographic findings. Duke Endocarditis Service. Am J Med 1994;96(3):200–9.

10. Li JS, Sexton DJ, Mick N, et al. Proposed modifications to the Duke criteria for the diagnosis of infective endocarditis. Clin Infect Dis 2000;30(4):633–8.

11. Rudasill SE, Sanaiha Y, Mardock AL, et al. Clinical outcomes of infective endocarditis in injection drug users. J Am Coll Cardiol 2019;73(5):559–70.

12. Rushani D, Kaufman JS, Ionescu-Ittu R, et al. Infective endocarditis in children with congenital heart disease: cumulative incidence and predictors. Circulation 2013;128(13):1412–9.

13. Rodbard S. Blood velocity and endocarditis. Circulation 1963;27:18–28.

14. Day MD, Gauvreau K, Shulman S, et al. Characteristics of children hospitalized with infective endocarditis. Circulation 2009;119(6):865–70.

15. Sharma A, Cote AT, Hosking MCK, et al. A systematic review of infective endocarditis in patients with bovine jugular vein valves compared with other valve types. JACC Cardiovasc Interv 2017;10(14):1449–58.

16. Abdelghani M, Nassif M, Blom NA, et al. Infective endocarditis after melody valve implantation in the pulmonary position: a systematic review. J Am Heart Assoc 2018;7(13):e008163.

17. Servy A, Valeyrie-Allanore L, Alla F, et al. Prognostic value of skin manifestations of infective endocarditis. JAMA Dermatol 2014;150(5):494–500.

18. Andrews MM, von Reyn CF. Patient selection criteria and management guidelines for outpatient parenteral antibiotic therapy for native valve infective endocarditis. Clin Infect Dis 2001;33(2):203–9.

19. Bayer AS, Bolger AF, Taubert KA, et al. Diagnosis and management of infective endocarditis and its complications. Circulation 1998;98(25):2936–48.

20. Nguyen MH, Nguyen ML, Yu VL, et al. Candida prosthetic valve endocarditis: prospective study of six cases and review of the literature. Clin Infect Dis 1996;22(2):262–7.

21. Tornos P, Iung B, Permanyer-Miralda G, et al. Infective endocarditis in Europe: lessons from the Euro heart survey. Heart 2005;91(5):571–5.

22. Prendergast BD, Tornos P. Surgery for infective endocarditis: who and when? Circulation 2010;121(9):1141–52.

23. Jones HR Jr, Siekert RG, Geraci JE. Neurologic manifestations of bacterial endocarditis. Ann Intern Med 1969;71(1):21–8.

24. Pasquali SK, He X, Mohamad Z, et al. Trends in endocarditis hospitalizations at US children's hospitals: impact of the 2007 American Heart Association Antibiotic prophylaxis guidelines. Am Heart J 2012;163(5):894–9.

25. Wilson W, Taubert KA, Gewitz M, et al. Prevention of infective endocarditis: guide-lines from the American Heart Association: a guideline from the American Heart Association Rheumatic Fever, Endocarditis, and Kawasaki Disease Committee, Council on Cardiovascular Disease in the Young, and the Council on Clinical Cardiology, Council on Cardiovascular Surgery and Anesthesia, and the Quality of Care and Outcomes Research Interdisciplinary Working Group. Circulation 2007;116(15):1736–54.

26. Iversen K, Ihlemann N, Gill SU, et al. Partial oral versus intravenous antibiotic treatment of endocarditis. N Engl J Med 2019;380(5):415–24.

27. Bundgaard H, Ihlemann N, Gill SU, et al. Long-term outcomes of partial oral treatment of endocarditis. N Engl J Med 2019;380(14):1373–4.

# Update of Pediatric Heart Failure

Kae Watanabe, MD[a,*], Renata Shih, MD[b]

## KEYWORDS

- Pediatric heart failure • Cardiomyopathy in infants and children
- Heart failure in congenital heart disease
- Heart failure in pediatric acquired heart disease

## KEY POINTS

- Pediatric heart failure diagnosis often is delayed because initial symptoms resemble common pediatric illness, such as the typical cold and gastrointestinal infections.
- The Ross heart failure classification is the main pediatric heart failure classification.
- Besides clinical symptoms, echocardiogram is the method of choice to monitor patients.
- Brain natriuretic peptide (BNP) and its precursor protein N-terminal prohormone of BNP are the most common prognostic biomarkers.
- Given the paucity of large pediatric multicenter studies, medications used to manage pediatric heart failure are based mostly on data extrapolated from adult literature.

## INTRODUCTION

Pediatric heart failure (PHF) data has wide variation due to the scarcity of large multicenter studies. Literature is based mostly on single-center publications. A systematic review by Shaddy and colleagues[1] observed primary heart failure (HF) rates ranging from 0.87/100,000 to 7.4/100,000, with 5-year mortality and/or heart transplant (HT) of 40% in pediatric dilated cardiomyopathy (DCM) patients.[2] A review by Mejia and colleagues[3] observed that emergency department admissions with a diagnosis of PHF had a high mortality rate, especially if associated with respiratory distress and kidney dysfunction.[4] This update reviews diagnosis, classifications, and causes of PHF. Lastly, clinical management with the latest medications and therapies published are discussed.

## DIAGNOSIS OF PEDIATRIC HEART FAILURE

Initial presentation often is overlooked by a long list of different diagnoses as upper respiratory and gastrointestinal infections.[5–7] Unfortunately, many patients with

[a] Northwestern University, 225 East Chicago Avenue, Box 21, Chicago, IL 60611-2605, USA;
[b] University of Florida, 1600 Southwest Archer Road PO Box 100296, Gainesville, FL 32610, USA
* Corresponding author.
*E-mail address:* kwatanabe@luriechildrens.org

Pediatr Clin N Am 67 (2020) 889–901
https://doi.org/10.1016/j.pcl.2020.06.004
0031-3955/20/© 2020 Elsevier Inc. All rights reserved.

PHF present to the emergency department in cardiogenic shock. The etiology list varies according to age and can determine different prognosis (**Table 1**). In infancy, the most common cause is congenital heart disease (CHD). After the first year of life, acquired heart disease and cardiomyopathies become the most common.[8]

## CLASSIFICATIONS OF PEDIATRIC HEART FAILURE

The New York Heart Association (NYHA) was established in 1928 and remained the only HF score for decades. NYHA is based on severity of symptoms and tracks progression of disease. In 1987, Ross developed a score tailored to symptoms of infants and younger children (see **Table 1**).[9] In 2002, Laer and colleagues[10] developed their own model based on age and 6 variables. By 2012, Ross[11] modified his own score to include age-based symptoms. The modified Ross score is comprehensive; however, it also is more cumbersome to validate due to multiple variants.

Other models for PHF classifications based on etiology include (1) cardiomyopathy; mainly distinguished as dilated, hypertrophic, restrictive, and left ventricular (LV) noncompaction; (2) CHD; and (3) acquired heart disease, including myocarditis, Kawasaki disease and endocarditis (**Box 1**). Another classification is based on systolic and diastolic dysfunction, referred to as HF with reduced ejection fraction (HFrEF) and HF with preserved ejection fraction (EF). Lastly, HF can be differentiated based on presentation: acute and chronic.

**Table 1**
**Heart failure classifications**

|  | New York Heart Association | Ross |
|---|---|---|
| Class I | No limitation of physical activity. Ordinary physical activity does not cause undue fatigue, palpitation, dyspnea (shortness of breath). | No limitations or symptoms |
| Class II | Slight limitation of physical activity. Comfortable at rest. Ordinary physical activity results in fatigue, palpitation, dyspnea (shortness of breath). | Mild tachypnea or diaphoresis with feeding |
| Class III | Marked limitation of physical activity. Comfortable at rest. Less than ordinary activity causes fatigue, palpitation, or dyspnea. | Infants with growth failure and marked tachypnea or diaphoresis with feedings, older children with marked dyspnea on exertion |
| Class IV | Marked limitation of physical activity. Comfortable at rest. Less than ordinary activity causes fatigue, palpitation, or dyspnea. | Symptoms at rest, such as tachypnea, retractions, grunting, and diaphoresis |

*Adapted from* Dolgin M, Association NYH, Fox AC, et al. New York Heart Association. Criteria Committee. Nomenclature and criteria for diagnosis of diseases of the heart and great vessels. 9th ed. Boston, MA: Lippincott Williams and Wilkins; March 1, 1994 and Ross RD, Daniels SR, Schwartz DC, et al. Plasma norepinephrine levels in infants and children with congestive heart failure. Am J Cardiol. 1987; 59: 911–914; with permission.

| **Box 1** |
| **Causes of pediatric heart failure** |

Primary cardiomyopathy
  DCM
  Hypertrophic cardiomyopathy
  Restrictive cardiomyopathy
  Arrhythmogenic right ventricular dysplasia
  LV noncompaction

Congenital heart disease
  Left-to-right shunting lesions (eg, VSD and PDA)
  Valvar disease (eg, aortic stenosis)
  Coarctation of the aorta
  Complex CHD (eg, systemic RV and SV)

Arrhythmia
  Tachycardia
  Bradycardia (eg, complete heart block)

Ischemia
  Coronary anomalies (eg, ALCAPA)
  Kawasaki disease

Infiltrative
  Malignancy
  Amyloidosis (rare in pediatrics)

Infection
  Myocarditis
  Acute rheumatic fever

Toxins
  Chemotherapy

Others
  Essential hypertension

*Abbreviations:* ALCAPA, anomalous left coronary artery from the pulmonary artery; PDA, patent ductus arteriosus; RV, right ventricle; VSD, ventricular septal defect.

## DIAGNOSTIC METHODS AND MONITORING
### Electrocardiogram and Holter Monitoring

Electrocardiogram might show signs of LV or biventricular hypertrophy (**Box 2**). QRS duration may be prolonged and there could be nonspecific ST segment changes representing strain. Holter monitoring might be indicated if a patient is symptomatic with palpitations or chest pain. Holter monitoring also can be helpful to reveal cardiomyopathies that occur secondary to arrhythmia, including arrhythmogenic right ventricular cardiomyopathy, frequent premature ventricular contractions, and heart block.

### Imaging

Echocardiogram is the most common method used for initial diagnosis and follow-up in HF. It is noninvasive and usually does not require sedation. The International Society for Heart and Lung Transplantation (ISHLT) guidelines for the management of PHF recommend monitoring measurements of LV dimension, LV wall thickness, and LV function, which is completed by calculating LVEF based on a well-standardized 2-dimensional method, which is level of evidence B for assessment of HF.[12]

---

**Box 2**
**Electrocardiogram findings in heart failure**

- Left atrial enlargement
- LV hypertrophy
- Low-voltage QRS in limb leads
- Intraventricular conduction delay, or left bundle branch block
- Abnormal ST segment changes, including depression and elevation
- T-wave inversions in lateral leads
- Supraventricular and ventricular arrhythmias

---

Cardiac magnetic resonance imaging (CMR) is a versatile imaging method in the HF population. CMR diagnostics are utilized for assisting myocarditis diagnosis, for risk stratification of sudden death in hypertrophic cardiomyopathy (HCM), in neuromuscular diseases such as Duchenne muscular dystrophy (DMD), and in diagnosis and assessment of HF in CHD.[13–18] Disadvantages include requiring general anesthesia in young children, involving a long scan time, being expensive, and not having established pediatric normative values. Recently, van der Ven and colleagues[19] published a multicenter study, including 141 patients with no cardiovascular history, suggesting normal CMR metrics for a wide pediatric age range. The advance of CMR technology will allow expansion of its use, especially in younger children.

### Cardiac Catheterization

Cardiac catheterization is applicable for assessing pulmonary vascular resistance and evaluating unexplained new onset of HF associated with hemodynamic compromise, per ISHLT recommendations.[12,20,21] It also allows performing endomyocardial biopsy, which can determine diagnosis, treatment, and prognosis of specific cardiac diseases, such as amyloidosis.[22]

### Biomarkers

In PHF, the most common biomarker is brain natriuretic peptide (BNP) and/or its precursor protein N-terminal prohormone of BNP (NT-proBNP). BNP is a hormone secreted by cardiomyocytes in the ventricles in response to stretching, caused by increase ventricular blood volume. BNP is used for diagnosis, treatment monitoring, and prognosis.[23] Their value varies according to age group and etiology of HF.

Auerbach and colleagues[24] performed a post hoc analysis of the Pediatric Carvedilol Trial, including patients with cardiomyopathy and CHD.[25] They observed a BNP cutoff of 140 pg/nL had sensitivity of 71% and specificity of 63% in predicting HF hospitalization, death, or HT but without distinction between single-ventricle (SV) or biventricular physiology. The cutoff value for BNP in SV population varies according to single-center studies and further studies on BNP are needed in this population. Current literature shows a cutoff greater than 30 pg/mL to 45 pg/mL regardless of the stage of palliation.[26–28] Butts and colleagues[29] identified the potential prognostic value of BNP by evaluating levels before and after superior cavopulmonary connection surgery. They observed that elevated BNP was associated with higher end systolic $z$ scores and increased atrioventricular valve regurgitation.[29]

After the PANORAMA trial for LCZ696, several pediatric centers have started using NT-proBNP as an alternative to BNP, because there is some evidence that the newer HF medication, sacubitril-valsartan, can affect BNP levels.[30,31] There are few single-center retrospective studies that have investigated the use of NT-proBNP, one including 36 PHF patients with HF secondary to DCM. This study showed that an NT-proBNP value above 1000 pg/mL identified more symptomatic patients.[32]

## PATHOPHYSIOLOGY OF PEDIATRIC HEART FAILURE

HF is the inability to maintain cardiac output to sustain metabolic demands. In response, metabolic and neurohumoral mechanisms are activated. There is activation of sympathetic nervous system (SNS) and the renin-angiotensin-aldosterone system (RAAS). Consequently, sodium and fluid retention occur in attempt to sustain preload and cardiac output (CO). The sympathetic nervous system and RAAS act in the peripheral vasculature causing vasoconstriction to raise blood pressure for vital organ perfusion. In response to changes in afterload and wall stress, there is myocardial cell growth and adaptation. These reactions lead to an increase in myocardial oxygen consumption, ventricular afterload due to eccentric hypertrophy, interstitial fibrosis, and reduction in capillary density. They also lead to changes in gene expression involving calcium handling in the sarcoplasmic reticulum and contractile proteins, resulting in direct cardiotoxicity[33] (**Fig. 1**).

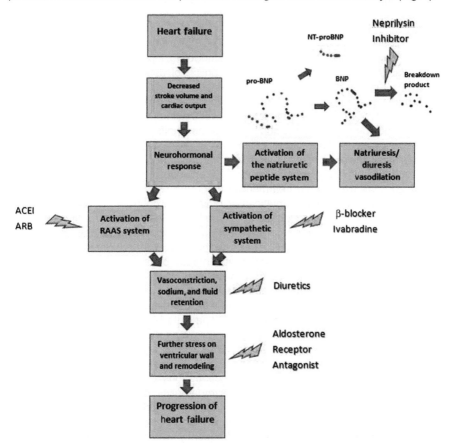

**Fig. 1.** Pathophysiology of HF and medication targets. ARB, angiotensin receptor blocker.

Distinctive research has been aimed at investigating the differences in pathophysiology of HF in adult and children. Miyamoto and colleagues[34] studied the difference in adrenergic receptor-mediated adaptation between adult and children with HF. Adults with DCM had down-regulation of only the $\beta_1$-adrenergic receptors whereas pediatric patients had down-regulation of $\beta_1$ and $\beta2$ receptors. Therefore, nonselective $\beta$-blockers, such as carvedilol, might cause a powerful adrenergic down regulation in the pediatric population. Myocardial fibrosis in adults with HF is well described. Woulfe and colleagues[35] described less fibrosis and fibrotic gene expression in pediatric patients with DCM in comparison with adults. Hence, antiremodeling agents, such as aldosterone antagonists, may not be as effective in PHF patients.

## MANAGEMENT OF PEDIATRIC HEART FAILURE
### Medications

Treatment in pediatrics is extrapolated mostly from the adult literature. The American College of Cardiology Foundation/American Heart Association guidelines base management recommendations on the NYHA class HF stage.[36] The pediatric cardiology taskforce has reviewed ISHLT guidelines in 2014 for management of PHF. Most of the recommendations are level of evidence B (based on a single randomized trial or multiple nonrandomized trials) or level of evidence C (based primarily on expert consensus opinion). Each class of medication is reviewed in conjugation with the most recent updates.[37]

Angiotensin-converting enzyme inhibitors (ACEIs) are the first-line treatment of HF. In adults, they have been shown to prevent remodeling, increased CO, and decreased hospitalization and mortality. Its dual mechanism of action includes prevention of myocardial remodeling and reducing afterload by inhibiting RAAS pathway. The largest pediatric cohort study is a randomized, double-blind, placebo-controlled trial conducted by the Pediatric Heart Network investigating the effects of enalapril in SV patients. It included 230 patients and there was no significant difference in HF severity whether or not they receive enalapril.[38] In another review by the Pediatric Health Information System, it was observed that ACEIs are prescribed by 69.6% of PHF patients discharged after an acute decompensated HF episode.[39]

$\beta$-Blockers are used in the treatment of moderate HF in adults. Shaddy and colleagues[25] published a pediatric, multicenter, randomized controlled double-blind study comparing carvedilol with a placebo in children with Ross class II to III. The results showed that carvedilol did not significantly improve clinical HF in children and adolescents with symptomatic systolic HF. The study, however, was thought to be underpowered or results were secondary to difference in pathophysiology.[25] Furthermore, the study combined a heterogeneous population with biventricular and SV physiology. Smaller pediatric cohorts with cardiomyopathies showed significant clinical and echocardiographic improvements with carvedilol.[40,41] Azeka and colleagues[42] published a double-blind placebo-controlled study with 22 patients listed for transplant secondary to DCM and 9 patients were delisted after EF improvement when treated with carvedilol.

Digoxin has been used since the late 1700s to manage HF. Digoxin inhibits the sodium-potassium ATPase pump of the myocardial cellular membrane, which increases sarcoplasmic reticulum calcium concentrations and creates positive inotropic effects.[43] It also increases vagal tone and sympatholytic effects, decreasing plasma norepinephrine levels and possibly an antagonist of aldosterone.[44,45] The ISHLT guidelines for PHF recommend use of digoxin for chronic HF, as level of evidence C.[12] In the pediatric population, digoxin frequently was used for congestive HF in left-to-right shunting lesions.[46]

Aldosterone receptor antagonists, such as spironolactone and eplerenone, act as blocking the RAAS in HF to avoid remodeling leading to myocardial fibrosis. The Randomized Aldactone Evaluation Study showed a 30% reduction in mortality, 35% lower rate of hospitalization, and significant improvement of symptoms in adults.[47] Eplerenone also has been shown beneficial in patients with HFrEF with mild symptoms.[48] Despite no pediatric studies providing evidence of aldosterone antagonists benefiting other than in the DMD population, it still is used frequently and well tolerated as a potassium-sparing diuretic.[49]

Diuretics are recommended in patients with fluid retention. They can act in different sites in the renal tubules: loop of Henle (such as bumetanide and furosemide) and distal portion of tubule (such as thiazides, metolazone, and potassium-sparing diuretics). The use of diuretics is a class I recommendation with level of evidence B or level of evidence C in the adults. There are no published clinical studies on effectiveness in reducing mortality or improving symptoms in pediatrics. Common long-term adverse outcomes are renal calcifications and osteoporosis.[50,51]

Ivabradine is hyperpolarization-activated cyclic nucleotide gated channel blocker. It acts by slowing the sinoatrial node without effects on inotropy, diastology, blood pressure, and vascular resistance.[52] Large randomized control studies in adults with HF due to coronary artery disease have shown mixed results.[53–57] In the SHIFT trial, the ivabradine group showed 18% reduction in cardiovascular death or hospital admission due worsening HF. Bonnet and colleagues[58] investigated the use of ivabradine in 116 children from ages 6 months to 18 years old with HF due to DCM. They observed improvement of LVEF, NYHA/Ross HF classification, and quality of life.

LCZ 696 is the angiotensin receptor neprilysin inhibitor and angiotensin receptor blocker valsartan. Angiotensin receptor neprilysin inhibitor is a class I recommendation for treatment of adult HF.[59] Neprilysin is a neutral endopeptidase that degrades endogenous vasoactive peptides, including natriuretic peptides, bradykinin, substance P, and adrenomedullin. Neprilysin inhibition causes increase of these peptides and negative feedback to neurohormonal activation, avoiding vasoconstriction, and remodeling. The PARADIGMA clinical trial demonstrated lower mortality and HF admissions compared with traditional ACEI therapy in the adult population.[60] The PANORAMA clinical trial currently is in progress and includes pediatric patients with biventricular physiology with decrease ventricular systolic function.[30] LCZ 696 has recently been Food and Drug Administration approved to be used for PHF.

## BEYOND MEDICAL MANAGEMENT

Cardiac resynchronization therapy is an established treatment in adults. It shows improved cardiac function and quality of life while decreasing mortality in patients with a left bundle branch block and an EF of less than 35%.[61] Despite not used frequently in pediatrics, a review by Motonga and Dubin[62] showed 11% to 23% of nonresponse rate to cardiac resynchronization therapy in pediatrics, better than the 30% rate seen in the adult population.

HT and ventricular-assist devices (VADs) should be considered in patients with severe HF. The Pediatric Interagency Registry for Mechanical Circulatory Support, a National Institutes of Health–sponsored US database, registered placement of 508 devices in 423 patients younger than 19 years from September 2012 to December 2017. The most common diagnosis was cardiomyopathy (61%), followed by CHD (20%) and myocarditis (11%).[63] There has been a significant increase in VADs over the past decade, with more than 20% of PHF being bridged to HT.[8]

Pulmonary artery banding has been studied over the years.[64] In 2018, Schranz and colleagues[65] showed improvement of heart function in 34 of 70 infant to toddler aged patients with end-stage DCM after pulmonary artery banding.

## DUCHENNE MUSCULAR DYSTROPHY

A 2014 National Institutes of Health working group recommends that all patients with DMD to start an ACEI or angiotensin receptor blocker by age 10, regardless of EF.[66–68] Mineralocorticoid receptor antagonists, such as aldactone and eplerenone, have been studied in DMD patients to slow the decline of EF in combination with ACEI.[69] Raman and colleagues[49] showed that adding eplerenone further attenuates the speed of decline in heart function within a 2-year period of use. In DMD patients who have failed medical management, the consideration for VADs and HT might be considered per individual and institutional bases.

## FUTURE OF PEDIATRIC HEART FAILURE MANAGEMENT

Micro-RNAs (miRNAs), known as short noncoding RNAs, work in gene modulation and potentially as a biomarker for PHF therapies.[70] Miyamoto and colleagues[71] identified singular miRNAs as being able to predict long-term outcomes in children with DCM. There is promising research with the use of pluripotent stem cell to manage RV failure in hypoplastic left heart syndrome.[72,73] New technologies with induced pluripotent stem cells and 3-dimensional printing are providing new directions toward a bio-artificial heart.[74–76]

## SUMMARY

HF in children is a rare occurrence. Unfortunately, initial diagnosis often is missed, which delays treatment until later stages of HF. Management is still extrapolated from adult literature but the increased collaboration among PHF services worldwide has allowed significant advances in PHF research. Hopefully, the discoveries of pathways, biomarkers, and medications might lead to improvement of the care of PHF patients.

## DISCLOSURE

The authors have nothing to disclose.

## REFERENCES

1. Shaddy RE, George AT, Jaecklin T, et al. Systematic literature review on the incidence and prevalence of heart failure in children and adolescents. Pediatr Cardiol 2018;39(3):415–36.
2. Towbin JA, Lowe AM, Colan SD, et al. Incidence, causes, and outcomes of dilated cardiomyopathy in children. JAMA 2006;296:1867–76.
3. Mejia EJ, O'Connor MJ, Lin KY, et al. Characteristics and outcomes of pediatric heart failure-related emergency department visits in the United States: a population-based study. J Pediatr 2018;193:114–8.
4. Rusconi P, Wilkinson JD, Sleeper LA, et al. Differences in presentation and outcomes between children with familial dilated cardiomyopathy and children with idiopathic dilated cardiomyopathy a report from the Pediatric Cardiomyopathy Registry Study Group. Circ Heart Fail 2017;10:e002637.

5. Kantor PF, Abraham JR, Dipchand AI, et al. The impact of changing medical therapy on transplantation-free survival in pediatric dilated cardiomyopathy. J Am Coll Cardiol 2010;55:1377–84.

6. Macicek SM, Macias CG, Jefferies JL, et al. Acute heart failure syndromes in the pediatric emergency department. Pediatrics 2009;124:e898–904.

7. Hollander SA, Addonizio LJ, Chin C, et al. Abdominal complaints as a common first presentation of heart failure in adolescents with dilated cardiomyopathy. Am J Emerg Med 2013;31(4):684–6.

8. Rossano JW, Cherikh WS, Chambers DC, et al. The registry of the international society for heart and lung transplantation: twentieth pediatric heart transplantation report-2017; focus theme: allograft ischemic time. J Heart Lung Transplant 2017;36:1060–9.

9. Ross RD, Daniels SR, Schwartz DC, et al. Plasma norepinephrine levels in infants and children with congestive heart failure. Am J Cardiol 1987;59:911–4.

10. Laer S, Mir TS, Behn F, et al. Carvedilol therapy in pediatric patients with congestive heart failure: a study investigating clinical and pharmacokinetic parameters. Am Heart J 2002;143:916–22.

11. Ross RD. The Ross classification for heart failure in children after 25 years: a review and an age-stratified revision. Pediatr Cardiol 2002;33:1295–300.

12. Kirk R, Dipchand A, Rosenthal DN, et al. The International Society for Heart and Lung Transplantation guidelines for the management of pediatric heart failure: executive summary. J Heart Lung Transplant 2014;33(9):888–909.

13. Friedrich MG, Sechtem U, Schulz-Menger J, et al. Cardiovascular magnetic resonance in myocarditis: a JACC white paper. J Am Coll Cardiol 2009;53(17):1475–87.

14. Silva MC, Meira ZM, Gurgel Giannetti J, et al. Myocardial delayed enhancement by magnetic resonance imaging in patients with muscular dystrophy. J Am Coll Cardiol 2007;49(18):1874–9.

15. Menon SC, Etheridge SP, Liesemer KN, et al. Predictive value of myocardial delayed enhancement in Duchenne muscular dystrophy. Pediatr Cardiol 2014;35(7):1279–85.

16. Florian A, Ludwig A, Engelen M, et al. Left ventricular systolic function and the pattern of late-gadolinium-enhancement independently and additively predict adverse cardiac events in muscular dystrophy patients. J Cardiovasc Magn Reson 2014;16:81.

17. Gersh BJ, Maron BJ, Bonow RO, et al. American College of Cardiology Foundation/American Heart Association Task Force on Practice; American Association for Thoracic Surgery; American Society of Echocardiography; American Society of Nuclear Cardiology; Heart Failure Society of America; Heart Rhythm Society; Society for Cardiovascular Angiography and Interventions; Society of Thoracic Surgeons. 2011 ACCF/AHA guideline for the diagnosis and treatment of hypertrophic cardiomyopathy: a report of the American College of Cardiology Foundation/American Heart Association Task Force on Practice Guidelines. J Thorac Cardiovasc Surg 2011;142(6):e153–203.

18. Elliott PM, Anastasakis A, Borger MA, et al. Authors/Task Force Members. 2014 ESC guidelines on diagnosis and management of hypertrophic cardiomyopathy: the Task Force for the Diagnosis and Management of Hypertrophic Cardiomyopathy of the European Society of Cardiology (ESC). Eur Heart J 2014;35(39):2733–79.

19. van der Ven JPG, Sadighy Z, Valsangiacomo Buechel ER, et al. Multicentre reference values for cardiac magnetic resonance imaging derived ventricular size

and function for children aged 0-18 years. Eur Heart J Cardiovasc Imaging 2019; 21(1):102–13.

20. Ofori-Amanfo G, Hsu D, Lamour JM, et al. Heart transplantation in children with markedly elevated pulmonary vascular resistance: Impact of right ventricular failure on outcome. J Heart Lung Transplant 2011;30:659–66.

21. Yilmaz B, Zuckerman WA, Lee TM, et al. Left ventricular assist device to avoid heart–lung transplant in an adolescent with dilated cardiomyopathy and severely elevated pulmonary vascular resistance. Pediatr Transplant 2013;17: E113–6.

22. Felker GM, Thompson RE, Hare JM, et al. Underlying causes and long-term survival in patients with initially unexplained cardiomyopathy. N Engl J Med 2000; 342:1077–84.

23. Cantinotti M, Law Y, Vittorini S, et al. The potential and limitations of plasma BNP measurement in the diagnosis, prognosis, and management of children with heart failure due to congenital cardiac disease: an update. Heart Fail Rev 2014;19(6):727–42.

24. Auerbach SR, Richmond ME, Lamour JM, et al. BNP levels predict outcome in pediatric heart failure patients post hoc analysis of the pediatric carvedilol trial. Circ Heart Fail 2010;3:606–11.

25. Shaddy RE, Boucek MM, Hsu DT, et al, For the Pediatric Carvedilol Study Group. Carvedilol for children and adolecents with heart failure. A randomized controlled trial. JAMA 2007;298(10):1171–9.

26. Lowenthal A, Camacho BV, Lowenthal S, et al. Usefulness of B-type Natriuretic Peptide and N-terminal Pro-B type natriuretic peptides biomarkers for heart failure in young children with single ventricle congenital heart disease. Am J Cardiol 2012;109(6):866–72.

27. Law YM, Ettedgui J, Beerman L. Comparison of plasma B-type natriuretic peptide levels in single ventricle patients with systemic ventricle heart failure versus isolated cavopulmonary failure. Am J Cardiol 2006;98:520–4.

28. Berry JG, Askovich B, Shaddy RE. Prognostic value of B-type natriuretic peptide in surgical palliation of children with single-ventricle congenital heart disease. Pediatr Cardiol 2008;29:70–5.

29. Butts RJ, Zak V, Hsu D. Factors associated with serum B-type natriuretic peptide in infants with single ventricles. Pediatr Cardiol 2014;35(5):879–87.

30. Shaddy R, Canter C, Halnon N, et al. Design for the sacubitril/valsartan (LCZ696) compared with enalapril study of pediatric patients with heart failure due to systemic left ventricle systolic dysfunction (PANORAMA-HF study). Am Heart J 2017; 193:23–34.

31. Myhre PL, Vaduganathan M, Claggett B, et al. B-type natriuretic peptide during treatment with sacubitril/valsartan. J Am Coll Cardiol 2019;73:1264–72.

32. Rusconi PG, Ludwig DA, Ratnasamy C, et al. Serial Measurements of Serum NT-proBNP as markers of left ventricular systolic function and remodeling in children with heart failure. Am Heart J 2010;160(4):776–83.

33. Jackson G, Gibbs CR, Davies MK, et al. ABC of heart failure. Pathophysiology. BMJ 2000;320:167–70.

34. Miyamoto SD, Stauffer BL, Nakano S, et al. Beta-adrenergic adaptation in paediatric idiopathic dilated cardiomyopathy. Eur Heart J 2014;35(1):33–41.

35. Woulfe KC, Siomos AK, Nguyen H, et al. Fibrosis and fibrotic gene expression in pediatric and adult patients with idiopathic dilated cardiomyopathy. J Card Fail 2017;23(4):314–24.

36. Yancy CW, Jessup M, Bozkurt B, et al. 2013 ACCF/AHA guideline for the management of heart failure: a report of the American College of Cardiology Foundation/American Heart Association Task Force on Practice Guidelines. J Am Coll Cardiol 2013;62:e147–239.

37. Kirk R, Dipchand AI, Rosenthal DN, editors. ISHLT guidelines for the management of pediatric heart failure. Birmingham (England): University of Alabama at Birmingham; 2014.

38. Hsu DT, Zak V, Mahony L, et al. Enalapril in infants with single ventricle results of a multicenter randomized trial. Circulation 2010;122:333–40.

39. Moffett BS, Price JF. National prescribing trends for heart failure medications in children. Congenit Heart Dis 2015;10:78–85.

40. Bruns LA, Chrisant MK, Lamour JM, et al. Carvedilol as therapy in pediatric heart failure: an initial multicenter experience. J Pediatr 2001;138:505–11.

41. Rusconi P, Gómez-Marín O, Rossique-González M, et al. Carvedilol in children with cardiomyopathy: 3-year experience at a single institution. J Heart Lung Transplant 2004;23:832–8.

42. Azeka E, Franchini Ramires JA, Valler C, et al. Delisting of infants and children from the heart transplantation waiting list after carvedilol treatment. J Am Coll Cardiol 2002;40:2034–8.

43. Hauptman PJ, Kelly RA. Digitalis. Circulation 1999;99:1265–70.

44. Ehle M, Patel C, Giugliano RP. Digoxin: Clinical highlights: A review of digoxin and Its use in contemporary medicine. Crit Pathw Cardiol 2011;10(2):93–8.

45. Gheorghiade M, Adams KF Jr, Colucci WS. Digoxin in the management of cardiovascular disorders. Circulation 2004;109(24):2959–64.

46. Berman W Jr, Yabek SM, Dillon T, et al. Effects of digoxin in infants with congested circulatory state due to a ventricular septal defect. N Engl J Med 1983;308(7):363–6.

47. Pitt B, Zannad F, Remme WJ, et al. Randomized Aldactone Evaluation Study Investigators. The effect of spironolactone on morbidity and mortality in patients with severe heart failure. N Engl J Med 1999;341:709–17.

48. Zannad F, McMurray JJ, Krum H, et al. Eplerenone in patients with systolic heart failure and mild symptoms. N Engl J Med 2011;364:11–21.

49. Raman SV, Hor KN, Mazur W, et al. Eplerenone for early cardiomyopathy in Duchenne muscular dystrophy: a randomised, double-blind, placebo-controlled trial. Lancet Neurol 2015;14(2):153–61.

50. Hufnagle KG, Khan SN, Penn D, et al. Renal calcifications: A complication of long-term furosemide therapy in preterm infants. Pediatrics 1982;70:360–3.

51. Heo JH, Rascati KL, Lopez KN, et al. Increased fracture risk with furosemide use in children with congenital heart disease. J Pediatr 2018;199:92–8.e10.

52. Koruth JS, Lala A, Pinney S, et al. The clinical use of Ivabradine. J Am Coll Cardiol 2017;70:1777–84.

53. Swedberg K, Komajda M, Böhm M, et al. SHIFT Investigators. Ivabradine and outcomes in chronic heart failure (SHIFT): a randomised placebo-controlled study. Lancet 2010;376:875–85.

54. Böhm M, Swedberg K, Komajda M, et al. SHIFT Investigators. Heart rate as a risk factor in chronic heart failure (SHIFT): the association between heart rate and outcomes in a randomised placebo- controlled trial. Lancet 2010;376:886–94.

55. Fox K, Ford I, Steg PG, et al. Ivabradine for patients with stable coronary artery disease and left- ventricular systolic dysfunction (BEAUTIFUL): a randomised, double-blind, placebo-controlled trial. Lancet 2008;372:807–16.

56. Fox K, Ford I, Steg PG, et al. Heart rate as a prognostic risk factor in patients with coronary artery disease and left-ventricular systolic dysfunction (BEAUTIFUL): a subgroup analysis of a randomised controlled trial. Lancet 2008;372:817–21.

57. Fox K, Ford I, Steg PG, et al. Ivabradine in stable coronary artery disease without clinical heart failure. N Engl J Med 2014;371:1091–9.

58. Bonnet D, Berger F, Jokinen E, et al. Ivabradine in children with dilated cardiomyopathy and symptomatic chronic heart failure. J Am Coll Cardiol 2017;70: 1262–72.

59. Yancy CW, Jessup M, Bozkurt B, et al. 2017 ACC/AHA/HFSA focused update of the 2013 ACCF/AHA guideline for the management of heart failure: a report of the American College of Cardiology/American Heart Association Task Force on Clinical Practice Guidelines and the Heart Failure Society of America. Circulation 2017;136:e137–61.

60. McMurray JJV, Packer M, Desai AS, et al. Angiotensin–Neprilysin Inhibition versus Enalapril in Heart Failure. N Engl J Med 2014;371:993–1004.

61. Abraham WT, Fisher WG, Smith AL, et al. Multicenter InSync Randomized Clinical Evaluation of Cardiac resynchronization in chronic heart failure. N Engl J Med 2002;346:1845–53.

62. Motonga KS, Dubin AM. Cardiac resynchronization therapy for pediatric patients with heart failure and congenital heart disease: A reappraisal of results. Circulation 2014;129:1879–91.

63. Morales DL, Rossano JW, VanderPluym C, et al. Third annual pediatric interagency registry for mechanical circulatory support (PediMACS) report: preimplant characteristics and outcomes. Ann Thorac Surg 2019;107:993–1004.

64. Schranz D, Rupp S, Muller M, et al. Pulmonary artery banding in infants and young children with left ventricular dilated cardio- myopathy: a novel therapeutic strategy before heart transplantation. J Heart Lung Transplant 2013;32:475–81.

65. Schranz D, Akintuerk H, Bailey L. . Pulmonary artery banding for functional regeneration of end-stage dilated cardiomyopathy in young children: world network report. Circulation 2018;137(13):1410–2.

66. Duboc D, Meune C, Lerebours G, et al. Effect of perindopril on the onset and progression of left ventricular dysfunction in Duchenne muscular dystrophy. J Am Coll Cardiol 2005;45:855–7.

67. Duboc D, Meune C, Pierre B, et al. Perindopril preventive treatment on mortality in Duchenne muscular dystrophy: 10 years' follow-up. Am Heart J 2007;154: 596–602.

68. Birnkrant DJ, Bushby K, Bann CM, et al. Diagnosis and Management of Duchenne Muscular Dystrophy part 2: respiratory, cardiac, bone, health and orthopaedic management. Lancet Neurol 2018;17(4):347–61.

69. McNally EM, Katman JR, Benson DW, et al. Contemporary cardiac issues in Duchenne's muscular dystrophy. Working Group of the National Heart, Lung and Blood Institute in collaboration with parent project muscular dystrophy. Circulation 2015;131:1590–8.

70. Stauffer BL, Russell G, Nunley K, et al. miRNA expression in pediatric failing human heart. J Mol Cell Cardiol 2013;57:43–6.

71. Miyamoto SD, Karimpour-Fard A, Peterson V, et al. Circulating microRNA as a biomarker for recovery in pediatric dilated cardiomyopathy. J Heart Lung Transplant 2015;34:724–33.

72. Ishigami S, Ohtsuki S, Eitoku T, et al. Intracoronary cardiac progenitor cells in single ventricle physiology: the PERSEUS (cardiac progenitor cell infusion to treat

univentricular heart disease) randomized phase 2 trial. Circ Res 2017;120: 1162–73.

73. Bittle GJ, Morales D, Deatrick KB, et al. Stem cell therapy for hypoplastic left heart syndrome: mechanism, clinical application, and future directions. Circ Res 2018;123:288–300.

74. Murphy SV, Atala A. 3D bioprinting of tissues and. Nat Biotechnol 2014;32: 773–85.

75. Ong CS, Fukunishi T, Zhang HT, et al. Biomaterial-free three-dimensional bio-printing of cardiac tissue using human induced pluripotent stem cell derived car-diomyocytes. Sci Rep 2017;7:4566.

76. Lundberg MS, Baldwin JT, Buxton DB. Building a bioartificial heart: Obstacles and opportunities. J Thorac Cardiovasc Surg 2017;153(4):748–50.

# Pediatric Pulmonary Arterial Hypertension

Benjamin S. Frank, MD*, D. Dunbar Ivy, MD

## KEYWORDS

- Pediatric pulmonary hypertension • Congenital heart disease
- Acute vasoreactivity testing • Operability • Atrial septal defect
- Pulmonary vasodilators

## KEY POINTS

- Proceedings published from the 2018 World Symposium on Pulmonary Hypertension updated the definition of pulmonary hypertension to include all adults and children with mean pulmonary artery pressure greater than 20 mm Hg.
- New therapies, approved in adults and used off-label in pediatric patients, have led to improved outcomes for affected children.
- Although multiple medications have been used off-label, in 2017 bosentan became the first targeted PAH therapy approved for use in children.
- Future studies focused on safe, effective, pediatric-specific strategies to improve outcomes are needed.

## INTRODUCTION

The natural history of pediatric pulmonary arterial hypertension (PAH) is associated with a poor prognosis. In the era before targeted therapy, the untreated median survival from diagnosis of idiopathic PAH (IPAH) was 10 months (adults from the same time period had a median survival of 2.8 years).[1] Without treatment, increase of pulmonary arterial pressure (PAP) and resistance in patients with PAH leads to right heart failure, clinical worsening, and death. Unlike with adult patients, however, PAH in children is linked to lung growth.[2] Because of this advantage, the child with PAH has greater potential to reverse the underlying pathologic condition with appropriate therapy. In the modern era, studies and guidelines offer tools for treating physicians to better risk stratify patients with PAH and improve selection of children with PAH for surgical repair of associated congenital heart disease.

As pediatric-specific evidence is deficient, management of children is largely based on clinical experience and follows an algorithm similar to the one used for

Department of Pediatrics, Section of Cardiology, University of Colorado School of Medicine, Aurora, CO, USA
* Corresponding author. 13123 East 16th Avenue Box B100, Aurora, CO 80045.
*E-mail address:* Benjamin.Frank@childrenscolorado.org

Pediatr Clin N Am 67 (2020) 903–921
https://doi.org/10.1016/j.pcl.2020.06.005
0031-3955/20/© 2020 Elsevier Inc. All rights reserved.

adult patients.[3–5] For patients whose disease progresses despite maximal medical therapy, invasive options exist including atrial septostomy, lung transplantation, and Potts shunt.[6]

## DEFINITION

In 2018, at the same time similar changes were introduced for adults, the definition of pulmonary hypertension (PH) in pediatric patients was updated to include any patient with a mean PAP greater than 20 mm Hg at rest by heart catheterization.[7] The term PAH was also updated to include the subset of children with PH who also have a pulmonary capillary wedge pressure less than 15 mm Hg as well as pulmonary vascular resistance index (PVRi) value greater than 3 Wood units (WU)•m$^2$.[3] The NICE classification, generated to cohort subjects by similar pathophysiology, is typically applied to both adults and children.[3,8] A specific classification for PAH associated with congenital heart disease (CHD-PAH) is also published (**Table 1**).[8,9] In younger children, for whom a normal systemic blood pressure is lower than for older children or adults, the ratio of mean PAP to mean systemic artery pressure can be used to diagnose PH, with a significant increase being a ratio greater than 0.5.

An exception to these definitions is the group of children with single-ventricle congenital heart disease (CHD). Because patients with either stage 2 (superior

**Table 1**
**Classification of pediatric patients with pulmonary arterial hypertension associated with congenital heart disease**

| | |
|---|---|
| 1. Eisenmenger syndrome | Includes all large intracardiac and extracardiac defects that begin as systemic-to-pulmonary shunts and progress with time to severe increase of pulmonary vascular resistance and to reversal (pulmonary-to-systemic) or bidirectional shunting; cyanosis, secondary erythrocytosis, and multiple organ involvement are usually present |
| 2. Left-to-right shunts | Includes moderate to large defects whereby pulmonary vascular resistance is mildly to moderately increased, systemic-to-pulmonary shunting is still present, and cyanosis is not a feature |
| 3. Pulmonary arterial hypertension with coincidental congenital heart disease | Marked increase in pulmonary vascular resistance in the presence of small cardiac defects, which themselves do not account for the development of increased pulmonary vascular resistance. The clinical picture is very similar to idiopathic pulmonary arterial hypertension |
| 4. Postoperative pulmonary arterial hypertension | Congenital heart disease is repaired but pulmonary arterial hypertension either persists immediately after surgery or recurs/develops months or years after surgery in the absence of significant residual lesions |

*Adapted from* Simonneau G, Gatzoulis MA, Adatia I, et al. Updated clinical classification of pulmonary hypertension. J Am Coll Cardiol. 2013;62(25 Suppl):D38; with permission.

cavopulmonary anastomosis) or stage 3 (total cavopulmonary connection) physiology rely on passive pulmonary blood flow, the pathophysiology of inadequate pulmonary blood flow resulting from increased pulmonary vascular resistance may adversely affect many patients despite mean PAP of less than 20 mm Hg and PVRi of less than 3 WU•m$^2$. In such patients, even very mild increase in PAP and PVRi can lead to circulatory failure and cause significant morbidity.[2]

## EPIDEMIOLOGY

National registries from the United Kingdom, the Netherlands, and Spain have all shown a lower incidence for IPAH in children than in adults. The incidence of IPAH in the national registry from the United Kingdom was 0.48 cases per million children per year and the prevalence was 2.1 cases per million.[10] In the Netherlands, annual incidence and point prevalence averaged 0.7 and 2.2 cases per million children, respectively.[11] Likewise, in the Spanish registry the incidence and prevalence were 0.49 and 2.9 cases per million children, respectively.[12] Recent national database studies from the United States have additionally suggested an increasing prevalence of hospitalized children with PAH as a comorbidity.[13,14]

## GENETICS

Abnormalities in bone morphogenetic protein receptor type 2 (BMPR2) are the most commonly identified mutations in children and adults with PAH.[15] The pattern of inheritance for those with heritable PAH and a BMPR2 mutation is autosomal dominant with variable penetrance of the PAH phenotype by gender—14% for males and 42% for females. Recently implicated as causative component of PAH, ALK-1 and TBX4 mutations are also common. Although the gene mutations for both ALK-1 and TBX4 can be inherited in an autosomal dominant fashion, the gene penetrance and potential epigenetic modifying factors are not yet well described. Advanced gene-sequencing methods have facilitated the discovery of additional, less common gene mutations implicated among those with PAH (SOX17, SMAD-9, CAV1, KCNK3, and EIF2AK4).[10,11,13,14]

## PROGNOSIS

Owing to wide variability in age at presentation, underlying etiology, and pathophysiology, prognosis varies significantly among children with PAH. CHD-PAH comprises a particularly heterogeneous population. The largest group of children with CHD and PH has a post-tricuspid systemic-to-pulmonary shunt with preoperative PAH followed by complete resolution after early shunt correction. This group has an excellent prognosis. A smaller group of patients with CHD and a post-tricuspid left-to-right shunt develop persistent or progressive PAH that does not resolve after shunt correction. This set of patients has a particularly poor prognosis.[16] Although it is not possible to predict exactly which patients will resolve PAH after repair and which patients will progress, progressive CHD-PAH does occur more frequently in children with genetic syndromes (genetic abnormalities were identified in 30% of patients with CHD-PAH in a recent analysis).[16,17] A recent report suggested that subjects with transposition of the great vessels who develop PAH after arterial switch operation may be at particularly high risk.[18]

## NONINVASIVE EVALUATION

A standardized approach to the initial evaluation, differential diagnosis, comprehensive evaluation, and initial management of a pediatric PH patient can be found in recently published guidelines (**Fig. 1**).[19] The Proceedings from the 6th World Symposium on Pulmonary Hypertension additionally provided guidance on risk stratification of patients with PAH (**Table 2**).

Echocardiography is a highly useful initial tool for evaluating patients suspected of having PH that is readily available in most facilities and does not require sedation or ionizing radiation.[20] An echocardiogram can define the cardiac anatomy (including the presence or absence of shunts), evaluate ventricular size, wall thickness, and function, demonstrate any valvar abnormalities, and evaluate the presence or absence of pericardial effusion. Using the simplified Bernoulli equation, Doppler interrogation of tricuspid valve insufficiency velocity (right ventricular systolic), pulmonary valve insufficiency (pulmonary artery diastolic and mean), and any systemic-to-pulmonary shunts can be used noninvasively to estimate important pressures.[21]

Although challenging because of the geometry and anterior location of the right ventricle, an assessment of right ventricular (RV) function by echocardiography is also important. Several measures are available to quantify RV performance including

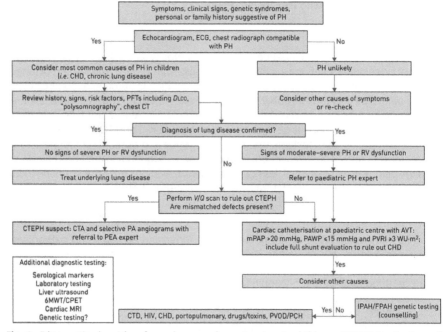

**Fig. 1.** Diagnostic algorithm for pulmonary hypertension in children. 6MWT, 6-minute walk test; AVT, acute vasodilator testing; CHD, congenital heart disease; CPET, cardiopulmonary exercise test; CT, computed tomography; CTA, computed tomography angiography; CTD, connective tissue disease; CTEPH, chronic thromboembolic pulmonary hypertension; DLCO, diffusing capacity of the lung for carbon monoxide; IPAH/FPAH, idiopathic/familial pulmonary arterial hypertension; mPAP, mean pulmonary arterial pressure; MRI, magnetic resonance imaging; PA, pulmonary artery; PAWP, pulmonary artery wedge pressure; PCH, pulmonary capillary hemangiomatosis; PEA, pulmonary endarterectomy; PFT, pulmonary function test; PVOD, pulmonary veno-occlusive disease; PVRI, pulmonary vascular resistance index; RV, right ventricular; V/Q, ventilation/perfusion; WU, Wood units. (Rosenzweig EB, Abman SH, Adatia I, et al. Paediatric pulmonary arterial hypertension: updates on definition, classification, diagnostics and management. Eur Respir J. 2019 53: 1801916; DOI: 10.1183/13993003.01916-2018. *Reproduced* with permission of the © ERS 2020.)

**Table 2**
**Risk stratification of patients with pediatric pulmonary arterial hypertension**

| Lower Risk | Risk Factor | Higher Risk |
|---|---|---|
| No | Clinical RV failure | Yes |
| No | Symptom progression | Yes |
| >350 m | 6-minute walk distance | <350 m |
| Normal | Growth | Failure to thrive |
| Minimally increased | BNP/NT-pro-BNP | Severely increased or rising |
| | Echocardiography | Severe RA/RV enlargement |
| | | Reduced LV size |
| | | Increased RV/LV ratio |
| | | Reduced RV function |
| | | Pericardial effusion |
| Cardiac index >3 L/min/m$^2$ | Catheterization | Cardiac index <2.5 L/min/m$^2$ |
| Systemic venous saturation >65% | | Mean RA pressure >10 mm Hg |
| Positive vasoreactivity testing | | PVR index >20 WU•m$^2$ |
| | | Systemic venous saturation <60% |
| | | PACI <0.85 mL/mm Hg/m$^2$ |

*Abbreviations*: BNP, brain natriuretic peptide; LV, left ventricle; PACI, pulmonary artery capacitance index; PVR, pulmonary vascular resistance; RA, right atrium; RV, right ventricle.

Rosenzweig EB, Abman SH, Adatia I, et al. Paediatric pulmonary arterial hypertension: updates on definition, classification, diagnostics and management. Eur Respir J. 2019 53: 1801916; DOI: 10.1183/13993003.01916-2018. *Reproduced* with permission of the © ERS 2020.

the RV Tei index (myocardial performance index), RV ejection fraction, RV fractional area change, and tricuspid annular plane systolic excursion (TAPSE).[19–22] Normal values for TAPSE have been recently published as a reference.[22,23] Three-dimensional (3D) echocardiography (including 3D RV ejection fraction) may improve assessment of RV function compared with 2D echocardiography alone.[24,25] Although beyond the scope of this review, recent data have identified emerging echocardiographic markers that can be helpful to track disease severity and, in some cases, predict clinical outcomes.[26]

Several additional noninvasive tests are commonly used to evaluate patients with PAH. These tests are particularly directed at defining a patient's functional status, disease severity, and prognosis. The 6-minute walk (6MW) test quantifies submaximal exercise capacity and documents saturations during activity in developmentally able children (typically those older than 7 years). There are now published pediatric normal values for 6MW distance (6MWD).[27–30] Of note, children with PAH tend to walk farther than their adult counterparts with the same World Health Organization (WHO) functional class. Although large registry studies have not consistently shown 6MWD to be a predictor of survival,[10,31] a recent single-center observational study suggested that, among children 7 to 18 years old, 6MWD less than 352 m and desaturation during the test (>5% for children with no shunt, >19% for children with a shunt) were associated with worse transplant-free survival.[32]

Cardiopulmonary exercise testing (CPET) can quantify both submaximal and peak exercise performance. Specifically, CPET can determine peak oxygen consumption ($Vo_{2max}$), ventilatory efficiency ($V_E/Vco_2$), the anaerobic threshold, and oxygen consumption at the anaerobic threshold ($Vo_2$ at AT).[33,34] $V_E/Vco_2$ is significantly higher in patients with PAH than in healthy controls and increases on average by 7.2 for each increase in WHO functional class.[35]

Among adult patients, measurement of brain natriuretic peptide (BNP) level is a useful tool to trend severity of disease, therapy response, and mortality risk.[36] Recent studies in children have suggested similar utility to trending BNP and N-terminal pro-BNP (NT-pro-BNP) levels, but confirmatory studies are ongoing.[37–39] In one study, an NT-pro-BNP >1200 ng/L conferred a poor prognosis.[26]

## INVASIVE EVALUATION

When clinically safe, cardiac catheterization is an important test in the evaluation of PH patients. Data from catheterization can be used to confirm the diagnosis of PAH via direct pressure measurement, quantify shunt lesions, calculate pulmonary vascular resistance (PVR) (using calculated or measured cardiac output), and perform acute vasoreactivity testing (AVT). Cardiac catheterization in pediatric PH patients carries a greater risk in those with baseline PAP greater than systemic compared with those with less severe PAH (odds ratio = 8.1).[40,41] One registry of PAH patients demonstrated a higher rate of catheterization complications in children compared with historical adult patients with PAH: this database recorded complications associated with heart catheterization in 5.9% of pediatric cases, including 5 deaths (0.6%).[42,43]

AVT during catheterization is an important step in risk-stratifying patients with PAH. A recent consensus statement published by the Pulmonary Vascular Research Institute has helped standardize the practice.[44] According to this statement, after baseline hemodynamic assessment, a short-acting vasodilator should be given, most commonly 20 to 40 parts per million of inhaled nitric oxide with or without high fractional inspired oxygen. Hemodynamics are then reassessed after a brief period of equilibration, typically 10 to 15 minutes.[45–47] Use of inhaled prostacyclin, inhaled milrinone, inhaled nitroglycerin, intravenous adenosine, and intravenous prostacyclin have also been reported.

Barst and colleagues[45] and Sitbon and colleagues[48] have each proposed strategies to classify patients as responders (positive test) or nonresponders (negative test), but consensus remains elusive. For a patient to be labeled a responder in the Barst criteria they must demonstrate a 20% or greater decrease in mean pulmonary artery (PA) pressure with decreased PVR/systemic vascular resistance (SVR) ratio and unchanged or increased cardiac index. For the Sitbon criteria, patients are labeled as vasoreactive if they show a decrease in mean PA pressure of greater than 10 mm Hg to a mean PA pressure less than 40 mm Hg with an unchanged or increased cardiac index. Depending on criteria used and patient population included, the percentage of patients with a new diagnosis of IPAH who are acute responders is between 6% and 20%.[49,50] A recent registry study suggested that the Sitbon criteria might be more sensitive in identifying pediatric subjects with a better prognosis.[51] A recent retrospective study using Barst criteria suggested that, among infants with PH secondary to bronchopulmonary dysplasia, children with positive AVT may have a decreased risk of adverse clinical outcomes.[52] Of note, the Barst and Sitbon criteria are used to determine therapy and prognosis in PAH but are not used to determine operability.

## SPECIAL CONSIDERATIONS FOR THE PATIENT WITH PULMONARY ARTERIAL HYPERTENSION ASSOCIATED WITH CONGENITAL HEART DISEASE

A common challenge facing physicians caring for children with CHD-PAH associated with a post-tricuspid systemic-to-pulmonary shunt (most commonly a ventricular septal defect or patent ductus arteriosus) is determining whether an individual patient is a candidate for defect closure. Optimal patient selection for defect closure is crucial: data suggest that patients with persistent PAH after CHD repair may have worse outcomes than those with unrepaired defects.[16] The recently published Proceedings of the 6th World Symposium on Pulmonary Hypertension suggest that a patient is likely a candidate for shunt closure if the calculated PVRi is <4 WU•m$^2$.[53] This report suggests that subjects are very high risk if PVRi is >8 WU•m$^2$ with an individualized decision based on specific lesion, age of patient, and comorbidities made when PVRi is between 4 and 8 WU•m$^2$. Guidelines for adults with CHD-PAH and systemic-to-pulmonary shunts are similar to the pediatrics guidelines (anatomic repair for PVRi of <4 WU•m$^2$, targeted PAH therapy, and re-evaluation for PVRi >8 WU•m$^2$), and add that repair may be considered in the "gray zone" of PVRi between 4 and 8 WU•m$^2$ when AVT is positive.[54] The American Heart Association/American Thoracic Society 2015 guidelines offer a treatment algorithm to guide operability of patients with "simple" shunts (**Fig. 2**).

The role of atrial septal defects (ASDs) in PAH poses a particular challenge. Among young children, patients with significant PAH and an isolated ASD are often classified as having PAH "incidental to" or "out of proportion to" their CHD.[55] Subjects in this group are thought to have outcomes and treatment response similar to those with IPAH or heritable PAH. However, data from adult patients suggest that the prevalence of preoperative PAH is between 29% and 73% of subjects with an ASD undergoing

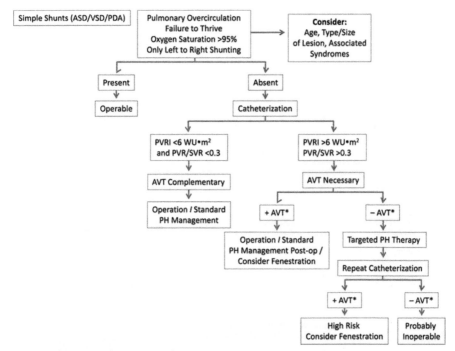

**Fig. 2.** Assessment of operability for shunt lesions in patients with congenital heart disease and pulmonary hypertension. ASD, atrial septal defect; AVT, acute vasoreactivity testing; PDA, patent ductus arteriosus; PVR, pulmonary vascular resistance; PVRI, pulmonary vascular resistance index; SVR, systemic vascular resistance; VSD, ventricular septal defect; WU, Wood units. (Lopes AA, Barst RJ. Daily practice revised: a proposed algorithm for management of patients with congenital cardiac defects associated with pulmonary hypertension.http://pvri. info. Reprinted with permission.)

closure. Persistent postoperative PAH is seen in 5% to 50% of patients.[56] Risk factors for developing PAH in the context of an ASD include residence at altitude, older age, female sex, and larger size of defect.[57] A recent retrospective study also suggested that the presence of an ASD may accelerate the progression of PAH in premature infants.[58] An experimental approach that can be considered for a patient with a large defect who is not a candidate for complete ASD closure based on PAH severity is fenestrated device closure to decrease shunt volume but allowing for intermittent right-to-left shunting as a pop-off during transient periods of increased PVR.[59]

## TARGETED PHARMACOLOGIC THERAPY FOR PULMONARY ARTERIAL HYPERTENSION

Three pathways have been extensively studied and yielded successful therapeutic targets for the treatment of PAH: prostacyclin, endothelin, and cyclic guanosine monophosphate (GMP). The recent proceedings of the World Symposium on Pulmonary Hypertension included an initial treatment algorithm (**Fig. 3**).[53] Prostanoids activate the prostacyclin pathway and stimulate cyclic adenosine monophosphate (epoprostenol, treprostinil, iloprost), endothelin receptor antagonists block endothelin signaling (bosentan, ambrisentan, macitentan), and phosphodiesterase inhibitors (sildenafil, tadalafil) and soluble guanylate cyclase stimulators (riociguat) increase intracellular cyclic GMP levels.

### *Prostacyclins*

It has been 30 years since the discovery that the biosynthesis of thromboxane $A_2$ and prostacyclin are altered in patients with PAH. This imbalance leads to insufficient prostacyclin activity.[60,61] Patients with severe PH also have decreased prostacyclin synthase expression at the level of their PAs.[62] Early studies demonstrated that prostacyclins administered chronically, using intravenous epoprostenol, improved survival and quality of life in adults and children with idiopathic PAH.[63–67]

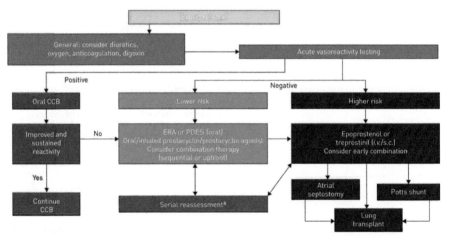

**Fig. 3.** Pediatric idiopathic/familial pulmonary arterial hypertension treatment algorithm. Hash mark indicates deterioration or not meeting treatment goals. CCB, calcium-channel blocker; ERA, endothelin receptor antagonist; PDE5i, phosphodiesterase type 5 inhibitor. (Rosenzweig EB, Abman SH, Adatia I, et al. Paediatric pulmonary arterial hypertension: updates on definition, classification, diagnostics and management. Eur Respir J. 2019 53: 1801916; DOI: 10.1183/13993003.01916-2018. *Reproduced* with permission of the © ERS 2020.)

The Food and Drug Administration (FDA) approved the prostacyclin analog treprostinil for subcutaneous use in 2002, followed by intravenous administration in 2004, inhaled administration in 2009, and oral therapy in 2013. Although subcutaneous treprostinil allows patients to receive parenteral therapy without a central venous catheter, it is associated with significant infusion-site pain for many. Intravenous treprostinil offers guaranteed drug delivery and avoids the infusion-site pain but requires central line access and a larger infusion pump than the one required for subcutaneous administration. Long-term efficacy of subcutaneous treprostinil[68] and intravenous treprostinil[69] has been shown in adults with PAH. Intravenous treprostinil has fewer side effects and a much longer half-life ($\sim$4 hours) than intravenous epoprostenol, making it a preferred option for many patients.[70] Subcutaneous treprostinil is well tolerated in many children of all ages, with tolerable side effects.[71,72] Although the regimen can be onerous, inhaled treprostinil is also available and is reasonably well tolerated by those who choose this route.[73]

Oral treprostinil has recently become available and is effective as monotherapy treatment in adult PAH[74] but may not be as add-on therapy, according to one report.[75] A different report noted improved 6MWT distance and decreased PVR after initiating therapy in adult patients.[76] Select pediatric patients may be able to transition from inhaled or subcutaneous or intravenous (SQ/IV) therapy to oral treprostinil, but side effects are frequent and challenging.[77,78] Recent reports have described early experience with the oral prostacyclin analog selexipag in pediatric patients,[76,79] noting 9 of 10 patients achieving goal dose and a trend toward improved hemodynamics.[79] A post hoc analysis of the Griphon trial conducted on adult patients with CHD-PAH demonstrated improved outcomes in patients treated with selexipag compared with placebo controls.[80] However, the long-term outcome of oral prostanoid therapy in pediatric patients with severe disease and the relative efficacy of oral therapy compared with IV/SQ delivery are not known.

### Endothelin Receptor Antagonists

Blocking the activity of the vasoconstrictor peptide endothelin (ET) is a well-established target for treatment of PAH.[81] ET-1 is a potent hormone produced primarily by vascular endothelial cells that causes pulmonary arteriolar vasoconstriction via endocrine and paracrine effects.[82]

Bosentan, the first ET-receptor antagonist to be approved (with activity against both receptors, $ET_A$ and $ET_B$), is known to decrease PAP, decrease PVR, and improve exercise capacity in adults with PAH.[81] FDA approved in 2001 for adults,[83] a series of pediatric trials demonstrating efficacy and safety led the FDA to approve bosentan for pediatric use in patients older than 3 years in September 2017.[84–88] One recent study demonstrated a wide dosing safety margin, favoring 2 mg/kg/dose twice per day as the goal dose.[89] Abnormal liver tests (most commonly increased aminotransferases) have been reported in 2.7% of children younger than 12 years compared with 7.8% of older patients. Because of this known toxicity, evaluation of monthly liver function is required for all patients on bosentan.

Macitentan, another dual ET-receptor antagonist with longer duration of action than bosentan (once daily dosing), achieved FDA approval for adult patients in 2013. Among adult patients, macitentan reduced the time to the first occurrence of a composite clinical worsening end point.[90] Pediatric-specific studies of macitentan are ongoing.

Selective $ET_A$ receptor blockade (with relative sparing of the vasodilator/clearance effects of $ET_B$) is hypothesized to offer therapeutic advantage over dual ET-receptor blockers. The $ET_A$-specific antagonist ambrisentan has been approved for use since June 2007. Adult patients with PAH showed significant improvements in 6MWD and increased time to first clinical worsening event on ambrisentan. The incidence of increased aminotransferase levels in adult patients was low at 2.8%.[83] Early experience with ambrisentan in children suggests that treatment is likely safe and effective for many patients, with pharmacokinetics and adverse reactions similar to those seen in adults.[91,92] There are no head-to-head trials comparing efficacy among the different available ET-receptor antagonists.

### Phosphodiesterase-5 Inhibitors and Soluble Guanylate Cyclase Stimulators

Phosphodiesterase-5 (PDE-5) is a membrane-bound protein found in vascular smooth muscle known to have increased activity in patients with PAH.[93] PDE-5 specific inhibitors sildenafil[94,95] and tadalafil[96–98] increase cyclic GMP levels, leading to pulmonary arteriolar vasodilation. On account of good efficacy and tolerability data, PDE-5 inhibitors are frequently used as first-line therapy for children with PAH in both the inpatient and outpatient settings.

Sildenafil is approved for the treatment of adult patients with WHO functional class II–IV PAH,[94] and has been well studied in children.[95,99,100] The STARTS-1 study was a randomized, double-blind, placebo-controlled trial of oral sildenafil in pediatric patients with PAH with 4 groups: low-, medium-, and high-dose sildenafil and placebo.[101] The trial did not meet its primary end point but did show a trend toward improved peak $V_{O_2}$ for all the sildenafil subjects combined in comparison with placebo.[101] After the initial 16-week study, subjects were enrolled in the STARTS-2 extension trial: patients in the sildenafil groups remained on their dose while patients on placebo were randomized to low, medium, or high dose.[102] At 3 years, the hazard ratio for mortality in STARTS-2 was 3.95 (95% confidence interval, 1.46–10.65) for high versus low dose. Patients who died disproportionately had idiopathic or heritable PAH (76% versus 33% overall) and baseline functional class III/IV disease (38% versus 15% overall). Three-year survival rates from the initiation of sildenafil therapy were 94%, 93%, and 88% for patients in the low-, medium-, and high-dose groups. Based on this information, the data monitoring committee recommended that all patients down-titrate from the high dose to medium dose. Review of the STARTS-1 and STARTS-2 studies by the FDA and the European Medicines Agency (EMA) resulted in highly disparate recommendations. Sildenafil was approved for pediatric patients by the EMA in 2011 with a subsequent warning against use of high-dose therapy. One year later, the FDA released a strong warning against the chronic use of sildenafil for pediatric patients. In 2014 the FDA amended the warning to state that there may be situations in which the risk-benefit profile may make sildenafil use acceptable in individual cases but that sildenafil is still not recommended in children with PAH. Most recently, a retrospective study of a mixed population of children with PAH treated with sildenafil therapy suggested that treatment was overall well tolerated with an acceptable side-effect profile.[55]

Tadalalfil is another PDE-5 inhibitor with a longer half-life than sildenafil, allowing for once daily dosing. There are no prospective, randomized pediatric PAH trials of tadalafil, and observational pediatric data are limited. In one study of 29 children with PAH switched from sildenafil to tadalafil for convenience of dosing, the change was generally well tolerated.[98] The average dose of sildenafil was 3.4 ± 1.1 mg/kg/d (divided among 3 doses) compared with tadalafil at 1.0 ± 0.4 mg/kg/d (given in one daily dose). For 14 of the 29 patients undergoing repeat catheterization, statistically significant improvements in PA pressure and PVR were observed after transition from sildenafil to tadalafil.

Riociguat is a direct soluble guanylate cyclase (sGC) stimulator that both increases the sensitivity of sGC to nitric oxide (NO) and augments cyclic GMP activity in a non–NO-dependent manner.[103] Both of these mechanisms are thought to contribute to its effect. Riociguat won FDA approval in 2013 for the treatment of adults with PAH and was the first medication with FDA approval for the treatment of chronic thromboembolic PH.[104] In the PATENT-1 and PATENT-2 trials, riociguat was well tolerated in adult patients with repaired CHD-PAH. In addition, subjects in the riociguat groups had improved PVR, 6MWD, WHO functional class, and NT-pro-BNP.[105] There are no published prospective or randomized studies of riociguat in children with PAH, and clinical experience to date is limited. A recent case report described a single patient with IPAH who experienced notable improvement in both PVR and WHO functional class after changing to riociguat from sildenafil.[106] A phase 3 safety and tolerability trial of riociguat is currently enrolling children.

### Calcium-Channel Blockers

Although not classically considered to be targeted PAH therapy, some children with PAH benefit from calcium-channel blocker therapy. In those patients who are acutely very responsive to either oxygen or NO (during AVT, based on Sitbon criteria stated earlier), common practice is to offer a trial of calcium-channel blocker monotherapy as first line. Children and adults treated with calcium-channel blockers may lose acute responsiveness over time and must be monitored carefully for continued efficacy.[67,107] In cases where patients initially respond but vasoreactivity is later lost on repeat testing and PAH persists, the authors favor a strategy of adding (but not discontinuing) PAH-targeted therapy to the calcium-channel blocker. Patients who do not have a positive acute vasodilator response during catheterization are unlikely to benefit from calcium-channel blocker therapy.[107] Eighty percent or more of children with severe PH are nonresponsive to AVT, and therefore require initiation of PAH-targeted therapy. Increased right atrial pressure and low cardiac output are contraindications to calcium-channel blockade in PAH.

### Combination Therapy

Early use of combination therapy—targeting 2 or more pathways with PAH-specific medications at treatment outset rather than starting monotherapy and adding additional therapy sequentially—is the treatment practice increasingly used for patients with moderate to severe disease and those with idiopathic or heritable PAH. In the randomized, controlled AMBITION trial of adult patients with PAH, the risk of a clinical worsening events was 50% lower among subjects who received initial combination therapy (ambrisentan + tadalafil) than among those on monotherapy with either medication.[5] Another retrospective study of 97 patients started on dual therapy (PDE-5 inhibitor + ET-receptor antagonist) at diagnosis demonstrated that this therapy was well tolerated and improved survival when compared with expected longevity derived from historical registry data.[108] A retrospective study comparing pediatric patients among 3 centers (2000–2010) showed that treatment with PAH-targeted combination therapy was independently and strongly associated with improved survival in comparison with monotherapy.[63]

### Adjunctive Therapy

Numerous adjunctive therapy options are used to treat RV failure and prevent the frequently encountered complications of PH. Digoxin has been tried in the presence of RV failure, although without positive data in children. Many providers maintain patients on warfarin or other antithrombotic agents to prevent thrombosis in situ, although specific data and indications in the pediatric population are lacking. Clinical experience dictates that anticoagulation is most often used in children with a hypercoagulable state, those with severe IPAH, and those with a central venous line for intravenous prostanoid therapy. In adults and children with IPAH who receive anticoagulation, warfarin is typically dosed to target an international normalized ratio of 1.5 to 2.[109] Diuretics are used to treat peripheral edema or ascites in the presence of right heart failure, but excessive diuresis should be avoided.

Preventive medicine is of particular importance for patients with severe disease. Careful attention to respiratory tract infections with good supportive care is required because pneumonitis may worsen alveolar hypoxia. Routine influenza vaccination and pneumococcal vaccination are recommended. The authors recommend against the use of decongestants with pseudoephedrine or other stimulant-type medications because these have been associated with PAH.[110] In children who require the use of oral contraceptive agents either for prevention of pregnancy or for regulation of menses, agents that have no estrogen content are recommended.

Among nonpharmacologic options, intermittent home pulse oximetry monitoring and polysomnography are indicated for patients with severe PH; chronic hypoxemia and nighttime desaturation should be aggressively treated. Although oxygen therapy is not used as a mainstay of therapy in children with normal daytime saturations, in the presence of resting hypoxemia chronic supplemental oxygen may be helpful.

## INVASIVE OPTIONS FOR REFRACTORY PULMONARY ARTERIAL HYPERTENSION

Atrial septostomy, performed during cardiac catheterization, can be considered for patients with severe PH, syncope, intractable heart failure refractory to chronic PAH-targeted therapy, and a symptomatic low cardiac output state.[111,112] Risks associated with this procedure include worsening of hypoxemia (secondary to right-to-left shunting), RV ischemia, increased left atrial pressure, and pulmonary edema. Contraindications include high right atrial pressure greater than 20 mm Hg and oxygen saturation at rest of less than 85%.[5] When selected for an individual patient, the authors favor serial balloon dilation under echocardiography and fluoroscopic guidance with saturation monitoring to determine the adequacy of shunting. Recent reports of a fenestrated ASD occlusion device (Occlutech) are intriguing, but more data are needed to demonstrate safety and efficacy.

Potts shunt—creating a connection between the left pulmonary artery and the descending aorta to provide a systolic "pop-off" and thereby decrease RV afterload—can be considered in cases of severe, refractory PAH with suprasystemic PAPs and adequate RV function. A Potts shunt offers the promise of an immediate reduction in RV afterload and may allow some patients to wean on targeted PAH therapy.[113–116] How to choose between atrial septostomy, Potts shunt, or initial lung transplantation for an individual patient failing medical therapy is a source of ongoing debate.

For patients whose disease is severe despite maximal medical and invasive therapy, lung transplantation should be considered.[117–119] Survival following pediatric lung transplant is similar to that encountered in adult patients, with recent registry data suggesting median survival of approximately 4.9 years.[120] The most common causes of early post-transplant death include graft failure, anatomic complications, and infection. Infection and bronchiolitis obliterans syndrome are the most common causes of late death after transplantation.

## SUMMARY

Pediatric PAH includes a highly heterogeneous group of children with diverse ages, disease severities, prognoses, and underlying causes. On diagnosis, it is important to complete a thorough evaluation for secondary causes of PAH and a cardiac catheterization with AVT. Although most treatment strategies for children with PAH are based on adult data and clinical experience, survival has improved significantly over recent decades as therapeutic options have increased. More pediatric-specific studies are needed to optimize therapy for affected children.

## ACKNOWLEDGMENTS

This review was supported by the Frederick and Margaret L. Weyerhaeuser Foundation, the Jayden de Luca Foundation, and NIH Grants R01HL114753 and U01HL121518. Supported by NIH/NCATS Colorado CTSA grant number UL1 TR002535.

## DISCLOSURE

The University of Colorado contracts with Actelion, Bayer, Janssen Lilly, and United Therapeutics for Dr Ivy to be a consultant and perform clinical research trials.

## REFERENCES

1. D'Alonzo GE, Barst RJ, Ayres SM, et al. Survival in patients with primary pulmonary hypertension. Results from a national prospective registry. Ann Intern Med 1991;115(5):343–9.
2. Cerro MJ, Abman S, Diaz G, et al. A consensus approach to the classification of pediatric pulmonary hypertensive vascular disease: Report from the PVRI Pediatric Taskforce, Panama 2011. Pulm Circ 2011;1(2):286–98.
3. Ivy DD, Abman SH, Barst RJ, et al. Pediatric pulmonary hypertension. J Am Coll Cardiol 2013;62(25 Suppl):D117–26.
4. Galie N, Corris PA, Frost A, et al. Updated treatment algorithm of pulmonary arterial hypertension. J Am Coll Cardiol 2013;62(25 Suppl):D60–72.
5. Galie N, Humbert M, Vachiery JL, et al. 2015 ESC/ERS Guidelines for the diagnosis and treatment of pulmonary hypertension: The Joint Task Force for the Diagnosis and Treatment of Pulmonary Hypertension of the European Society of Cardiology (ESC) and the European Respiratory Society (ERS): Endorsed by: Association for European Paediatric and Congenital Cardiology (AEPC), International Society for Heart and Lung Transplantation (ISHLT). Eur Respir J 2015;12:26.
6. Potts WJ, Smith S, Gibson S. Anastomosis of the aorta to a pulmonary artery; certain types in congenital heart disease. J Am Med Assoc 1946;132(11): 627–31.
7. Simonneau G, Montani D, Celermajer DS, et al. Haemodynamic definitions and updated clinical classification of pulmonary hypertension. Eur Respir J 2019; 53(1):1801913.
8. Simonneau G, Gatzoulis MA, Adatia I, et al. Updated clinical classification of pulmonary hypertension. J Am Coll Cardiol 2013;62(25 Suppl):D34–41.
9. Zijlstra WM, Douwes JM, Ploegstra MJ, et al. Clinical classification in pediatric pulmonary arterial hypertension associated with congenital heart disease. Pulm Circ 2016;6(3):302–12.
10. Moledina S, Hislop AA, Foster H, et al. Childhood idiopathic pulmonary arterial hypertension: a national cohort study. Heart 2010;96(17):1401–6.
11. van Loon RL, Roofthooft MT, Hillege HL, et al. Pediatric pulmonary hypertension in the Netherlands: epidemiology and characterization during the period 1991 to 2005. Circulation 2011;124(16):1755–64.

12. Cerro Marin MJ, Sabate Rotes A, Rodriguez Ogando A, et al. Assessing pulmonary hypertensive vascular disease in childhood: data from the Spanish registry. Am J Respir Crit Care Med 2014;190(12):1421–9.

13. Frank DB, Crystal MA, Morales DL, et al. Trends in pediatric pulmonary hypertension-related hospitalizations in the United States from 2000-2009. Pulm Circ 2015;5(2):339–48.

14. Maxwell BG, Nies MK, Ajuba-Iwuji CC, et al. Trends in hospitalization for pediatric pulmonary hypertension. Pediatrics 2015;136(2):241–50.

15. Southgate L, Machado R, Graf S, et al. Molecular genetic framework underlying pulmonary arterial hypertension. Nat Rev Cardiol 2020;17(2):85–95.

16. Haworth SG, Hislop AA. Treatment and survival in children with pulmonary arterial hypertension: the UK Pulmonary Hypertension Service for Children 2001-2006. Heart 2009;95(4):312–7.

17. Berger RM, Beghetti M, Humpl T, et al. Clinical features of paediatric pulmonary hypertension: a registry study. Lancet 2012;379(9815):537–46.

18. Zijlstra WMH, Ploegstra MJ, Vissia-Kazemier T, et al. Physical activity in pediatric pulmonary arterial hypertension measured by accelerometry. a candidate clinical endpoint. Am J Respir Crit Care Med 2017;196(2):220–7.

19. Abman SH, Hansmann G, Archer SL, et al. Pediatric pulmonary hypertension: guidelines from the American Heart Association and American Thoracic Society. Circulation 2015;132(21):2037–99.

20. Jone PN, Ivy DD. Echocardiography in pediatric pulmonary hypertension. Front Pediatr 2014;2:124.

21. Masuyama T, Kodama K, Kitabatake A, et al. Continuous-wave Doppler echocardiographic detection of pulmonary regurgitation and its application to noninvasive estimation of pulmonary artery pressure. Circulation 1986;74(3):484–92.

22. Koestenberger M, Ravekes W, Everett AD, et al. Right ventricular function in infants, children and adolescents: reference values of the tricuspid annular plane systolic excursion (TAPSE) in 640 healthy patients and calculation of z score values. J Am Soc Echocardiogr 2009;22(6):715–9.

23. Kurath-Koller S, Avian A, Cantinotti M, et al. Normal pediatric values of the subcostal tricuspid annular plane systolic excursion (S-TAPSE) and its value in pediatric pulmonary hypertension. Can J Cardiol 2019;35(7):899–906.

24. Jone PN, Schafer M, Pan Z, et al. 3D echocardiographic evaluation of right ventricular function and strain: a prognostic study in paediatric pulmonary hypertension. Eur Heart J Cardiovasc Imaging 2018;19(9):1026–33.

25. Jone PN, Patel SS, Cassidy C, et al. Three-dimensional echocardiography of right ventricular function correlates with severity of pediatric pulmonary hypertension. Congenit Heart Dis 2016;11(6):562–9.

26. Ploegstra MJ, Douwes JM, Roofthooft MT, et al. Identification of treatment goals in paediatric pulmonary arterial hypertension. Eur Respir J 2014;44(6):1616–26.

27. Geiger R, Strasak A, Treml B, et al. Six-minute walk test in children and adolescents. J Pediatr 2007;150(4):395–9 .e1-2.

28. Lammers AE, Hislop AA, Flynn Y, et al. The 6-minute walk test: normal values for children of 4-11 years of age. Arch Dis Child 2008;93(6):464–8.

29. Lesser DJ, Fleming MM, Maher CA, et al. Does the 6-min walk test correlate with the exercise stress test in children? Pediatr pulmonology 2010;45(2):135–40.

30. Li AM, Yin J, Au JT, et al. Standard reference for the six-minute-walk test in healthy children aged 7 to 16 years. Am J Respir Crit Care Med 2007;176(2): 174–80.

31. van Loon RL, Roofthooft MT, Delhaas T, et al. Outcome of pediatric patients with pulmonary arterial hypertension in the era of new medical therapies. Am J Cardiol 2010;106(1):117–24.
32. Douwes JM, Hegeman AK, van der Krieke MB, et al. Six-minute walking distance and decrease in oxygen saturation during the six-minute walk test in pediatric pulmonary arterial hypertension. Int J Cardiol 2015;202:34–9.
33. Garofano RP, Barst RJ. Exercise testing in children with primary pulmonary hypertension. Pediatr Cardiol 1999;20(1):61–4 [discussion: 65].
34. Yetman AT, Taylor AL, Doran A, et al. Utility of cardiopulmonary stress testing in assessing disease severity in children with pulmonary arterial hypertension. Am J Cardiol 2005;95(5):697–9.
35. Rausch CM, Taylor AL, Ross H, et al. Ventilatory efficiency slope correlates with functional capacity, outcomes, and disease severity in pediatric patients with pulmonary hypertension. Int J Cardiol 2013;169(6):445–8.
36. Nagaya N, Nishikimi T, Uematsu M, et al. Plasma brain natriuretic peptide as a prognostic indicator in patients with primary pulmonary hypertension. Circulation 2000;102(8):865–70.
37. Bernus A, Wagner BD, Accurso F, et al. Brain natriuretic peptide levels in managing pediatric patients with pulmonary arterial hypertension. Chest 2009; 135(3):745–51.
38. Lammers AE, Hislop AA, Haworth SG. Prognostic value of B-type natriuretic peptide in children with pulmonary hypertension. Int J Cardiol 2009;135(1):21–6.
39. Van Albada ME, Loot FG, Fokkema R, et al. Biological serum markers in the management of pediatric pulmonary arterial hypertension. Pediatr Res 2008; 63(3):321–7.
40. Carmosino MJ, Friesen RH, Doran A, et al. Perioperative complications in children with pulmonary hypertension undergoing noncardiac surgery or cardiac catheterization. Anesth Analg 2007;104(3):521–7.
41. Friesen RH, Williams GD. Anesthetic management of children with pulmonary arterial hypertension. Paediatr Anaesth 2008;18(3):208–16.
42. Beghetti M, Berger RM, Schulze-Neick I, et al. Diagnostic evaluation of paediatric pulmonary hypertension in current clinical practice. Eur Respir J 2013;42(3): 689–700.
43. Beghetti M, Schulze-Neick I, Berger RM, et al. Haemodynamic characterisation and heart catheterisation complications in children with pulmonary hypertension: Insights from the Global TOPP Registry (tracking outcomes and practice in paediatric pulmonary hypertension). Int J Cardiol 2015;203:325–30.
44. Del Cerro MJ, Moledina S, Haworth SG, et al. Cardiac catheterization in children with pulmonary hypertensive vascular disease: consensus statement from the Pulmonary Vascular Research Institute, Pediatric and Congenital Heart Disease Task Forces. Pulm Circ 2016;6(1):118–25.
45. Barst RJ, Maislin G, Fishman AP. Vasodilator therapy for primary pulmonary hypertension in children. Circulation 1999;99(9):1197–208.
46. Beghetti M. Current treatment options in children with pulmonary arterial hypertension and experiences with oral bosentan. Eur J Clin Invest 2006;36(Suppl 3): 16–24.
47. Rosenzweig EB, Barst RJ. Pulmonary arterial hypertension: a comprehensive review of pharmacological treatment. Treat Respir Med 2006;5(2):117–27.
48. Sitbon O, Humbert M, Jais X, et al. Long-term response to calcium channel blockers in idiopathic pulmonary arterial hypertension. Circulation 2005; 111(23):3105–11.

49. Douwes JM, van Loon RL, Hoendermis ES, et al. Acute pulmonary vasodilator response in paediatric and adult pulmonary arterial hypertension: occurrence and prognostic value when comparing three response criteria. Eur Heart J 2011;32(24):3137–46.

50. Barst RJ, McGoon MD, Elliott CG, et al. Survival in childhood pulmonary arterial hypertension: insights from the registry to evaluate early and long-term pulmonary arterial hypertension disease management. Circulation 2012;125(1): 113–22.

51. Douwes JM, Humpl T, Bonnet D, et al. Acute vasodilator response in pediatric pulmonary arterial hypertension: current clinical practice from the TOPP registry. J Am Coll Cardiol 2016;67(11):1312–23.

52. Frank BS, Schafer M, Grenolds A, et al. Acute vasoreactivity testing during cardiac catheterization of neonates with bronchopulmonary dysplasia-associated pulmonary hypertension. J Pediatr 2019;208:127–33.

53. Rosenzweig EB, Abman SH, Adatia I, et al. Paediatric pulmonary arterial hypertension: updates on definition, classification, diagnostics and management. Eur Respir J 2019;53(1):1801916.

54. Kaemmerer H, Apitz C, Brockmeier K, et al. Pulmonary hypertension in adults with congenital heart disease: Updated recommendations from the Cologne Consensus Conference 2018. Int J Cardiol 2018;272S:79–88.

55. Cohen JL, Nees SN, Valencia GA, et al. Sildenafil use in children with pulmonary hypertension. J Pediatr 2019;205:29–34 e21.

56. Zwijnenburg RD, Baggen VJM, Geenen LW, et al. The prevalence of pulmonary arterial hypertension before and after atrial septal defect closure at adult age: a systematic review. Am Heart J 2018;201:63–71.

57. Mullen MP. Challenges in the patient with pulmonary hypertension and atrial septal defect: understanding when and how to close the defect. Adv Pulm Hypertens 2019;18(1):10–3.

58. Vyas-Read S, Guglani L, Shankar P, et al. Atrial septal defects accelerate pulmonary hypertension diagnoses in premature infants. Front Pediatr 2018;6:342.

59. Kaley V, Dahdah N, El-Sisi A, et al. Atrial septal defect-associated pulmonary hypertension: outcomes of closure with a fenestrated device. Adv Pulm Hypertens 2019;18(1):4–9.

60. Adatia I, Barrow SE, Stratton PD, et al. Thromboxane A2 and prostacyclin biosynthesis in children and adolescents with pulmonary vascular disease. Circulation 1993;88(5 Pt 1):2117–22.

61. Christman BW, McPherson CD, Newman JH, et al. An imbalance between the excretion of thromboxane and prostacyclin metabolites in pulmonary hypertension. N Engl J Med 1992;327(2):70–5.

62. Tuder RM, Cool CD, Geraci MW, et al. Prostacyclin synthase expression is decreased in lungs from patients with severe pulmonary hypertension. Am J Respir Crit Care Med 1999;159(6):1925–32.

63. Zijlstra WMH, Douwes JM, Rosenzweig EB, et al. Survival differences in pediatric pulmonary arterial hypertension: clues to a better understanding of outcome and optimal treatment strategies. J Am Coll Cardiol 2014;63(20):2159–69.

64. Ivy DD, Doran A, Claussen L, et al. Weaning and discontinuation of epoprostenol in children with idiopathic pulmonary arterial hypertension receiving concomitant bosentan. Am J Cardiol 2004;93(7):943–6.

65. Lammers AE, Hislop AA, Flynn Y, et al. Epoprostenol treatment in children with severe pulmonary hypertension. Heart 2007;93(6):739–43.

66. Siehr SL, Ivy DD, Miller-Reed K, et al. Children with pulmonary arterial hypertension and prostanoid therapy: long-term hemodynamics. J Heart Lung Transplant 2013;32(5):546–52.
67. Yung D, Widlitz AC, Rosenzweig EB, et al. Outcomes in children with idiopathic pulmonary arterial hypertension. Circulation 2004;110(6):660–5.
68. Barst RJ, Galie N, Naeije R, et al. Long-term outcome in pulmonary arterial hypertension patients treated with subcutaneous treprostinil. Eur Respir J 2006; 28(6):1195–203.
69. Gomberg-Maitland M, Tapson VF, Benza RL, et al. Transition from intravenous epoprostenol to intravenous treprostinil in pulmonary hypertension. Am J Respir Crit Care Med 2005;172(12):1586–9.
70. Ivy DD, Claussen L, Doran A. Transition of stable pediatric patients with pulmonary arterial hypertension from intravenous epoprostenol to intravenous treprostinil. Am J Cardiol 2007;99(5):696–8.
71. Doran AK, Ivy DD, Barst RJ, et al. Guidelines for the prevention of central venous catheter-related blood stream infections with prostanoid therapy for pulmonary arterial hypertension. Int J Clin Pract Suppl 2008;(160):5–9.
72. Ferdman DJ, Rosenzweig EB, Zuckerman WA, et al. Subcutaneous treprostinil for pulmonary hypertension in chronic lung disease of infancy. Pediatrics 2014;134(1):e274–8.
73. Krishnan U, Takatsuki S, Ivy DD, et al. Effectiveness and safety of inhaled treprostinil for the treatment of pulmonary arterial hypertension in children. Am J Cardiol 2012;110(11):1704–9.
74. Jing ZC, Parikh K, Pulido T, et al. Efficacy and safety of oral treprostinil monotherapy for the treatment of pulmonary arterial hypertension: a randomized, controlled trial. Circulation 2013;127(5):624–33.
75. Tapson VF, Jing ZC, Xu KF, et al. Oral treprostinil for the treatment of pulmonary arterial hypertension in patients receiving background endothelin receptor antagonist and phosphodiesterase type 5 inhibitor therapy (the FREEDOM-C2 study): a randomized controlled trial. Chest 2013;144(3):952–8.
76. Tanabe N, Ikeda S, Tahara N, et al. Efficacy and safety of an orally administered selective prostacyclin receptor agonist, selexipag, in Japanese patients with pulmonary arterial hypertension. Circ J 2017;81(9):1360–7.
77. Ivy DD, Feinstein JA, Yung D, et al. Oral treprostinil in transition or as add-on therapy in pediatric pulmonary arterial hypertension. Pulm Circ 2019;9(3). https://doi.org/10.1177/2045894019856471.
78. Kanaan U, Varghese NP, Coleman RD, et al. Oral treprostinil use in children: a multicenter, observational experience. Pulm Circ 2019;9(3). https://doi.org/10.1177/2045894019862138.
79. Gallotti R, Drogalis-Kim DE, Satou G, et al. Single-center experience using selexipag in a pediatric population. Pediatr Cardiol 2017;38(7):1405–9.
80. Beghetti M, Channick RN, Chin KM, et al. Selexipag treatment for pulmonary arterial hypertension associated with congenital heart disease after defect correction: insights from the randomised controlled GRIPHON study. Eur J Heart Fail 2019;21(3):352–9.
81. Rubin LJ, Badesch DB, Barst RJ, et al. Bosentan therapy for pulmonary arterial hypertension. N Engl J Med 2002;346(12):896–903.
82. Vignon-Zellweger N, Heiden S, Miyauchi T, et al. Endothelin and endothelin receptors in the renal and cardiovascular systems. Life Sci 2012;91(13-14): 490–500.

83. Galie N, Olschewski H, Oudiz RJ, et al. Ambrisentan for the treatment of pulmonary arterial hypertension: results of the ambrisentan in pulmonary arterial hypertension, randomized, double-blind, placebo-controlled, multicenter, efficacy (ARIES) study 1 and 2. Circulation 2008;117(23):3010–9.

84. Barst RJ, Ivy D, Dingemanse J, et al. Pharmacokinetics, safety, and efficacy of bosentan in pediatric patients with pulmonary arterial hypertension. Clin Pharmacol Ther 2003;73(4):372–82.

85. Beghetti M. Bosentan in pediatric patients with pulmonary arterial hypertension. Curr Vasc Pharmacol 2009;7(2):225–33.

86. Hislop AA, Moledina S, Foster H, et al. Long-term efficacy of bosentan in treatment of pulmonary arterial hypertension in children. Eur Respir J 2011; 38(1):70–7.

87. Maiya S, Hislop AA, Flynn Y, et al. Response to bosentan in children with pulmonary hypertension. Heart 2006;92(5):664–70.

88. Rosenzweig EB, Ivy DD, Widlitz A, et al. Effects of long-term bosentan in children with pulmonary arterial hypertension. J Am Coll Cardiol 2005;46(4): 697–704.

89. Berger RMF, Gehin M, Beghetti M, et al. A bosentan pharmacokinetic study to investigate dosing regimens in paediatric patients with pulmonary arterial hypertension: FUTURE-3. Br J Clin Pharmacol 2017;83(8):1734–44.

90. Pulido T, Adzerikho I, Channick RN, et al. Macitentan and morbidity and mortality in pulmonary arterial hypertension. N Engl J Med 2013;369(9):809–18.

91. Zuckerman WA, Leaderer D, Rowan CA, et al. Ambrisentan for pulmonary arterial hypertension due to congenital heart disease. Am J Cardiol 2011;107(9): 1381–5.

92. Takatsuki S, Rosenzweig EB, Zuckerman W, et al. Clinical safety, pharmacokinetics, and efficacy of ambrisentan therapy in children with pulmonary arterial hypertension. Pediatr Pulmonol 2013;48(1):27–34.

93. Hanson KA, Ziegler JW, Rybalkin SD, et al. Chronic pulmonary hypertension increases fetal lung cGMP phosphodiesterase activity. Am J Physiol 1998;275(5 Pt 1):L931–41.

94. Galie N, Ghofrani HA, Torbicki A, et al. Sildenafil citrate therapy for pulmonary arterial hypertension. N Engl J Med 2005;353(20):2148–57.

95. Humpl T, Reyes JT, Holtby H, et al. Beneficial effect of oral sildenafil therapy on childhood pulmonary arterial hypertension: twelve-month clinical trial of a single-drug, open-label, pilot study. Circulation 2005;111(24):3274–80.

96. Pettit RS, Johnson CE, Caruthers RL. Stability of an extemporaneously prepared tadalafil suspension. Am J Health Syst Pharm 2012;69(7):592–4.

97. Rosenzweig EB. Tadalafil for the treatment of pulmonary arterial hypertension. Expert Opin Pharmacother 2010;11(1):127–32.

98. Takatsuki S, Calderbank M, Ivy DD. Initial experience with tadalafil in pediatric pulmonary arterial hypertension. Pediatr Cardiol 2012;33(5):683–8.

99. Karatza AA, Bush A, Magee AG. Safety and efficacy of sildenafil therapy in children with pulmonary hypertension. Int J Cardiol 2005;100(2):267–73.

100. Mourani PM, Sontag MK, Ivy DD, et al. Effects of long-term sildenafil treatment for pulmonary hypertension in infants with chronic lung disease. J Pediatr 2009; 154(3):379–84, 384.e1-2.

101. Barst RJ, Ivy DD, Gaitan G, et al. A randomized, double-blind, placebo-controlled, dose-ranging study of oral sildenafil citrate in treatment-naive children with pulmonary arterial hypertension. Circulation 2012;125(2):324–34.

102. Barst RJ, Beghetti M, Pulido T, et al. STARTS-2: long-term survival with oral sildenafil monotherapy in treatment-naive pediatric pulmonary arterial hypertension. Circulation 2014;129(19):1914–23.
103. Schermuly RT, Janssen W, Weissmann N, et al. Riociguat for the treatment of pulmonary hypertension. Expert Opin Investig Drugs 2011;20(4):567–76.
104. Ghofrani HA, D'Armini AM, Grimminger F, et al. Riociguat for the treatment of chronic thromboembolic pulmonary hypertension. N Engl J Med 2013;369(4):319–29.
105. Rosenkranz S, Ghofrani HA, Beghetti M, et al. Riociguat for pulmonary arterial hypertension associated with congenital heart disease. Heart 2015;101(22):1792–9.
106. Spreemann T, Bertram H, Happel CM, et al. First-in-child use of the oral soluble guanylate cyclase stimulator riociguat in pulmonary arterial hypertension. Pulm Circ 2018;8(1). https://doi.org/10.1177/2045893217743123.
107. Barst RJ. Recent advances in the treatment of pediatric pulmonary artery hypertension. Pediatr Clin North Am 1999;46(2):331–45.
108. Sitbon O, Sattler C, Bertoletti L, et al. Initial dual oral combination therapy in pulmonary arterial hypertension. Eur Respir J 2016;47(6):1727–36.
109. Olsson KM, Delcroix M, Ghofrani HA, et al. Anticoagulation and survival in pulmonary arterial hypertension: results from the Comparative, Prospective Registry of Newly Initiated Therapies for Pulmonary Hypertension (COMPERA). Circulation 2014;129(1):57–65.
110. Barst RJ, Abenhaim L. Fatal pulmonary arterial hypertension associated with phenylpropanolamine exposure. Heart 2004;90(7):e42.
111. Chiu JS, Zuckerman WA, Turner ME, et al. Balloon atrial septostomy in pulmonary arterial hypertension: effect on survival and associated outcomes. J Heart Lung Transplant 2015;34(3):376–80.
112. Sandoval J, Gaspar J, Pulido T, et al. Graded balloon dilation atrial septostomy in severe primary pulmonary hypertension. A therapeutic alternative for patients nonresponsive to vasodilator treatment. J Am Coll Cardiol 1998;32(2):297–304.
113. Baruteau AE, Belli E, Boudjemline Y, et al. Palliative Potts shunt for the treatment of children with drug-refractory pulmonary arterial hypertension: updated data from the first 24 patients. Eur J Cardiothorac Surg 2015;47(3):e105–10.
114. Baruteau AE, Serraf A, Levy M, et al. Potts shunt in children with idiopathic pulmonary arterial hypertension: long-term results. Ann Thorac Surg 2012;94(3):817–24.
115. Blanc J, Vouhe P, Bonnet D. Potts shunt in patients with pulmonary hypertension. N Engl J Med 2004;350(6):623.
116. Grady RM, Eghtesady P. Potts shunt and pediatric pulmonary hypertension: what we have learned. Ann Thorac Surg 2015;101(4):1539–43.
117. Aurora P, Boucek MM, Christie J, et al. Registry of the International Society for Heart and Lung Transplantation: tenth official pediatric lung and heart/lung transplantation report–2007. J Heart Lung Transplant 2007;26(12):1223–8.
118. Mallory GB, Spray TL. Paediatric lung transplantation. Eur Respir J 2004;24(5):839–45.
119. Toyoda Y, Thacker J, Santos R, et al. Long-term outcome of lung and heart-lung transplantation for idiopathic pulmonary arterial hypertension. Ann Thorac Surg 2008;86(4):1116–22.
120. Hill C, Maxwell B, Boulate D, et al. Heart-lung vs. double-lung transplantation for idiopathic pulmonary arterial hypertension. Clin Transplant 2015;29(12):1067–75.

# Update on Preventive Cardiology

Sarah B. Clauss, MD[a],*, Sarah D. de Ferranti, MD, MPH[b]

## KEYWORDS

- Hypercholesterolemia • Hypertension • Diabetes • Tobacco • Obesity • Child
- Prevention • Cardiovascular disease

## KEY POINTS

- Dyslipidemias can be diagnosed as early as age 2 years; statins may be used as early as age 8 years if low-density lipoprotein levels are high and unresponsive to lifestyle.
- Pediatric hypertension is increasing in prevalence, and poor blood pressure control accounts for 62% of cerebrovascular disease and 49% of ischemic heart disease in adults.
- Obesity affects 18.5% of US youth and has long-term sequelae of metabolic syndrome, type 2 diabetes mellitus, premature cardiovascular disease (CVD), and all-cause mortality.
- Diabetes mellitus leads to premature CVD; better glycemic control and treatment of associated risk factors is associated with lower CVD risk.
- Primary and secondary nicotine exposure in combustible formats is associated with CVD events; the emerging health effects of vaporized nicotine products are adverse.

## INTRODUCTION

Rates of cardiovascular disease (CVD) mortality had been improving over the past decades, but in recent years the positive trend has reversed. CVD is the most common cause of mortality in US women and in men, and youth represent the future of CVD prevention. CVD has been shown to have its origins in childhood.[1,2] Furthermore, many risk factors are known to track reasonably well from youth to adulthood, particularly at the extremes of the distribution. Because CVD and its risk factors are present early, it is important to identify and mitigate these risk factors during childhood, to the greatest extent possible.[3–8] The American Heart Association has defined ideal cardiovascular health based on 4 behaviors and 3 risk factors (Life's Simple 7), many of which people can improve through lifestyle changes: smoking status, physical activity, diet, weight, blood glucose, cholesterol, and blood pressure. This article reviews dyslipidemia, obesity, hypertension, diabetes, and smoking because these all contribute

a Children's National Medical Center, George Washington School of Medicine, 111 Michigan Avenue NW, Washington DC 20010, USA; b Boston Children's Hospital, Harvard School of Medicine, 300 Longwood Avenue, Boston, MA 02115, USA
* Corresponding author.
E-mail address: sclauss@childrensnational.org

Pediatr Clin N Am 67 (2020) 923–944
https://doi.org/10.1016/j.pcl.2020.06.006
0031-3955/20/© 2020 Elsevier Inc. All rights reserved.

to lifetime CVD burden. It discusses the prevalence, diagnosis, treatment, and cardio-vascular complications of these risk factors.

## HYPERCHOLESTEROLEMIA

Pathology, epidemiology, and genetic studies show that CVD risk factors begin in childhood and adolescence, forming the basis of atherosclerosis, and support the argument that treatment should begin early in life.[1] There is a growing body of litera-ture suggesting that earlier treatment, through lifestyle changes and pharmaco-therapy, can help reduce this risk.[9,10] Universal lipid screening is recommended between 9 and 11 years of age and again between 17 and 18 years.[11] This time frame is recommended because total cholesterol and low-density lipoprotein cholesterol (LDL-C) may decrease by 10% to 20% or more during adolescence.[12] Selective screening between the ages of 2 and 9 years and between 11 and 17 years of age is recommended if there are other CVD risk factors or a family history of premature CVD or significant hypercholesterolemia (**Table 1**). Other conditions associated with increased CVD include a history of cancer or congenital heart disease (especially coarctation of aorta and d-transposition of the great arteries), passive smoke expo-sure, and an unknown family history.[11] Cut points to define normative cholesterol values in children and adolescents are shown in **Table 2**. Dyslipidemia is present if 1 or more of these lipid, lipoprotein, or apolipoprotein factors are abnormal.

Dyslipidemias can be primary or secondary; secondary causes must be excluded in children with abnormal lipid values. Blood tests, including glucose level and renal, liver, and thyroid function, should be drawn. In secondary dyslipidemia, the associated disorder producing the dyslipidemia should be treated first in an attempt to normalize lipoprotein levels; however, if the dyslipidemia persists (eg, as it often does in diabetes

| Table 1 |
|---|
| **Disease stratification by risk** |

| Category | Condition |
|---|---|
| High risk | Homozygous FH, T2DM, end-stage renal disease, T1DM, Kawasaki disease with persistent aneurysms, solid-organ transplant vasculopathy, childhood cancer survivor (stem cell recipient) |
| Moderate risk | Severe obesity, heterozygous FH, confirmed hypertension, coarctation, lipoprotein (a), predialysis CKD, aortic stenosis, childhood cancer survivor (chest radiation) |
| At risk | Obesity, insulin resistance with comorbidities (dyslipidemia, NAFLD, PCOS), white-coat hypertension, hypertrophic cardiomyopathy and other cardiomyopathies, pulmonary hypertension, chronic inflammatory conditions (JIA, SLE, IBD, HIV), after coronary artery translocation for anomalous coronary arteries or transposition of the great arteries, childhood cancer (cardiotoxic chemotherapy only), Kawasaki disease with regressed aneurysms (zMax $\geq$ 5) |

*Abbreviations:* CKD, chronic kidney disease; FH, familial hypercholesterolemia; HIV, human immu-nodeficiency virus; IBD, inflammatory bowel disease; JIA, juvenile idiopathic arthritis; NAFLD, nonalcoholic fatty liver disease; PCOS, polycystic ovary syndrome; SLE, systemic lupus erythemato-sus; T1DM, type 1 diabetes mellitus; T2DM, type 2 diabetes mellitus.

*From* de Ferranti, SD, Steiberger J, Ameduri R, et al. Cardiovascular Risk Reduction in High-Risk Pediatric Patients: A Scientific Statement From the American Heart Association. Reprinted with permission Circulation.2019;139:e603-e634 ©2019 American Heart Association, Inc.

**Table 2**
**Cholesterol values (Units for TC, TG, HDL, non HDL and LDL= mg/dl; units for ApoB nmol/L)**

| Category | Acceptable | Borderline | High + |
|---|---|---|---|
| Total cholesterol | <170 | 170–199 | ≥200 |
| LDL-C | <110 | 110–129 | ≥130 |
| Non–HDL-C | <123 | 123–143 | ≥144 |
| Apolipoprotein B | <90 | 90–109 | ≥110 |
| Triglycerides | | | |
| 0–9 y | <75 | 75–99 | ≥100 |
| 10–19 y | <90 | 90–129 | ≥130 |

*Abbreviation:* HDL-C, high-density lipoprotein cholesterol.

mellitus [DM] and nephrotic syndrome), the patient will require dietary treatment, and, if indicated, drug therapy.

Most dyslipidemias are caused by a combination of genetic and environmental factors such as obesity, diet, and lack of exercise. However, there are patients who are more severely affected and who carry 1 or more mutant alleles resulting in dyslipidemia. Further, there are some inherited disorders of dyslipidemia that are prevalent, such as familial hypercholesterolemia (FH) and familial combined hyperlipidemia.

### Lifestyle Recommendations to Improve Dyslipidemia

For any child or adolescent who presents with dyslipidemia, implementing lifestyle changes is the first step in management.[13,14] Dietary recommendations should be tailored to the identified abnormality. The National Heart, Lung, and Blood Institute expert panel developed the Cardiovascular Health Integrated Lifestyle Diet (CHILD), which is specific for children and adolescents with dyslipidemia and increased risk for CVD.[11] This approach limits caloric intake, sodium, cholesterol, and refined carbohydrates. A diet high in fiber from fruits and vegetables, whole grains, polyunsaturated and monounsaturated fats, low in saturated fats, and without trans fats is recommended. In general, youth should obtain greater than 5 h/wk of moderate to vigorous physical activity.[15] However, there is conflicting evidence that physical activity modifies lipid values even with documented improvements in fitness.[16–18]

### Pharmacologic Therapy for Dyslipidemia

There are 6 main classes of lipid-altering drugs (**Table 3**): (1) inhibitors of hydroxymethylglutaryl coenzyme A reductase (the statins), (2) bile acid sequestrants, (3) cholesterol absorption inhibitors, (4) niacin (nicotinic acid), (5) omega-3 fatty acids (eicosapentaenoic acid and docosahexaenoic acid), and (6) fibric acid derivatives. Drug treatment to reduce LDL-C level is initiated when the post–dietary intervention LDL-C is greater than or equal to 190 mg/dL and there is a negative or unobtainable family history of premature CVD. If low-density lipoprotein (LDL) level is greater than or equal to 160 mg/dL after implementing dietary changes and there is a family history of premature CVD, or 2 or more risk factors for CVD, or the metabolic syndrome is present, drug treatment is recommended beginning at 10 years of age.[19] Lower cut points may be used in individuals with other conditions that significantly increase CVD risk.[15]

In most cases of dyslipidemia, statins are the first-line pharmaceutical therapy. As of 2020, the US Food and Drug Administration (FDA) has approved 5 statins for children and adolescents. Four of them (lovastatin, simvastatin, atorvastatin, and rosuvastatin)

**Table 3**
**Classes of medications used in the treatment of dyslipidemia in children and adolescents**

| Type | Mechanism of Action | Effects | Adverse Effects |
|---|---|---|---|
| HMG CoA reductase inhibitor (statin) | Inhibits HMG CoA reductase, which increases synthesis of LDL | ↓ LDL-C<br>↓ TG<br>↑ HDL-C | Rhabdomyolysis<br>Myopathy |
| Cholesterol absorption inhibitor (ezetimibe) | Upregulation of hepatic LDL receptors<br>Inhibition of intestinal cholesterol absorption | ↓ LDL-C | Myopathy (rare)<br>Gastrointestinal distress<br>Headache |
| Bile acid sequestrant | Binding of bile acids<br>Interruption of enterohepatic circulation | ↓ LDL-C<br>Variable changes in TG | Gastrointestinal distress |
| PCSK9 inhibitors | Inhibit PCSK9 from degrading LDL receptors | ↓ LDL-C<br>↓ TG<br>↓ lipoprotein (a) | Myopathy<br>Upper respiratory tract infections<br>Influenzalike symptoms |
| Lomitapide[a] | Inhibits MTP from transferring triglycerides to apoB for the production of VLDL | ↓ LDL-C<br>↓ lipoprotein(a) | Gastrointestinal distress<br>Hepatotoxicity |
| Mipomersen[a] | Disrupts the production of the structurally important apoB-100 lipoprotein | ↓ LDL-C<br>↓ TG<br>↓ lipoprotein (a) | Injection site reactions<br>Influenzalike symptoms<br>Hepatotoxicity |

*Abbreviations:* HMG CoA, hydroxymethylglutaryl coenzyme A; MTP, microsomal triglyceride transfer protein; PCSK9, proprotein convertase subtilisin kexin 9; TG, triglycerides; VLDL, very-low-density lipoprotein.

[a] Available under the FDA Risk Evaluation and Mitigation Strategy program.

*From* Hartz J, Clauss S. Treatment Strategies for Hypercholesterolemia. Curr Pediatr Rev. 2017;13(4):243-254. https://doi.org/10.2174/1573396314666180111143900; with permission.

are approved for children more than the age of 10 years, whereas pravastatin is approved for children aged 8 years and older.[20]

In addition to decreasing LDL-C and increasing high-density lipoprotein cholesterol (HDL-C), statins have been shown to improve endothelial function, stabilize developing atherogenic plaques, decrease inflammation, and inhibit the thrombogenic response.[21–24] An increased risk for DM with statin use was first noted in the Justification for the Use of Statins in Prevention: an Intervention Trial Evaluating Rosuvastatin (JUPITER) trial.[25] Although this has not been well studied in children, 1 study specifically of pediatric patients with FH did not find an increased risk for diabetes in patients after starting a statin; those with FH also have a lower risk of developing diabetes while on statin therapy.[26] The risk in the general population of developing diabetes after starting statin therapy is concentrated in those with additional risk factors for diabetes.[27,28]

One of the most promising new therapies for hypercholesterolemia is the proprotein convertase subtilisin kexin 9 (PCSK9) inhibitors. PCSK9 is a protease found primarily in the liver that directs LDL receptors to the lysosome for degradation, subsequently decreasing the availability of the LDL receptor to remove circulating LDL-C. Two PCSK9 inhibitors have been approved by the FDA: alirocumab and evolocumab. Both are monoclonal antibodies that are currently available only as subcutaneous injections administered every 2 to 4 weeks. Evolocumab is approved for adolescents more than 13 years old with homozygous FH, given as a subcutaneous injection of 420 mg every 4 weeks. Alirocumab does not have pediatric indication.[29,30] The efficacy of PCSK9 inhibitors depends on the presence of at least 1 (partially) functioning LDL receptor, making them ineffective in individuals with double null homozygous FH.

Lomitapide and mipomersen are indicated for use in patients with homozygous FH. Both are available only through the FDA Risk Evaluation and Mitigation Strategy. Lomitapide inhibits the microsomal triglyceride transfer protein from transferring triglycerides to apolipoprotein B (apoB) for the production hepatic very-low-density lipoproteins (VLDLs) and enterocyte-derived chylomicrons. Because of its mechanism of action, it should be given at least 2 hours after a meal for maximum effectiveness and to reduce the incidence and severity of adverse effects. Mipomersen is a single-stranded antisense oligonucleotide that disrupts the production of the apoB-100 lipoprotein, which is the main structural component of LDL and VLDL. It has been shown to have similar efficacy to lomitapide and decreases LDL-C level up to 61% and triglyceride (TG) levels up to 53%.[31] Both drugs have as adverse effects steatohepatitis, which is dose related, requires regular monitoring, and may be a reason to discontinue therapy in some individuals.

Hypertriglyceridemia can result from either increased TG production or reduced TG clearance. The cause is often multifactorial and is often associated with obesity or diabetes. Diet and lifestyle changes are an important therapeutic intervention. If the TG levels are severely increased, fibrates, omega-3 fatty acid supplementation ($\sim$4 g eicosapentaenoic acid/docosahexaenoic acid), or statins (if non-HDL or apoB level is increased) may be indicated.[15] The REDUCE-IT [Reduction of Cardiovascular Events with Icosapent Ethyl–Intervention Trial] study of adults with hypertriglyceridemia showed that patients had significantly lower risk of ischemic events if they were taking 4 g of icosapent ethyl twice a day regardless of the use of statin.[32] There is no current pediatric indication to empirically use omega-3 supplementation in pediatric patients. In addition to prescription formulations, they are available over the counter in a variety of concentrations; if they are used, care should be taken to use high-concentration formulations.

## OBESITY

Body mass index (BMI) is a measure used to determine childhood overweight and obesity. Note that BMI does not measure body fat directly, and does not indicate excess adiposity in every patient. Overweight is defined as a BMI at or more than the 85th percentile and less than the 95th percentile for children; obesity is defined as a BMI at or more than the 95th percentile for children and teens of the same age and sex. Because children's body composition varies as they age and varies between boys and girls, BMI levels need to be expressed relative to other children of the same age and sex. An alternate measure of adiposity is waist circumference (WC). WC is a simple measurement that has been well recognized in adults to be a useful risk indicator, independent of BMI.[33,34] The WC is obtained by measuring the waist circumference on bare skin measured just above the iliac crest. In a study in Mississippi, children with a WC greater than or equal to the 75th percentile or a waist/height ratio greater than 0.50 had excess adiposity that was an indicator of obesity-related health risk.[35]

National Health and Nutrition Examination Survey (NHANES) data from 2015 to 2016 showed that the prevalence of obesity among US youth was 18.5%; this is an increase from the previously prevalence of 17%.[36,37] Adolescents have the highest prevalence of obesity, followed by school-aged children and then preschoolers: 20.6%, 18.4%, and 13.9% respectively. Boys and girls were equally obese. The prevalence of obesity among non-Hispanic Asian youth is 11%, in non-Hispanic white youth 14.1%, non-Hispanic black youth 22%, and 25.8% in Hispanic youth (https://www.cdc.gov/obesity/data/childhood.html). In addition, three-quarters of overweight adolescents become obese adults.[36,38,39]

### Complications of Obesity

Specific morbidities associated with obesity include hypertension, insulin resistance, type 2 diabetes mellitus (T2DM), dyslipidemia, nonalcoholic fatty liver disease (NAFLD), and obstructive sleep apnea (OSA). Further, in obese individuals, the clustering of dyslipidemia, hypertension, and impaired glucose tolerance/insulin resistance is referred to as the metabolic syndrome, which further increases the risk of atherosclerotic heart disease.[40,41]

In 1 study of obese children undergoing polysomnography, 46% had OSA.[42] The presence of OSA may promote leptin resistance and enhance ghrelin levels, both of which can perpetuate the tendency for obesogenic behaviors.[43,44] In addition, sleepiness reduces the likelihood of engaging in physical activity and enhances obesogenic eating behaviors that favor calorie-dense foods, particularly in those children at risk for obesity. In addition, OSA is a chronic low-grade inflammatory disease that interacts with and potentiates obesity-induced inflammatory processes.[45–48]

NAFLD is defined as hepatic fat infiltration in greater than 5% of hepatocytes with no evidence of hepatocellular injury on liver biopsy and no history of alcohol intake. NAFLD is highly correlated with obesity, affecting at least 38% of obese adolescents in autopsy series and ~50% in epidemiologic surveys.[49,50] On evaluation, the most common findings are hepatomegaly and mild to moderate increase in serum alanine aminotransferase (ALT) level.[51–53] Hepatic fat deposition usually occurs in the context of generalized obesity but reflects much more strongly the presence of increased visceral adiposity, which can be seen by an increased WC.[54]

Increased insulin levels are associated with obesity and insulin resistance (IR) and lead to the onset of diabetes. Combined dyslipidemia of obesity (CDO) results from IR. Increased TG levels and low HDL levels are diagnostic of CDO. LDL level is not significantly increased; however, smaller dense LDL particles are present secondary to hepatic lipase activity. Hepatic VLDL production is increased in insulin-resistant states because of the excess of free fatty acids. Lipoprotein lipase activity is impaired, resulting in decreased clearance of TG-rich particles. HDL becomes TG rich, which then is broken down by hepatic lipase, resulting in smaller HDL, which causes degradation of the particle and less renal uptake, leading to lower total HDL-C levels.

### Lifestyle Recommendations to Treat Obesity

Lifestyle management is the mainstay of prevention and treatment of obesity. Dietary, physical activity, and behavioral changes should be recommended in an age-appropriate, culturally sensitive, family-centered manner. Dietary recommendations are similar to those with increased lipid levels, with an additional emphasis on decreased consumption of added sugar, sugar-sweetened beverages, high-fructose corn syrup, and processed and fast foods.[55] Increased physical activity, healthy sleep habits, and reduced screen time are key as well. Providers should assess and treat for psychosocial comorbidities. A recent study by Lloyd-

Richardson and colleagues[56] showed sustained weight-loss success with long-term behavioral therapy. Formal behavioral therapy may not be reimbursed, requires considerable time from the family, and therefore may be a barrier to its success outside the research arena. Behavior strategies that can be done independently include self-monitoring (eg, food diaries, exercise logs), education, goal setting, and participating in a support group.

Obesity is associated with an increased risk of mortality. Franks and colleagues[57] studied obese American Indians from Arizona and showed increased risk of death before age 55 years. In the highest BMI group, the rate of death was more than double that of the lowest BMI group. In addition, individuals with an impaired oral glucose tolerance test in childhood had a 73% higher rate of death caused by complications of obesity/CVD. The investigators concluded that increased premature death in adulthood of individuals who were obese as children may be mediated by early glucose intolerance and hypertension in childhood.[57] Other investigators have shown a 50% increase in heart failure in obese individuals 18 to 34 years olds (1987–2006) and increased risk of kidney failure in the presence of obesity.[58–60]

### Pharmacologic Therapy for Obesity

Pharmacotherapy is indicated for adolescents with obesity only if intensive lifestyle modifications are not successful and the BMI is greater than or equal to 30 kg/m$^2$, or if there is at least 1 comorbidity and the BMI is greater than or equal to 27 kg/m$^2$.[55] Medications should be discontinued if the patient does not experience at least a 0.4% BMI/BMI z score reduction after taking antiobesity medication for 12 weeks at the medication's full dosage.[61]

FDA-approved pharmacotherapy in the pediatric age group is limited. Orlistat is the only FDA-approved medication for obesity treatment of youth aged 12 to 16 years. Orlistat reduces adolescents' fat absorption by 30% and therefore can affect the absorption of fat-soluble vitamins.[62] Orlistat reduces BMI significantly in adolescents, by 0.7 to 1.7 kg/m$^2$, but treatment is associated with significant gastrointestinal side effects.[63,64] Orlistat must be taken with each meal, thus reducing its utility in school-attending adolescents. In 1 trial, 50% of pediatric patients prescribed orlistat discontinued it within 1 month, 75% stopped using it by 3 months, and only 10% remained on orlistat after 6 months.[65,66]

Metformin is not FDA approved for obesity treatment. However, metformin reduces hepatic glucose production, increases peripheral insulin sensitivity, and may reduce appetite.[67] Metformin resulted in a mean decrease of only 1.16 kg/m$^2$ over 6 to 12 months.[68] Metformin may also be useful in combating the weight gain observed in children and adolescents who are taking atypical psychotropic medications or who have polycystic ovary syndrome.[69–72] Given its limited weight-loss efficacy, metformin is not a considered a weight-loss treatment.

Other newer pharmacologic agents are on the horizon for the treatment of obesity. Kelly and colleagues[73] conducted a 6-month open-label study of exenatide on 12 obese children and teenagers. This glucagonlike peptide-1 (GLP-1) receptor agonist is used in adults with T2DM and has been found to reduce BMI, body weight, and body fat through its ability to increase feelings of satiety and suppress appetite.[74,75] Kelly and colleagues[73] found that exenatide reduced BMI, body weight, and fasting insulin level. The drug was well tolerated, with the most common adverse event being mild nausea. Topiramate has been associated with weight loss when used for epilepsy; therefore, it has been used as a weight-loss drug in adults. In a small pediatric study, topiramate showed weight loss without significant adverse events.[76] The mechanism of action is not well understood, and higher doses of medications are associated with adverse side effects in adults.[77,78] Further research needs to be performed on pharmacologic weight-loss agents to provide additional options for obese children and teenagers, particularly when viewed as an alternative to bariatric surgery.

### Bariatric Surgery

Bariatric surgery is recommended only after the patient has attained Tanner 4 or 5 pubertal development and final or near-final adult height. Eligible patients usually have a BMI of greater than or equal to 40 kg/m$^2$ or a BMI of greater than or equal to 35 kg/m$^2$ and significant, extreme comorbidities despite compliance with a formal program of lifestyle modification, with or without pharmacotherapy. Patients must be seen by a psychologist, have a stable home life, and agree to long-term compliance with follow-up.[79,80] Although there are no studies evaluating the effect of bariatric surgery on adolescent mortality, a Swedish study of adults with obesity showed a sustained 67% weight loss; reduced relative risk of death of 89%; and decreased CVD, cancer, endocrine disorders, psychiatric complications, and health costs.[81] Bariatric surgery can result in macronutrient and micronutrient deficiency, therefore supplements are required. Teenagers are at risk for noncompliance, therefore vitamin level monitoring is recommended. In addition, reoperation may be necessary because of a complication from the procedure or if there is inadequate weight loss or persistence of comorbidities.[82]

## HYPERTENSION

Childhood hypertension tracks into adulthood and is a risk factor for CVD in adulthood, because it has been associated with increased left ventricular mass, increased carotid intima media thickness (cIMT), decreased endothelial function, and increased arterial stiffness.[83–87] In 2017, "Clinical Practice Guideline for Screening and Management of High Blood Pressure in Children and Adolescents" (CPG) was published as an update to the previous 2004 report (**Box 1** provides a synopsis of the updates).[88,89] Children greater than or equal to 3 years old who are seen in a medical setting should have their blood pressure measured. If the averaged oscillometric reading is greater than or equal to the 90th percentile, 2 auscultatory measurements should be taken and averaged to define the blood pressure category for that day. Readings on 3 or more days are required to diagnose hypertension. Correct measurement requires a cuff that is appropriate to the size of the child's upper arm. Unlike the tables in the fourth report, the blood pressure values in CPG are derived from a population of children and adolescents without overweight or obesity (ie, those with a BMI <85th percentile); therefore, they represent normative blood pressure values for normal-weight youth. Blood pressure values in the new update are several millimeters of mercury lower than similar tables in the fourth report (**Table 4**). Recommended testing when hypertension is present is shown in **Box 2**. Primary hypertension is thought to be the cause for hypertension in most cases in children older than 6 years of age.[90–92] Younger children with an abnormal serum creatinine level, renal ultrasonography, or echocardiography findings tend to have secondary hypertension.[91]

Hypertension in childhood can lead to target organ damage and is a risk factor for future CVD.[93] The only testing currently routinely recommended in pediatrics is echocardiogram to evaluate for left ventricular mass for patients being treated with antihypertensive medication. However, studies of children and adolescents with hypertension show vascular changes related to hypertension, such as increased cIMT and arterial stiffness, which are associated with increased risk of premature CVD in adults. Litwin and colleagues[94] showed that reducing blood pressure in

---

**Box 1**
**Clinical practice guideline for screening and management of high blood pressure in children and adolescents: synopsis of changes from fourth report**

1. Replacement of the term prehypertension with the term "elevated blood pressure"

2. New normative pediatric blood pressure tables based on normal-weight children; blood pressure values in new update several millimeters of mercury lower than similar tables in the fourth report

3. Simplified screening table for identifying blood pressures needing further evaluation

4. Simplified blood pressure classification in adolescents greater than or equal to 13 years of age that aligns with the American Heart Association and American College of Cardiology adult blood pressure guidelines.

---

children with a mean age of 14 yeas decreased intima media thickness measurements. Furthermore, data from the Cardiovascular Risk in Young Finns Study, Childhood Determinants of Adult Healthy Study, the Bogalusa Heart Study, and the Muscatine Study show that increased systolic blood pressure after age 6 years is associated with increased cIMT and, importantly, with a risk for premature CVD.[84]

### Lifestyle Modifications to Reduce Blood Pressure

Lifestyle changes are recommended as initial treatment of all children and adolescents with hypertension. A Dietary Approaches to Stop Hypertension (DASH) diet is recommended; this is high in fruits, vegetables, low-fat milk products, whole grains, fish, poultry, nuts, and lean meats, and low in sugar, sweets, and sodium, and is a proven dietary intervention in adults that has been associated with lower blood pressure.[95,96] A 10-year study showed lower childhood blood pressure and a 36% lower risk of high blood pressure in late adolescence in 2000 girls who consumed greater than or equal to 2 servings of dairy and greater than or equal to 3 servings of fruits and vegetables daily.[97] Physical activity should be encouraged, with a minimum of 30 to 60 minutes of moderate to vigorous physical activity at least 3 to 5 d/wk. A study conducted in adults who participated in 8 hours of sports training over 1 year showed a decrease in blood pressure of approximately 15 mm Hg systolic and approximately 4 mm Hg diastolic after training.[98] Although pediatric data are limited, a review of physical activity

**Table 4**
**Staging of hypertension according to current guidelines**

|  | 1–13 y Old | ≥13 y Old |
|---|---|---|
| Normal | <90th percentile | <120/<80 mm Hg |
| Increased blood pressure | ≥90th to 95th percentile, or 120/80 mm Hg to <95th percentile (whichever is lower) | 120/<80–129/<80 mm Hg |
| Stage 1 hypertension | ≥95th to 95th percentile + 12 mm Hg or 130/80–139/89 mm Hg (whichever is lower) | 130/80–139/89 mm Hg |
| Stage 2 hypertension | ≥ 95th percentile + 12 mm Hg or ≥140/90 mm Hg (whichever is lower) | ≥140/90 mm Hg |

---

**Box 2**
**Recommended testing after diagnosis of hypertension**

Recommended for all
1. Blood test for electrolytes, urea nitrogen, creatinine
2. Lipid profile
3. Urinalysis: presence of hematuria or proteinuria
   Renal ultrasonography in patients less than 6 years of age or those with abnormal urinalysis or renal function

Optional testing
1. In obese children: hemoglobin A1c, aspartate transaminase, ALT, fasting lipid panel
2. Thyroid-stimulating hormone
3. Fasting serum glucose for patients at high risk for DM
4. Drug screen
5. Sleep study
6. Complete blood count (patients with growth delay or abnormal renal function)

---

interventions in overweight children and adolescents showed that at least 40 minutes of moderate to vigorous aerobic physical activity 3 to 5 d/wk improved systolic blood pressure by an average of 6.6 mm Hg and prevented vascular dysfunction.[99] In addition, stress reduction has been shown to reduce blood pressure. A mindfulness-based stress reduction program at the University of Massachusetts Memorial Medical Center, conducted in 175 African American teenagers, led to a reduction in daytime, nighttime, and 24-hour systolic and diastolic blood pressures.[100]

### Pharmacologic Therapy

Pharmacologic therapy should be initiated in children who remain hypertensive despite a trial of lifestyle modifications or who have symptomatic hypertension, stage 2 hypertension without a clearly modifiable factor (eg, obesity), or any stage of hypertension associated with chronic kidney disease or DM.[88] Therapy should be initiated with a single medication at the low end of the dosing range. Medication options include angiotensin-converting enzyme inhibitors (ACEi), long-acting calcium channel blockers (CCBs), angiotensin receptor blockers (ARBs), and thiazide diuretics (**Table 5**). In general, these medications have few side effects.[101,102] There are few studies that compare agents head to head; there seems to be no significant difference in the amount of blood pressure reduction between medications.[103] African Americans may require a higher dose of ACEi.[104,105] In addition, based on adult data, β-blockers are not recommended for treatment of hypertension in children. The CPG recommends a target blood pressure of less than the 90th percentile for children and adolescents with primary hypertension.[88]

### Diabetes and prediabetes

DM, caused by either absolute insulin deficiency, as seen in type 1 DM (T1DM), or by IR and relative impaired insulin secretion, as seen in type 2, is increasingly common in children and adolescents. Diabetes affects 9.4% of the US population overall (30.3 million), with 1.25 million children and adults having T1DM. Incidence rates of T2DM are increasing with the epidemic in childhood obesity; in contrast with the adult epidemiology, most patients newly diagnosed with diabetes have T1DM but T2DM is becoming a bigger proportion of childhood-onset diabetes.[106] T1DM incidence is around 20 per 1000,000, and 1 more recent study suggests that the incidence is holding steady in recent years.[107] The incidence of type 2 during childhood, as reported in the SEARCH study, ranges more widely, between 3.9 and 46.5 per 100,000, with the

**Table 5**
**Pharmacotherapy used for the treatment of hypertension**

| Type | Contraindications | Common Adverse Effects | Serious Adverse Effects |
|---|---|---|---|
| ACEi<br>• Benazepril<br>• Captopril<br>• Enalapril<br>• Fosinopril<br>• Lisinopril<br>• Ramipril<br>• Quinapril | Pregnancy, angioedema | Cough, headache, dizziness, asthenia | Hyperkalemia, acute kidney injury, angioedema, fetal toxicity |
| ARBs<br>• Candesartan<br>• Irbesartan<br>• Dimesartan<br>• Valsartan | Pregnancy | Headaches, dizziness | Hyperkalemia, acute kidney injury, fetal toxicity |
| Thiazide diuretics<br>• Chlorotrialidone<br>• Chlorothiazide<br>• Hydrochlorothiazide | Anuria | Dizziness, hypokalemia | Cardiac dysrhythmias, cholestatic jaundice, new-onset DM, pancreatitis |
| CCBs<br>• Amlodipine<br>• Felodipine<br>• Isradipine<br>• Nifedipine ER | Hypersensitivity to CCBs | Flushing, peripheral edema, dizziness | Angioedema |

*Abbreviation:* ER, extended release.
*From* Flynn JT., Kaelber DC., Baker-Smith CM., et al. Clinical practice guideline for screening and management of high blood pressure in children and adolescents. Pediatrics 2017. https://doi.org/10.1542/peds.2017-1904; with permission.

highest rates seen in non-Hispanic black people and Native Americans.[108] Incidence rates of type 2 are increasing year by year by ~2% or more as rates of severe obesity in childhood increase; at least 5000 youth develop type 2 every year.[109] Risk factors for T2DM include obesity, notably central adiposity, sedentary lifestyle and poor diet, exposure to maternal diabetes in utero, low birth weight, polycystic ovary syndrome, as well as female gender and a parent with diabetes.

The increase in the incidence of DM, particularly T2DM, is concerning because of its association with premature CVD, including coronary artery disease, heart failure, and cerebrovascular disease. Rates of CVD in adults with DM are 3.6-fold higher in men and 7 times higher in women compared with the general population. The degree to which DM increases the future risk for CVD is not well quantified, but vascular assessments for subclinical atherosclerosis show stiffer vasculature in children with T1DM compared with children without diabetes.[110–112] Individuals with DM also have autonomic dysfunction. Both types of diabetes are characterized by both hyperglycemia and hyperinsulinemia, either exogenous or exogenous (as treatment) or both. Worse clinical outcomes are seen in patients with more advanced disease, either poorly controlled or of longer duration.

**Cardiovascular perspective on the management of diabetes mellitus** The specific management of T1DM and T2DM are beyond the scope of this article and are well described elsewhere.[113] However, glycemic control, even in adolescence, is a key factor in reducing CVD risk, as shown in the Diabetes Control and Complications Trial (DCCT) and other studies.[114,115] Therefore, an important modality for reducing CVD risk is to focus on treating the primary diagnosis, DM. A secondary but also important area of focus is to minimize diabetic nephropathy, a complication of DM that is associated with worse CVD outcomes because of proteinuria and hypertension.

### Lifestyle Modification

Physical activity is advised by the American Diabetes Association, specifically 60 min/d of moderate to vigorous aerobic activity plus muscle-strengthening and bone-strengthening activities at least 3 d/wk. Care needs to be taken with regard to hypo-glycemia during and after exercise; consultation with the patient's pediatric endocrinologist is advised. Optimizing diet is associated with improved outcomes, even in T1DM, and ongoing consultation with a diabetes nurse educator or dietitian is advised.[113,116–119]

### Pharmacotherapy

Insulin is the mainstay of treatment of T1DM and is an important therapy for youth with T2DM. Children with type 1 may benefit from continuous insulin delivery.[119] Frequent glucose monitoring is advised and continuous glucose monitoring may be helpful to bring the hemoglobin A1c level down. More frequent blood glucose monitoring can result in better glycemic control, and therefore reduce the risk for microvascular and macrovascular complications.[113,120] When assessing glycemic control in the context of cardiovascular risk it may be helpful to inquire about the frequency of glucose monitoring, the patient's awareness of goal hemoglobin A1c level, and how far the patient is from that goal. Goal hemoglobin A1c varies from 6.5% up to 8% depending on frequency and self-awareness of hypoglycemia; targets on the lower end of this range can be used for children with T2DM, given the low risk of hypoglycemia in this population.[113] Lower hemoglobin A1c level during adolescence can result in fewer complications, including heart disease.[114,120–122] An important effect of intensive insulin regimens is weight gain.

Insulin-sensitizing therapy, most often metformin, should be initiated in those youth with T2DM with normal renal function. Insulin should be used in symptomatic patients to get glycemia under control. Choices of glucose-modulating therapy have broadened, with some newer agents having additional beneficial effects related to reducing cardiovascular risk. Thus, if these 2 agents are not sufficient, both SGLT2 inhibitors (empagliflozin, canagliflozin, dapagliflozin) and GLP-1 receptor agonists (liraglutide, albiglutide, semaglutide, and dulaglutide) have been shown to reduce the risk of CVD events in adults with T2DM and CVD, or CVD risk factors. Liraglutide may be trialed in children aged 10 years and older.

### Additional Cardiovascular Risk Factors in Youth with Diabetes Mellitus

In addition to optimizing glycemic control, identifying and treating other cardiovascular risks is key to reducing future CVD.[123–125] This point is important because children with diabetes are more likely to have additional CVD risk factors than their peers without diabetes; between 14% and 45% of youth with T1DM have at least 2 risk factors for CVD in addition to diabetes. Higher prevalence is seen in older youth, girls more than boys, and in racial and ethnic minorities. Screening for lipid disorders every year and measuring blood pressure at least every 6 months is recommended.[124,125]

The treatment of hypertension and hyperlipidemia in patients with diabetes includes the same approaches as used in children without diabetes, but the presence of diabetes should prompt a truncation in the trial of lifestyle modification alone, and the use of lower cut points to trigger treatment. Pharmacotherapy should be started alongside lifestyle modification if the level of the risk factor is high, in contrast with children without diabetes, where lifestyle alone is generally the first line of defense. Specifically, with regard to blood pressure in youth with diabetes, blood pressures greater than or equal to the 90th percentile or, for youth 13 years of age and older, greater than or equal to 120/80 mm Hg should prompt the initiation of antihypertensive therapy with an ACEi or an ARB.[113] Antihypertensive pharmacotherapy should start alongside lifestyle modification advice in youth with systolic or diastolic blood pressure consistently greater than or equal to the 95th percentile for age, sex, and height or greater than or equal to 140/90 mm Hg in adolescents greater than or equal to 13 years of age. In the case of hyperlipidemia, lipid cut points and the timeline for initiating pharmacotherapy are reduced compared with youth without diabetes. Dietary modification and optimizing glycemic control are first recommended, followed by pharmacotherapy if lifestyle change has not been sufficiently effective to reduce LDL level to less than 130 mg/dL, aiming to bring it to less than 100 mg/dL if possible, and TG level less than 150 mg/dL. Fenofibrates should be considered if TG level is greater than 400 mg/dL. Goals of therapy also differ, with the intention being to reduce blood pressure and LDL level more, to consider non-HDL as an indication for more statin, and to use an ACEi in patients with proteinuria even if blood pressure is not greatly increased. Screening and diabetes treatment recommendations are described yearly by the American Diabetes Association.[113]

### Nicotine

Cigarette smoking is a major risk factor for CVD, explaining the largest proportion of coronary artery disease, heart failure, and stroke. According to NHANES data, 8.8% of high school and 1.8% of middle school students reported to be smoking cigarettes in the past 30 days used combustible nicotine.[37] Secondhand smoke exposure increases the risk of coronary heart disease and stroke in nonsmokers by 20% to 30%.[37] Subclinical vascular dysfunction has been shown in youth exposed to secondhand smoke.[126] The adverse clinical outcomes in adults and subclinical abnormalities in childhood have led to policies banning smoking in the workplace and other locations where secondhand exposure is possible.

Other methods of nicotine delivery using electronic delivery methods have been introduced into the market in recent years, raising concerns about negative CVD effects. Although these products may have initially been conceived of as a way to quit smoking, along the lines of nicotine patches and nicotine gum, their introduction to the market has led to an epidemic of new users of nicotine products, particularly in youth.[127] This field is rapidly evolving but recent data show that 27.5% of high school students and 10.5% of middle school students currently use e-cigarettes.[128] Understanding of the adverse effects of these nicotine products is still evolving, but they are known to contain chemicals that may increase risks of addiction and disease, and their use has been connected to more than 2000 lung injury cases and at least 42 deaths in the United States (as of November 2019). Some of these serious pulmonary conditions are thought to be related to home preparations or additives. An unintended and serious adverse consequence of the introduction of inhaled nicotine products is the ingestion by toddlers of the concentrated liquid, which contains very large amounts of nicotine, and this has led to significant morbidity and even mortality. Part of the attractiveness of these products to toddlers, and to teens as well, seems to lie in the flavorings, which smell like foods (eg, mango). These high-profile events and severe health outcomes have prompted some states to ban or significantly curtail the availability of these products for public sale until more is learned. CVD outcomes are likely longer term, and little is known about long-term effects of vaporized nicotine. Research is complicated by the variety of proprietary formulas, making it challenging to compare Juul with Puff Bar in terms of long-term health effects. In addition to the specific negative effect on youth, there are concerns about other health disparities. Menthol nicotine products are more often chosen by African Americans.

Cessation programs for combustible nicotine products have been used to help adult smokers quit smoking. Successful quit rates in adults are 3% to 5% without support and 30% to 50% as part of an organized program with behavioral and nicotine substitution products such as patches or gum. Most successful quitters try multiple times before they succeed. Cessation efforts in youth have shown modest efficacy.[129] There is no published experience on e-cigarette cessation in youth; this is an area of urgent need, as championed by the American Heart Association, the Centers for Disease Control and Prevention, and others. Public health campaigns have included messaging around both serious (death, tracheostomy, chronic lung disease) and more cosmetic (stained teeth and fingers) adverse effects. Labeling of cigarettes with direct messaging about adverse health outcomes has been a long-standing strategy.

## SUMMARY

The decades-long trend showing deceasing rates of CVD mortality have been reversed in recent years. Identification and treatment of risk factors in childhood is paramount to reducing CVD in adulthood. Clinicians can mitigate future disease through advising their patients and families to follow heart-healthy behaviors, such as healthful eating, increased physical activity, and avoidance of tobacco products. Furthermore, screening of blood pressures, lipid values, and anthropologic measurements can identify children at high risk of CVD. Early identification and treatment of risk factors, laboratory abnormalities, or vital signs can ideally lead to corrections to improve lifetime cardiovascular health.

## REFERENCES

1. McGill HC, McMahan CA. Determinants of atherosclerosis in the young. Pathobiological Determinants of Atherosclerosis in Youth (PDAY) Research Group. Am J Cardiol 1998;82(10B):30T–6T.

2. Berenson GS, Srinivasan SR, Bao W, et al. Association between multiple cardiovascular risk factors and atherosclerosis in children and young adults. The Bogalusa Heart Study. N Engl J Med 1998. https://doi.org/10.1056/NEJM199806043382302.

3. Chen X, Wang Y. Tracking of blood pressure from childhood to adulthood: a systematic review and meta-regression analysis. Circulation 2008. https://doi.org/10.1161/CIRCULATIONAHA.107.730366.

4. Juhola J, Magnussen CG, Viikari JSA, et al. Tracking of serum lipid levels, blood pressure, and body mass index from childhood to adulthood: the cardiovascular risk in young Finns study. J Pediatr 2011. https://doi.org/10.1016/j.jpeds.2011.03.021.

5. Baker JL, Olsen LW, Sørensen TIA. Childhood body-mass index and the risk of coronary heart disease in adulthood. N Engl J Med 2007. https://doi.org/10.1056/NEJMoa072515.

6. Morrison JA, Glueck CJ, Horn PS, et al. Pediatric triglycerides predict cardio-vascular disease events in the fourth to fifth decade of life. Metabolism 2009. https://doi.org/10.1016/j.metabol.2009.04.009.

7. Morrison JA, Glueck CJ, Wang P. Childhood risk factors predict cardiovascular disease, impaired fasting glucose plus type 2 diabetes mellitus, and high blood pressure 26 years later at a mean age of 38 years: the Princeton-lipid research clinics follow-up study. Metabolism 2012. https://doi.org/10.1016/j.metabol.2011.08.010.

8. Gunnell DJ, Frankel SJ, Nanchahal K, et al. Childhood obesity and adult cardio-vascular mortality: a 57-y follow-up study based on the Boyd Orr cohort. Am J Clin Nutr 1998. https://doi.org/10.1093/ajcn/67.6.1111.

9. Juonala M, Viikari JSA, Raitakari OT. Main findings from the prospective Cardio-vascular Risk in Young Finns Study. Curr Opin Lipidol 2013. https://doi.org/10.1097/MOL.0b013e32835a7ed4.

10. McGill HC Jr, McMahan CA, Herderick EE, et al. Obesity accelerates the pro-gression of coronary atherosclerosis in young men. Circulation 2002;105(23):2712–8.

11. Expert panel on integrated guidelines for cardiovascular health and risk reduc-tion in children and adolescents: summary report. Pediatrics 2011. https://doi.org/10.1542/peds.2009-2107c.

12. Berger S, Raman G, Vishwanathan R, et al. Dietary cholesterol and cardiovas-cular disease: a systematic review and meta-analysis. Am J Clin Nutr 2015;276–94. https://doi.org/10.3945/ajcn.114.100305.

13. Hu FB, Willett WC. Optimal diets for prevention of coronary heart disease. J Am Med Assoc 2002. https://doi.org/10.1001/jama.288.20.2569.

14. Mente A, De Koning L, Shannon HS, et al. A systematic review of the evidence supporting a causal link between dietary factors and coronary heart disease. Arch Intern Med 2009. https://doi.org/10.1001/archinternmed.2009.38.

15. De Ferranti SD, Steinberger J, Ameduri R, et al. Cardiovascular risk reduction in high-risk pediatric patients: a scientific statement from the American Heart As-sociation. Circulation 2019. https://doi.org/10.1161/CIR.0000000000000618.

16. Stavnsbo M, Aadland E, Anderssen SA, et al. Effects of the Active Smarter Kids (ASK) physical activity intervention on cardiometabolic risk factors in children: a cluster-randomized controlled trial. Prev Med (Baltim) 2020. https://doi.org/10.1016/j.ypmed.2019.105868.

17. Crouter SE, De Ferranti SD, Whiteley J, et al. Effect on physical activity of a ran-domized afterschool intervention for Inner City Children in 3rd to 5th grade. PLoS One 2015. https://doi.org/10.1371/journal.pone.0141584.

18. Sun C, Pezic A, Tikellis G, et al. Effects of school-based interventions for direct delivery of physical activity on fitness and cardiometabolic markers in children and adolescents: a systematic review of randomized controlled trials. Obes Rev 2013. https://doi.org/10.1111/obr.12047.

19. Lauer RM, Barness LA, Clark R, et al. National Cholesterol Education Program (NCEP): highlights of the report of the expert panel on blood cholesterol levels in children and adolescents. Pediatrics 1992;89(3):495–501.

20. Kusters DM, Vissers MN, Wiegman A, et al. Treatment of dyslipidaemia in child-hood. Expert Opin Pharmacother 2010. https://doi.org/10.1517/14656561003592169.

21. De Jongh S, Lilien MR, Op'T Roodt J, et al. Early statin therapy restores endo-thelial function in children with familial hypercholesterolemia. J Am Coll Cardiol 2002. https://doi.org/10.1016/S0735-1097(02)02593-7.

22. Araujo DB, Bertolami MC, Ferreira WP, et al. Pleiotropic effects with equivalent low-density lipoprotein cholesterol reduction: comparative study between simvastatin and simvastatin/ezetimibe coadministration. J Cardiovasc Pharmacol 2010. https://doi.org/10.1097/FJC.0b013e3181bfb1a2.

23. Lahera V, Goicoechea M, Garcia de Vinuesa S, et al. Endothelial dysfunction, oxidative stress and inflammation in atherosclerosis: beneficial effects of statins. Curr Med Chem 2006. https://doi.org/10.2174/092986707779313381.

24. Wang CY, Liu PY, Liao JK. Pleiotropic effects of statin therapy: molecular mechanisms and clinical results. Trends Mol Med 2008. https://doi.org/10.1016/j.molmed.2007.11.004.

25. Ridker PM, Pradhan A, MacFadyen JG, et al. Cardiovascular benefits and diabetes risks of statin therapy in primary prevention: an analysis from the JUPITER trial. Lancet 2012. https://doi.org/10.1016/S0140-6736(12)61190-8.

26. Joyce NR, Zachariah JP, Eaton CB, et al. Statin use and the risk of type 2 diabetes mellitus in children and adolescents. Acad Pediatr 2017. https://doi.org/10.1016/j.acap.2017.02.006.

27. Collins R, Reith C, Emberson J, et al. Interpretation of the evidence for the efficacy and safety of statin therapy. Lancet 2016. https://doi.org/10.1016/S0140-6736(16)31357-5.

28. Skoumas J, Liontou C, Chrysohoou C, et al. Statin therapy and risk of diabetes in patients with heterozygous familial hypercholesterolemia or familial combined hyperlipidemia. Atherosclerosis 2014. https://doi.org/10.1016/j.atherosclerosis.2014.08.047.

29. Latimer J, Batty JA, Neely RDG, et al. PCSK9 inhibitors in the prevention of cardiovascular disease. J Thromb Thrombolysis 2016. https://doi.org/10.1007/s11239-016-1364-1.

30. Gouni-Berthold I. PCSK9 antibodies: a new class of lipid-lowering drugs. Atheroscler Suppl 2015. https://doi.org/10.1016/j.atherosclerosissup.2015.02.003.

31. Akdim F, Tribble DL, Flaim JD, et al. Efficacy of apolipoprotein B synthesis inhibition in subjects with mild-to-moderate hyperlipidaemia. Eur Heart J 2011. https://doi.org/10.1093/eurheartj/ehr148.

32. Bhatt DL, Steg PG, Miller M, et al. Cardiovascular risk reduction with icosapent ethyl for hypertriglyceridemia. N Engl J Med 2019. https://doi.org/10.1056/NEJMoa1812792.

33. Janiszewski PM, Janssen I, Ross R. Does waist circumference predict diabetes and cardiovascular disease beyond commonly evaluated cardiometabolic risk factors? Diabetes Care 2007. https://doi.org/10.2337/dc07-0945.

34. Klein S, Allison DB, Heymsfield SB, et al. Waist circumference and cardiometabolic risk: a consensus statement from shaping America's health: Association for weight management and obesity prevention; NAASO, the obesity society; the American society for nutrition; and the American diabetes association. Obesity 2007. https://doi.org/10.1038/oby.2007.632.

35. Gamble A, Waddell D, Allison Ford M, et al. Obesity and health risk of children in the Mississippi Delta. J Sch Health 2012. https://doi.org/10.1111/j.1746-1561.2012.00725.x.

36. Ogden CL, Carroll MD, Fryar CD, et al. Prevalence of obesity among adults and youth: United States, 2011-2014. NCHS Data Brief; 2015. Available at: https://www.cdc.gov/nchs/data/databriefs/db219.pdf.

37. Virani SS, Alonso A, Benjamin EJ, et al. Heart disease and stroke statistics—2020 update. Circulation 2020. https://doi.org/10.1161/cir.0000000000000757.

38. Freedman DS, Mei Z, Srinivasan SR, et al. Cardiovascular risk factors and excess adiposity among overweight children and adolescents: the Bogalusa Heart Study. J Pediatr 2007;150(1):12–7.e2.
39. Deshmukh-Taskar P, Nicklas TA, Morales M, et al. Tracking of overweight status from childhood to young adulthood: the Bogalusa Heart Study. Eur J Clin Nutr 2006. https://doi.org/10.1038/sj.ejcn.1602266.
40. Whitaker RC, Wright JA, Pepe MS, et al. Predicting obesity in young adulthood from childhood and parental obesity. N Engl J Med 1997. https://doi.org/10.1056/NEJM199709253371301.
41. Daniels SR, Arnett DK, Eckel RH, et al. Overweight in children and adolescents: pathophysiology, consequences, prevention, and treatment. Circulation 2005. https://doi.org/10.1161/01.CIR.0000161369.71722.10.
42. Marcus CL, Curtis S, Koerner CB, et al. Evaluation of pulmonary function and polysomnography in obese children and adolescents. Pediatr Pulmonol 1996. https://doi.org/10.1002/(SICI)1099-0496(199603)21:3<176::AID-PPUL5>3.0.CO;2-O.
43. Tauman R, Serpero LD, Capdevila OS, et al. Adipokines in children with sleep disordered breathing. Sleep 2007. https://doi.org/10.1093/sleep/30.4.443.
44. Spruyt K, Capdevila OS, Serpero LD, et al. Dietary and physical activity patterns in children with obstructive sleep apnea. J Pediatr 2010. https://doi.org/10.1016/j.jpeds.2009.11.010.
45. Gozal D, Serpero LD, Sans Capdevila O, et al. Systemic inflammation in non-obese children with obstructive sleep apnea. Sleep Med 2008. https://doi.org/10.1016/j.sleep.2007.04.013.
46. Kim J, Bhattacharjee R, Snow AB, et al. Myeloid-related protein 8/14 levels in children with obstructive sleep apnoea. Eur Respir J 2010. https://doi.org/10.1183/09031936.00075409.
47. Spruyt K, Gozal D. A mediation model linking body weight, cognition, and sleep-disordered breathing. Am J Respir Crit Care Med 2012. https://doi.org/10.1164/rccm.201104-0721OC.
48. Bhattacharjee R, Kim J, Alotaibi WH, et al. Endothelial dysfunction in children without hypertension: potential contributions of obesity and obstructive sleep apnea. Chest 2012. https://doi.org/10.1378/chest.11-1777.
49. Giorgio V, Prono F, Graziano F, et al. Pediatric non alcoholic fatty liver disease: old and new concepts on development, progression, metabolic insight and potential treatment targets. BMC Pediatr 2013. https://doi.org/10.1186/1471-2431-13-40.
50. Berardis S, Sokal E. Pediatric non-alcoholic fatty liver disease: an increasing public health issue. Eur J Pediatr 2014. https://doi.org/10.1007/s00431-013-2157-6.
51. Vajro P, Lenta S, Socha P, et al. Diagnosis of nonalcoholic fatty liver disease in children and adolescents: position paper of the ESPGHAN hepatology committee. J Pediatr Gastroenterol Nutr 2012;54(5):700–13.
52. Molleston JP, Schwimmer JB, Yates KP, et al. Histological abnormalities in children with nonalcoholic fatty liver disease and normal or mildly elevated alanine aminotransferase levels. J Pediatr 2014. https://doi.org/10.1016/j.jpeds.2013.10.071.
53. Mann JP, Goonetilleke R, McKiernan P. Paediatric non-alcoholic fatty liver disease: a practical overview for non-specialists. Arch Dis Child 2015. https://doi.org/10.1136/archdischild-2014-307985.

54. Fusillo S, Rudolph B. Nonalcoholic fatty liver disease. Pediatr Rev 2015. https://doi.org/10.1542/pir.36-5-198.

55. Styne DM, Arslanian SA, Connor EL, et al. Pediatric obesity-assessment, treatment, and prevention: an endocrine society clinical practice guideline. J Clin Endocrinol Metab 2017. https://doi.org/10.1210/jc.2016-2573.

56. Lloyd-Richardson EE, Jelalian E, Sato AF, et al. Two-year follow-up of an adolescent behavioral weight control intervention. Pediatrics 2012. https://doi.org/10.1542/peds.2011-3283.

57. Franks PW, Hanson RL, Knowler WC, et al. Childhood obesity, other cardiovascular risk factors, and premature death. N Engl J Med 2010;362(6):485–93. https://doi.org/10.1056/NEJMoa0904130.

58. Koskinen J, Juonala M, Dwyer T, et al. Impact of lipid measurements in youth in addition to conventional clinic-based risk factors on predicting preclinical atherosclerosis in adulthood international childhood cardiovascular cohort consortium. Circulation 2018. https://doi.org/10.1161/CIRCULATIONAHA.117.029726.

59. Barasa A, Schaufelberger M, Lappas G, et al. Heart failure in young adults: 20-year trends in hospitalization, aetiology, and case fatality in Sweden. Eur Heart J 2014. https://doi.org/10.1093/eurheartj/eht278.

60. Vivante A, Golan E, Tzur D, et al. Body mass index in 1.2 million adolescents and risk for end-stage renal disease. Arch Intern Med 2012. https://doi.org/10.1001/2013.jamainternmed.85.

61. Chanoine JP, Richard M. Early weight loss and outcome at one year in obese adolescents treated with orlistat or placebo. Int J Pediatr Obes 2011. https://doi.org/10.3109/17477166.2010.519387.

62. McDuffie JR, Calis KA, Uwaifo GI, et al. Three-month tolerability of orlistat in adolescents with obesity-related comorbid conditions. Obes Res 2002. https://doi.org/10.1038/oby.2002.87.

63. Weng SF, Redsell SA, Swift JA, et al. Systematic review and meta-analyses of risk factors for childhood overweight identifiable during infancy. Arch Dis Child 2012. https://doi.org/10.1136/archdischild-2012-302263.

64. Czernichow S, Lee CMY, Barzi F, et al. Efficacy of weight loss drugs on obesity and cardiovascular risk factors in obese adolescents: a meta-analysis of randomized controlled trials. Obes Rev 2010. https://doi.org/10.1111/j.1467-789X.2009.00620.x.

65. Viner RM, Hsia Y, Neubert A, et al. Rise in antiobesity drug prescribing for children and adolescents in the UK: a population-based study. Br J Clin Pharmacol 2009. https://doi.org/10.1111/j.1365-2125.2009.03528.x.

66. Sun AP, Kirby B, Black C, et al. Unplanned medication discontinuation as a potential pharmacovigilance signal: a nested young person cohort study. BMC Pharmacol Toxicol 2014. https://doi.org/10.1186/2050-6511-15-11.

67. Adeyemo MA, Mcduffie JR, Kozlosky M, et al. Effects of metformin on energy intake and satiety in obese children. Diabetes Obes Metab 2015. https://doi.org/10.1111/dom.12426.

68. McDonagh MS, Selph S, Ozpinar A, et al. Systematic review of the benefits and risks ofmetformin in treating obesity in children aged 18 years and younger. JAMA Pediatr 2014. https://doi.org/10.1001/jamapediatrics.2013.4200.

69. Klein DJ, Cottingham EM, Sorter M, et al. A randomized, double-blind, placebo-controlled trial of metformin treatment of weight gain associated with initiation of atypical antipsychotic therapy in children and adolescents. Am J Psychiatry 2006. https://doi.org/10.1176/ajp.2006.163.12.2072.

70. Morrison JA, Cottingham EM, Barton BA. Metformin for weight loss in pediatric patients taking psychotropic drugs. Am J Psychiatry 2002. https://doi.org/10.1176/appi.ajp.159.4.655.

71. Allen HF, Mazzoni C, Heptulla RA, et al. Randomized controlled trial evaluating response to metformin versus standard therapy in the treatment of adolescents with polycystic ovary syndrome. J Pediatr Endocrinol Metab 2005. https://doi.org/10.1515/JPEM.2005.18.8.761.

72. Hoeger K, Davidson K, Kochman L, et al. The impact of metformin, oral contraceptives, and lifestyle modification on polycystic ovary syndrome in obese adolescent women in two randomized, placebo-controlled clinical trials. J Clin Endocrinol Metab 2008. https://doi.org/10.1210/jc.2008-0461.

73. Kelly AS, Rudser KD, Nathan BM, et al. The effect of glucagon-like peptide-1 receptor agonist therapy on body mass index in adolescents with severe obesity. JAMA Pediatr 2013. https://doi.org/10.1001/jamapediatrics.2013.1045.

74. Buse JB, Drucker DJ, Taylor KL, et al. DURATION-1: exenatide once weekly produces sustained glycemic control and weight loss over 52 weeks. Diabetes Care 2010. https://doi.org/10.2337/dc09-1914.

75. Rosenstock J, Klaff LJ, Schwartz S, et al. Effects of exenatide and lifestyle modification on body weight and glucose tolerance in obese subjects with and without pre-diabetes. Diabetes Care 2010. https://doi.org/10.2337/dc09-1203.

76. Fox CK, Marlatt KL, Rudser KD, et al. Topiramate for weight reduction in adolescents with severe obesity. Clin Pediatr (Phila) 2015. https://doi.org/10.1177/0009922814542481.

77. Astrup A, Caterson I, Zelissen P, et al. Topiramate: long-term maintenance of weight loss induced by a low-calorie diet in obese subjects. Obes Res 2004. https://doi.org/10.1038/oby.2004.206.

78. Bray GA, Hollander P, Klein S, et al. A 6-month randomized, placebo-controlled, dose-ranging trial of topiramate for weight loss in obesity. Obes Res 2003. https://doi.org/10.1038/oby.2003.102.

79. Pate RR, Davis MG, Robinson TN, et al. Promoting physical activity in children and youth: a leadership role for schools - A scientific statement from the American Heart Association Council on Nutrition, Physical Activity, and Metabolism (Physical Activity Committee) in collaboration with the C. Circulation 2006. https://doi.org/10.1161/CIRCULATIONAHA.106.177052.

80. Hsia DS, Fallon SC, Brandt ML. Adolescent bariatric surgery. Arch Pediatr Adolesc Med 2012. https://doi.org/10.1001/archpediatrics.2012.1011.

81. Christou NV, Sampalis JS, Liberman M, et al. Surgery decreases long-term mortality, morbidity, and health care use in morbidly obese patients. Ann Surg 2004; 240(3):416–23.

82. Pratt JSA, Browne A, Browne NT, et al. ASMBS pediatric metabolic and bariatric surgery guidelines, 2018. Surg Obes Relat Dis 2018. https://doi.org/10.1016/j.soard.2018.03.019.

83. Sun SS, Grave GD, Siervogel RM, et al. Systolic blood pressure in childhood predicts hypertension and metabolic syndrome later in life. Pediatrics 2007. https://doi.org/10.1542/peds.2006-2543.

84. Juonala M, Magnussen CG, Venn A, et al. Influence of age on associations between childhood risk factors and carotid intima-media thickness in adulthood: the cardiovascular risk in young finns study, the childhood determinants of adult health study, the bogalusa heart study, and the muscatine study for the International Childhood Cardiovascular Cohort (i3C) Consortium. Circulation 2010. https://doi.org/10.1161/CIRCULATIONAHA.110.966465.

85. Shen W, Zhang T, Li S, et al. Race and sex differences of long-term blood pressure profiles from childhood and adult hypertension: the Bogalusa Heart Study. Hypertension 2017. https://doi.org/10.1161/HYPERTENSIONAHA.117.09537.

86. Urbina EM, Khoury PR, Mccoy C, et al. Cardiac and vascular consequences of pre-hypertension in youth. J Clin Hypertens 2011. https://doi.org/10.1111/j.1751-7176.2011.00471.x.

87. Garanty-Bogacka B, Syrenicz M, Syrenicz A, et al. Serum markers of inflammation and endothelial activation in children with obesity-related hypertension. Neuroendocrinol Lett 2005.

88. Flynn JT, Kaelber DC, Baker-Smith CM, et al. Clinical practice guideline for screening and management of high blood pressure in children and adolescents. Pediatrics 2017. https://doi.org/10.1542/peds.2017-1904.

89. Falkner B, Daniels SR, Flynn JT, et al. The fourth report on the diagnosis, evaluation, and treatment of high blood pressure in children and adolescents. Pediatrics 2004. https://doi.org/10.1542/peds.114.2.S2.555.

90. Patel HP, Mitsnefes M. Advances in the pathogenesis and management of hypertensive crisis. Curr Opin Pediatr 2005. https://doi.org/10.1097/01.mop.0000150769.38484.b3.

91. Flynn JT. Evaluation and management of hypertension in childhood. Prog Pediatr Cardiol 2001. https://doi.org/10.1016/S1058-9813(00)00071-0.

92. Seeman T, Dušek J, Vondřichová H, et al. Ambulatory blood pressure correlates with renal volume and number of renal cysts in children with autosomal dominant polycystic kidney disease. Blood Press Monit 2003. https://doi.org/10.1097/00126097-200306000-00003.

93. Hanevold C, Waller J, Daniels S, et al. The effects of obesity, gender, and ethnic group on left ventricular hypertrophy and geometry in hypertensive children: a collaborative study of the international pediatric hypertension association. Pediatrics 2004. https://doi.org/10.1542/peds.113.2.328.

94. Litwin M, Niemirska A, Śladowska-Kozlowska J, et al. Regression of target organ damage in children and adolescents with primary hypertension. Pediatr Nephrol 2010. https://doi.org/10.1007/s00467-010-1626-7.

95. Damasceno MMC, De Araújo MFM, Freire de Freitas RWJ, et al. The association between blood pressure in adolescents and the consumption of fruits, vegetables and fruit juice - an exploratory study. J Clin Nurs 2011. https://doi.org/10.1111/j.1365-2702.2010.03608.x.

96. Yuan WL, Kakinami L, Gray-Donald K, et al. Influence of dairy product consumption on children's blood pressure: results from the QUALITY cohort. J Acad Nutr Diet 2013. https://doi.org/10.1016/j.jand.2013.03.010.

97. Moore LL, Bradlee ML, Singer MR, et al. Dietary approaches to stop hypertension (DASH) eating pattern and risk of elevated blood pressure in adolescent girls. Br J Nutr 2012. https://doi.org/10.1017/S000711451100715X.

98. Chen YL, Liu YF, Huang CY, et al. Normalization effect of sports training on blood pressure in hypertensives. J Sports Sci 2010. https://doi.org/10.1080/02640410903508862.

99. Torrance B, McGuire KA, Lewanczuk R, et al. Overweight, physical activity and high blood pressure in children: a review of the literature. Vasc Health Risk Manag 2007;3(1):139–49.

100. Gregoski MJ, Barnes VA, Tingen MS, et al. Breathing awareness meditation and lifeskills training programs influence upon ambulatory blood pressure and sodium excretion among African American adolescents. J Adolesc Health 2011. https://doi.org/10.1016/j.jadohealth.2010.05.019.

101. Trachtman H, Hainer JW, Sugg J, et al. Efficacy, safety, and pharmacokinetics of candesartan cilexetil in hypertensive children aged 6 to 17 years. J Clin Hypertens 2008. https://doi.org/10.1111/j.1751-7176.2008.00022.x.

102. Herder SD, Weber E, Winkemann A, et al. Efficacy and safety of angiotensin II receptor type 1 antagonists in children and adolescents. Pediatr Nephrol 2010. https://doi.org/10.1007/s00467-009-1346-z.

103. Gartenmann AC, Fossali E, Von Vigier RO, et al. Better renoprotective effect of angiotensin II antagonist compared to dihydropyridine calcium channel blocker in childhood. Kidney Int 2003. https://doi.org/10.1046/j.1523-1755.2003.00238.x.

104. Menon S, Berezny KY, Kilaru R, et al. Racial differences are seen in blood pressure response to fosinopril in hypertensive children. Am Heart J 2006. https://doi.org/10.1016/j.ahj.2005.12.025.

105. Li JS, Baker-Smith CM, Smith PB, et al. Racial differences in blood pressure response to angiotensin-converting enzyme inhibitors in children: a meta-analysis. Clin Pharmacol Ther 2008. https://doi.org/10.1038/clpt.2008.113.

106. Duncan GE. Prevalence of diabetes and impaired fasting glucose levels among US adolescents. Arch Pediatr Adolesc Med 2006. https://doi.org/10.1001/archpedi.160.5.523.

107. Rush T, McGeary M, Sicignano N, et al. A plateau in new onset type 1 diabetes: incidence of pediatric diabetes in the United States Military Health System. Pediatr Diabetes 2018. https://doi.org/10.1111/pedi.12659.

108. Mayer-Davis EJ, Lawrence JM, Dabelea D, et al. Incidence trends of type 1 and type 2 diabetes among youths, 2002-2012. N Engl J Med 2017. https://doi.org/10.1056/NEJMoa1610187.

109. Lawrence JM, Imperatore G, Dabelea D, et al. Trends in incidence of type 1 diabetes among non-hispanic white youth in the U.S., 2002-2009. Diabetes 2014. https://doi.org/10.2337/db13-1891.

110. Singh TP, Groehn H, Kazmers A. Vascular function and carotid intimal-medial thickness in children with insulin-dependent diabetes mellitus. J Am Coll Cardiol 2003. https://doi.org/10.1016/S0735-1097(02)02894-2.

111. Haller MJ, Stein J, Shuster J, et al. Peripheral artery tonometry demonstrates altered endothelial function in children with type 1 diabetes. Pediatr Diabetes 2007. https://doi.org/10.1111/j.1399-5448.2007.00246.x.

112. Urbina EM, Wadwa RP, Davis C, et al. Prevalence of increased arterial stiffness in children with type 1 diabetes mellitus differs by measurement site and sex: the SEARCH for diabetes in youth study. J Pediatr 2010. https://doi.org/10.1016/j.jpeds.2009.11.011.

113. American Diabetes Association. 13. Children and adolescents: standards of medical care in diabetes-2020. Diabetes Care 2020. https://doi.org/10.2337/dc20-S013.

114. Effect of intensive diabetes treatment on the development and progression of long-term complications in adolescents with insulin-dependent diabetes mellitus: diabetes control and complications trial. Diabetes Control and Complications Trial Research Group. J Pediatr 1994. https://doi.org/10.1016/S0022-3476(94)70190-3.

115. Orchard TJ, Nathan DM, Zinman B, et al. Association between 7 years of intensive treatment of type 1 diabetes and long-Term mortality. JAMA 2015. https://doi.org/10.1001/jama.2014.16107.

116. Mehta SN, Volkening LK, Anderson BJ, et al. Dietary behaviors predict glycemic control in youth with type 1 diabetes. Diabetes Care 2008. https://doi.org/10.2337/dc07-2435.

117. Cameron FJ, de Beaufort C, Aanstoot HJ, et al. Lessons from the Hvidoere International Study Group on childhood diabetes: be dogmatic about outcome and flexible in approach. Pediatr Diabetes 2013. https://doi.org/10.1111/pedi.12036.

118. Nimri R, Weintrob N, Benzaquen H, et al. Insulin pump therapy in youth with type 1 diabetes: a retrospective paired study. Pediatrics 2006. https://doi.org/10.1542/peds.2005-2621.

119. Doyle EA, Weinzimer SA, Steffen AT, et al. A randomized, prospective trial comparing the efficacy of continuous subcutaneous insulin infusion with multiple daily injections using insulin glargine. Diabetes Care 2004. https://doi.org/10.2337/diacare.27.7.1554.

120. White NH, Cleary PA, Dahms W, et al. Beneficial effects of intensive therapy of diabetes during adolescence: outcomes after the conclusion of the Diabetes Control and Complications Trial (DCCT). J Pediatr 2001. https://doi.org/10.1067/mpd.2001.118887.

121. Samuelsson U, Steineck I, Gubbjornsdottir S. A high mean-HbA1c value 3-15months after diagnosis of type 1 diabetes in childhood is related to metabolic control, macroalbuminuria, and retinopathy in early adulthood-a pilot study using two nation-wide population based quality registries. Pediatr Diabetes 2014. https://doi.org/10.1111/pedi.12085.

122. Carlsen S, Skrivarhaug T, Thue G, et al. Glycemic control and complications in patients with type 1 diabetes – a registry-based longitudinal study of adolescents and young adults. Pediatr Diabetes 2017. https://doi.org/10.1111/pedi.12372.

123. Rodriguez BL, Fujimoto WY, Mayer-Davis EJ, et al. Prevalence of cardiovascular disease risk factors in U.S. children and adolescents with diabetes: the SEARCH for Diabetes in Youth Study. Diabetes Care 2006. https://doi.org/10.2337/dc06-0310.

124. Margeirsdottir HD, Larsen JR, Brunborg C, et al. High prevalence of cardiovascular risk factors in children and adolescents with type 1 diabetes: a population-based study. Diabetologia 2008. https://doi.org/10.1007/s00125-007-0921-8.

125. Schwab KO, Doerfer J, Hecker W, et al. Spectrum and prevalence of atherogenic risk factors in 27,358 children, adolescents, and young adults with type 1 diabetes: cross-sectional data from the German diabetes documentation and quality management system (DPV). Diabetes Care 2006. https://doi.org/10.2337/diacare.29.02.06.dc05-0724.

126. Kallio K, Jokinen E, Hämäläinen M, et al. Decreased aortic elasticity in healthy 11-year-old children exposed to tobacco smoke. Pediatrics 2009. https://doi.org/10.1542/peds.2008-2659.

127. Gibson-Young LM. Juuling: what kids don't know will hurt them. Contemp Pediatr 2018.

128. Cullen KA, Gentzke AS, Sawdey MD, et al. e-Cigarette use among youth in the United States, 2019. JAMA 2019. https://doi.org/10.1001/jama.2019.18387.

129. Pbert L, Farber H, Horn K, et al. State-of-the-art office-based interventions to eliminate youth tobacco use: the past decade. Pediatrics 2015. https://doi.org/10.1542/peds.2014-2037.

# Outcomes in Hypoplastic Left Heart Syndrome

Meghan Kiley Metcalf, MD[a,b], Jack Rychik, MD[a,b],*

## KEYWORDS

- Hypoplastic left heart syndrome • Outcomes for congenital heart disease
- Congenital heart surgery • Fetal echocardiography
- Neurocognitive deficits in congenital heart disease

## KEY POINTS

- Hypoplastic left heart syndrome (HLHS) is one of the most severe forms of congenital heart disease, one of the most difficult to treat, and today still is one of the most discussed and debated of congenital cardiovascular conditions.
- A pathway for survival is possible utilizing 3 stages of surgical reconstruction, in which the right ventricle is assigned systemic perfusion, the aortic outflow rebuilt, and systemic venous return channeled into the pulmonary circulation.
- A majority of newborns operated on for HLHS today survive, with two-thirds alive after third-stage Fontan operation, with approximately 70% to 80% surviving up to 20 years thereafter.
- Prenatal diagnosis, improved newborn care, advanced surgical skill, specialized postoperative care and innovative interstage monitoring all are contributing to continued improvements in outcomes.
- Young adults with HLHS demonstrate the next realm of challenges. End-organ consequences as well as mental health challenges are an increasingly focused area of care for survivors.

## INTRODUCTION

Congenital heart defects occur in 8 per 1000 live births, with anomalies ranging from minor septal defects to major structural abnormalities of the great vessels or ventricles. Why focus on hypoplastic left heart syndrome (HLHS)? Arguably, HLHS is one of the most severe forms of congenital heart disease, one of the most difficult to treat, and, still today, one of the most discussed and debated of congenital cardiovascular conditions.[1] Perhaps for no other form of congenital

[a] Division of Cardiology, The Children's Hospital of Philadelphia, 3401 Civic Center Boulevard, Philadelphia, PA 19104, USA; [b] Department of Pediatrics, Perelman School of Medicine at the University of Pennsylvania, Philadelphia, PA, USA
* Corresponding author. Division of Cardiology, The Children's Hospital of Philadelphia, 3401 Civic Center Boulevard, Philadelphia, PA 19104.
E-mail address: rychik@email.chop.edu

Pediatr Clin N Am 67 (2020) 945–962
https://doi.org/10.1016/j.pcl.2020.06.008
0031-3955/20/© 2020 Elsevier Inc. All rights reserved.

pediatric.theclinics.com

heart disease is the promise of a normal quality and duration of life so far than for HLHS. Loosely defined, it is a categorical diagnosis of structural deficiency and insufficiency in the capacity of the left ventricle (LV) to support and provide for systemic perfusion. HLHS incorporates a fairly large group of congenital cardiovascular malformations. The condition includes anomalies, such as mitral atresia with aortic atresia, in which there may be no identifiable LV at all, to mitral stenosis or mitral hypoplasia with aortic atresia or aortic stenosis, in which a small but inadequate LV is present (**Fig. 1**). In addition, conditions, such as severely unbalanced atrioventricular canal defect to the right or complex forms of double-outlet right ventricle (RV) with small LV, also are possible.

What all these conditions share is an inability for the LV to perform its natural intended duty of providing for systemic perfusion. Without intervention, HLHS is lethal. Through a series of complex surgeries, a pathway for survival is possible today for most patients, with outcome data for over 30 years now available. Treatment is not a cure, because it results in a rerouting of the circulation with success based on the viability of the remaining RV to function as the systemic ventricle and for passive systemic venous return to make its way through the pulmonary vasculature without the benefit of a ventricular pump. Despite this, survival with reasonable quality of life is quite possible for most. This review discusses the diagnosis and pathophysiology of HLHS, the current treatment strategies, the outcomes of these strategies, and the challenges and uncertainties patients and families face as they head into the future.

## Hypoplastic Left Heart Syndrome (HLHS)

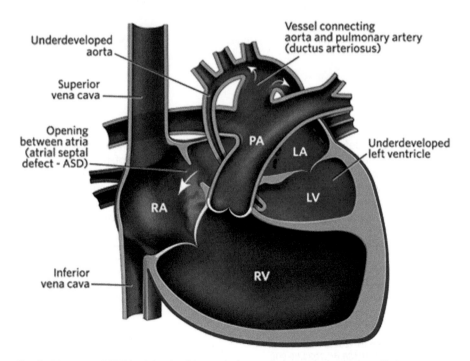

**Fig. 1.** Diagram of HLHS with mitral hypoplasia, aortic hypoplasia, and small LV.

## PRENATAL DIAGNOSIS AND FETAL CARE OF HYPOPLASTIC LEFT HEART SYNDROME

The fetus with HLHS is very stable. In utero demise in highly unusual but, if it occurs, is often in association with a genetic or chromosomal anomaly. The single RV in HLHS typically performs well and propels the combination of fetal systemic venous return as well as placental umbilical venous return through the fetoplacental circulation. The presence of HLHS is often suspected or diagnosed by an obstetrician at the 20-week gestation obstetric ultrasound scan. The 4-chamber view readily reveals the abnormality (**Fig. 2**). Additional features of importance in utero include a careful evaluation via fetal echocardiography of the flow across the atrial septum and analysis of flow patterns of pulmonary venous return. Approximately 5% to 6% of fetuses with HLHS have an important restriction at the atrial septum. If this is present, then blood egress from the left atrium and pulmonary venous circulation is obstructed, resulting in pulmonary vasculopathy and damaged lungs. Such fetuses once born are at incredibly high risk for poor oxygenation due to obstruction of pulmonary venous return as well as developmental abnormalities of the pulmonary vasculature.[2] A highly restrictive or intact atrial septum in HLHS is an important risk factor for survival.[3] Additional prenatal risk factors for postnatal survival include tricuspid valve regurgitation; genetic, chromosomal, or syndromic anomalies; additional extracardiac anomalies (eg, diaphragmatic hernia); and prematurity at less than 34 weeks' gestation.[4] If possible, these features are important to ascertain in order to provide families with proper prenatal counseling. Such findings may influence decision making toward timely termination of pregnancy or for palliative care without intervention at birth. In a large series of more than 500 fetuses with single-ventricle heart disease, including HLHS, the authors reported the likelihood of survival from the point of prenatal diagnosis through all stages of surgery, when there is intention to treat, as approximately 67%.[5]

## NEWBORN PHYSIOLOGY

Today, the vast majority of HLHS is detected prenatally. This allows for before-birth counseling of the family as well as for preparative planning for delivery and postnatal care by the obstetric and cardiology teams. Rarely, infants with HLHS are born undiagnosed. These newborns can remain stable for a period of time. The stability of a newborn with HLHS depends on the natural patency of the ductus arteriosus, the

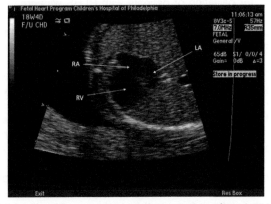

**Fig. 2.** Image of fetal echocardiogram at 18 weeks' gestation. There is HLHS with mitral and aortic atresia. No LV of any significance is noted. LA, left atrium; RA, right atrium.

pulmonary vascular resistance, the size of the atrial communication, and other variables related to intrinsic cardiac structure and function, such as valve regurgitation and function of the RV.

Shortly after birth, while pulmonary vascular resistance is relatively high and the ductus arteriosus remains wide open, infants may have a "normal" physical examination, with adequate oxygenation and systemic perfusion. A balance is achieved between the amount of blood flow making its way to the pulmonary circulation for oxygenation versus the amount that is being delivered to the systemic circulation and body. As pulmonary vascular resistance naturally falls, however, more blood is shunted across the pulmonary vascular bed at the expense of the systemic circulation, leading to tachypnea, relative hypotension, and development of acidosis. As the ductus arteriosus begins to close, systemic perfusion becomes further compromised. Such undiagnosed newborns typically can present at the first few hours of life or at 2 days to 3 days of age with feeding difficulties and respiratory distress, and, without intervention, they progress rapidly to heart failure and shock. Early initiation of continuous intravenous prostaglandin E1 infusion to maintain ductal patency is key to initial survival. Infants can be stabilized and remain on prostaglandin infusion for days to weeks while awaiting therapy, as long as the balance between pulmonary and systemic circulations is maintained.

An important subgroup of patients with HLHS may have inadequate mixing of blood at the atrial level due to a restrictive, or small, atrial septal defect or interatrial communication. In these patients, blood returning from the lungs has little to no egress and can back up in the left atrium, leading to left atrial hypertension. Chest radiograph in these patients demonstrates pulmonary venous congestion. These infants may demonstrate profound hypoxemia and early respiratory distress, and they may progress rapidly to acidosis and shock. Rapid detection of this finding, or prenatal detection, can allow for preparation for urgent cardiac catheterization to enlarge the interatrial communication, typically via stenting procedure. Such stent placement has been performed in utero.[6] Overall outcomes for HLHS with an intact or highly restrictive atrial septum are still very poor, because, despite opening of the restriction, pulmonary vascular damage already may have occurred that is not reversible by the time this intervention takes place.

## FIRST-STAGE OPERATION

A surgical pathway for palliation of patients with HLHS was created approximately 40 years ago,[7] and the basic elements employed in this initial surgical pathway remain utilized today. Because creation of a LV is not possible, surgical intervention for HLHS is not curative. Instead, the goal is to create a circulation that can mimic the functions of a normal heart.

The first stage, or stage I, operation in HLHS begins with the Norwood procedure. This is performed in the neonatal period, typically within the first week of life. The goal of this operation is to augment systemic oxygen delivery and organ perfusion. This is accomplished by reconstructing the aorta and establishing a connection between it and the RV, by ensuring adequate intracardiac mixing through the atrial communication, and by providing a reliable but restrictive supply of blood flow to the lungs through a conduit or shunt (**Fig. 3**).

The Norwood operation consists of several parts. An atrial septectomy is performed, removing as much of the atrial septum as possible to create a large communication between the left and right atrium. A reconstruction of a neoaorta is undertaken, in which the pulmonary artery (PA) and small aorta are joined above the

## Hypoplastic Left Heart Syndrome (HLHS)
## Stage 1 - Norwood

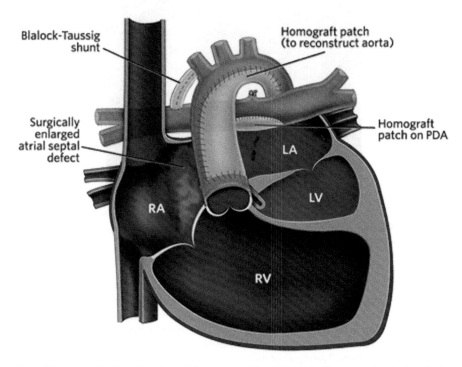

**Fig. 3.** Diagram of HLHS after stage I Norwood with a BTS. Note the reconstructed aorta includes 3 elements—the native aorta incised along its length, the proximal PA, and homograft patch material used to properly refashion the aortic arch in an unobstructed manner.

level of the valves. The native aorta is often very hypoplastic (**Fig. 4**). The PA is transected proximally and connected to the incised small aorta with augmentation using pulmonary homograft patch material to fashion a smooth, curved, new aortic arch. This allows for unobstructed egress from the RV to make its way to the systemic circulation and provides for cardiac output. After transection of the main PA, pulmonary blood flow must be established. This can occur in 1 of 2 ways, either through a Blalock-Taussig shunt (BTS), or through an RV-to-PA conduit, otherwise known as a Sano shunt. A BTS is a tube graft, typically 3.5 mm or 4 mm in diameter, placed from the innominate or subclavian artery to the PA. With this type of shunt, blood flows continuously into the pulmonary arteries during both systole and diastole, which can lead to diastolic retrograde flow in the descending aorta as well as continuous runoff from the ascending aorta. Because the coronary arteries are perfused in diastole, this theoretically can lead to coronary artery steal, particularly in patients with atresia of the aortic valve where there is no antegrade aortic flow. Given this concern, the RV-PA conduit often is preferred in patients with this anatomy. This is a conduit that passes from the RV cavity to the distal PA, resulting in blood flow to the pulmonary circulation during systole. Although this may help to eliminate this aortic steal phenomenon, there are additional morbidities that may be associated with this procedure, including RV

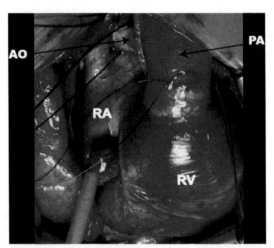

**Fig. 4.** Intraoperative image of HLHS with aortic atresia. Note the extremely hypoplastic aorta then will need to be incorporated into a newly rebuilt aortic arch. The native aorta ultimately will serve as the common coronary artery as it will feed the coronary arteries coming off at the base. AO, aorta; RA, right atrium.

dysfunction due to the need for an incision in the systemic RV for conduit placement. A randomized clinical trial, the Single Ventricle Reconstruction (SVR) trial, sponsored by the National Institutes of Health Pediatric Heart Network, looked at outcomes in patients undergoing BTS versus RV-PA conduit and found a slight survival advantage at 12 months in the RV-PA conduit group; however, there was no survival advantage after 12 months of age.[8] Analysis of the cohorts now up to 6 years of age continues to show no differences in transplant-free survival with unique complications noted in both the BTS and RV-PA conduit groups.[9]

Because the Norwood procedure involves augmentation of the aortic arch and surgical intervention within the heart chambers, cardiopulmonary bypass (CPB) is required. In patients with HLHS who may be considered too unstable for CPB or who are unable to undergo a Norwood procedure for a variety of other reasons, another option, known as a hybrid procedure, may be performed.[10] The goals of this procedure are the same as for the stage I operation—to provide a sufficient pathway for systemic cardiac output and to provide for sufficient, but limited, pulmonary blood flow to avoid pulmonary overcirculation and heart failure. This is accomplished with a combined cardiac catheterization and surgical procedure, in which a stent is placed in the ductus arteriosus via cardiac catheterization, and surgical bands are placed around the right and left branch pulmonary arteries. Alternatively, if a patient is unable to receive anticoagulation, which is required to maintain patency of the ductal stent, or if a stent cannot be placed in the ductus arteriosus due to anatomic considerations, PA bands may be placed, and the patient may remain on prostaglandin E1 infusion for ductal patency. The atrial communication also is assessed at the time of catheterization, and, if necessary, widening of this communication with a balloon septostomy or with placement of an atrial septal stent may be performed.

After a Norwood or hybrid procedure, there is complete intracardiac mixing and pulmonary blood flow is limited. Typical systemic arterial oxygen saturations are in the 75% to 85% range. The newborn then enters the interstage period, which is a closely monitored time frame with goals of sustained adequate growth in face of this fragile circulation, until the next stage can be safely undertaken.

## Early Outcomes

Prior to the advent of neonatal intervention, HLHS was a uniformly fatal disease, with 95% of affected newborns dying within the first month of life.[11] Survival to hospital discharge after the Norwood procedure has continued to improve over the past 30 years, with survival rates of up to over 85% in certain eras.[12] A secondary analysis in the SVR trial found a 16% mortality rate during hospitalization for the Norwood procedure and a 30-day mortality rate of 12%. This trial found low birthweight, associated genetic abnormalities, and factors related to the surgical procedure itself (including duration of circulatory arrest and the need for extracorporeal membrane oxygenation after CPB) to be associated with mortality.[13] Although surgical and critical care advances have greatly improved survival, HLHS remains one of the most common congenital birth defects, resulting in death within the first year of life.

## MONITORING DURING THE HIGH-RISK INTERSTAGE PERIOD

The interstage period refers to the period of time between the stage I procedure and stage II procedure in a patient with HLHS. This time period is associated with a significant risk of morbidity, growth failure, and mortality, with centers reporting mortality rates of approximately 10% to 15% in this period.[14] After hospital discharge, the development of the concept of infant single-ventricle interstage monitoring programs (ISVMPs) has greatly improved survival to stage II palliation. Interstage monitoring programs were first introduced in the early 2000s, and standardization of these programs by the National Pediatric Cardiology Quality Improvement Collaborative has led to their adoption in the majority of centers caring for interstage patients.[15,16] The components of these programs include standardization of hospital discharge criteria, parental education prior to discharge, and a standardized discharge process. Families are provided with a pulse oximeter and with a weight scale and are instructed to monitor oxygen levels and weights daily. Weekly home nursing visit or electronic encounters are performed to document how the infant is feeding, weight gain, and oxygen saturations, and weekly calls to parents from a dedicated member of the program document this information and address any parental concerns. Biweekly cardiology visits with echocardiograms are performed, and these visits alternate with biweekly visits to the pediatrician for an examination and assessment of vital signs and weight. Patients followed by ISVMP programs are reviewed weekly by the specialized dedicated teams of physicians and nurses, with high-risk patients flagged with concerns addressed.

A critical component of parental and provider education is identification of specific red flag symptoms. These are symptoms that may be indicative of cardiopulmonary or nutritional decompensation and include fussiness or irritability, parental assessment of change in behavior from the norm, increased diarrhea or vomiting, poor feeding, change in color, decreased $O_2$ levels, change in breathing pattern, increased sleepiness, fever or cold symptoms, significant weight loss, or failure to gain an average of 20 g/d over 3 days.

Interstage mortality rates have been as high as 15% in the past. With the advent of interstage monitoring programs, mortality rate has been reduced significantly, and in the authors' large-volume cardiac center, an ISVMP participant was reported to have had a nearly 30% decrease in predicted probability of death compared with historical controls.[17] Interstage monitoring as well as various proactive interventions, including anticongestive medications,[18] have contributed to a substantial improvement in outcomes.

## STAGE II: SUPERIOR CAVOPULMONARY CONNECTION

The stage II procedure, known as the superior cavopulmonary anastomosis or the bidirectional Glenn operation, typically is performed at approximately 3 months to 6 months of age. This procedure is associated with low perioperative and late mortality. The goal is to begin the separation of systemic and pulmonary venous blood flow by allowing blood returning from the superior vena cava (SVC) to enter directly into the pulmonary circulation (**Fig. 5**). This is accomplished by transecting the SVC prior to its insertion into the right atrium and connecting the SVC with the right PA, end to side. The previous source of pulmonary blood flow (BTS or RV-PA conduit) is taken down. Alternatively, a variation called a hemi-Fontan operation can be performed, in which the SVC is not disconnected from the right atrium but instead a patch is sewn over its entrance within the right atrium and an anastomosis is made with the

## Hypoplastic Left Heart Syndrome (HLHS)
## Stage 2 - Bidirectional Glenn

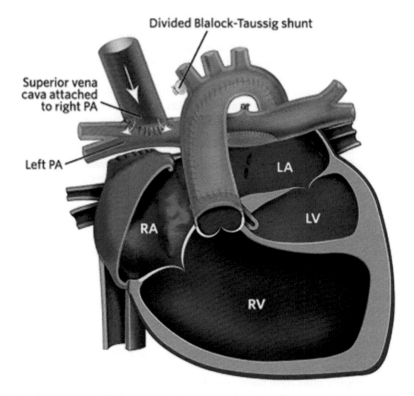

**Fig. 5.** Diagram of the bidirectional Glenn operation. SVC flow now drains directly into the PA, supplying pulmonary blood flow. The IVC flow continues to drain into the right atrium; hence, patients after this operation still are moderately cyanosed with saturations of approximately 85%.

PA posteriorly, with generous patch augmentation of the pulmonary arteries.[19] This operation typically is done no sooner than 3 months of life because this is the earliest time developmentally when the pulmonary vasculature has matured and can accept a reasonable amount of passive systemic venous return without the benefit of systolic thrust from a ventricle.

After the stage II operation, infants often demonstrate improved activity levels due to improved physiologic reserve. Oxygen saturations tend to increase slightly and typically settle in the 80% to 90% range. With increasing growth of the lower body and increasing oxygen consumption with increased activity levels as the child advances in age, however, progressive cyanosis occurs and leads to the need for completion of the stage III procedure, or the Fontan.

### Stage II Outcomes

When breaking down outcomes based on each individual operation, compared with stage I palliation, survival outcomes after the stage II operation are quite high.[20] A single-center study that compared infants who underwent bidirectional Glenn operation with or without CPB found similar mortality and morbidity among each group, with a 0.9% operative mortality rate and a complication rate of 16%. The 5-year survival among these patients was 93%.[21]

## STAGE III: THE FONTAN OPERATION

The Fontan procedure is the last anticipated procedure in patients with HLHS and typically is performed between 18 months and 4 years of age. During this surgery, the inferior vena cava (IVC) is connected to the pulmonary arteries in order to complete the separation of systemic and pulmonary circulations (**Fig. 6**). In patients in whom a bidirectional Glenn operation was performed, the Fontan operation typically is done using an extracardiac conduit, in which a conduit tube-graft of 16 mm to 20 mm in diameter is connected from the IVC to the right PA outside the perimeter of the heart. If a patient underwent a prior hemi-Fontan, a lateral-tunnel Fontan completion usually is performed, in which the patch placed over the entrance of the SVC to the right atrium is removed, the IVC is left connected in situ to the right atrium and an intra-atrial baffle channels IVC blood through the heart into the PA. In both cases, a window, or fenestration, often is created, which is a small hole that connects the Fontan pathway (systemic venous chamber) to the right atrium (pulmonary venous chamber), which allows for desaturated venous blood to enter the systemic circulation. This also allows for a residual small right-to-left shunt and results in slightly lower than normal oxygen saturations in the range of 90% to 95%. Fenestration placement is deemed to offer benefits by reducing venous congestion and optimizing oxygen delivery, which is the product of oxygen saturation and cardiac output. A fenestration, by slightly reducing oxygen saturation, actually improves ventricular filling such that stroke volume is increased and oxygen delivery optimized.[22,23]

Determinants of pulmonary blood flow in a Fontan circulation include the PA pressures, pulmonary vascular resistance, and architecture of the pulmonary arteries. Downstream, the compliance of the ventricle in diastole is important, but perhaps as important, if not more important, is the systolic performance of the ventricle. Descent of the atrioventricular valve (AVV) toward the apex of the heart causes enlargement of the atrium, a sucking effect on pulmonary venous blood and thus draws blood forward in an active manner across the pulmonary vascular bed and forward in the SVC and IVC.[24] It is important for patients with a Fontan circulation to stay well hydrated and to maintain good intravascular volume, in order to ensure high central venous pressure

## Hypoplastic Left Heart Syndrome (HLHS)
## Stage 3 - Extracardiac Fenestrated Fontan

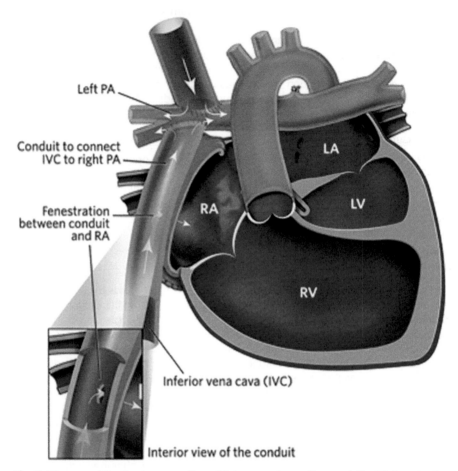

Left PA

Conduit to connect
IVC to right PA

Fenestration
between conduit
and RA

RA

LA

LV

RV

Inferior vena cava (IVC)

Interior view of the conduit

**Fig. 6.** Diagram of the Fontan operation utilizing an extracardiac conduit with fenestration. Nearly all of the systemic venous return superior and inferior and now drain passively into the lungs. The fenestration allows for some right-to-left shunting. Oxygen saturations are in the low 90% range. The RV serves as the systemic ventricle delivering the oxygenated blood to the body, while systemic venous return is channeled to the lungs without the benefit of a pump. This is the final anticipated stage of palliation.

to properly drive pulmonary blood flow. Additionally, respiratory mechanics with inspiratory negative pressure play a vital role in Fontan circulatory physiology.[25]

### Fontan Operation Outcomes for Hypoplastic Left Heart Syndrome

In 2018, the number living with a Fontan circulation was estimated to have grown to up to 70,000 people around the globe.[26] Despite the ever-increasing number of Fontan patients surviving to adulthood, however, life span still remains limited and quality of life often suffers due to multiorgan system dysfunction. A recent single-center study that looked at long-term survival with an intact Fontan circulation found survival rates of 94% at 1 year, 90% at 10 years, 85% at 15 years, and 74% at 20 years post-Fontan, with a risk of transplant of 8% at 20 years.[27] For those surviving to 1 year after Fontan operation, as a reflection of the relatively healthy standard/low-risk cohort, survival up to 20 years is approximately 80%. This study included all patients with Fontan palliation regardless of underlying anatomy, and, although slightly lower at the later years, survival in those with HLHS and a single RV was not statistically different from those with single ventricle of LV morphology (**Fig. 7**).

A pathway for survival for those with HLHS is possible. It has become clear that although lifesaving, the Fontan procedure is far from a perfect solution, and it results in physiologic disturbances that can lead to significant health challenges. Adults with the Fontan circulation may be faced with symptoms of heart failure, arrhythmia, end-organ dysfunction, and mental health issues, such as anxiety and concern for their future health. Because survival outcomes have improved significantly in recent years in this population, focus has now shifted to developing strategies and improvements for the betterment of quality of life.

## HOW ARE PATIENTS WITH HYPOPLASTIC LEFT HEART SYNDROME DOING?

The story of HLHS is a true testimony to the wonders of modern medicine. Through rigorous human surgical trial and error in the era of the 1970s to 1980s, a strategy creating a pathway to survival has emerged. There now is a generation of human beings with a unique cardiovascular physiology who never before have walked the face of the earth. How are these individuals faring? This is a growing focus of attention, as new challenges and complications emerge.

### Cardiovascular Outcomes

The principal limitation in the Fontan circulation is the lack of a subpulmonary ventricle. In the normal circulation, the normal RV serves to pump blood in a pulsatile manner through the pulmonary bed, which further serves to increase cardiac output and keep venous and right atrial pressures low. In the Fontan circulation, pulmonary blood

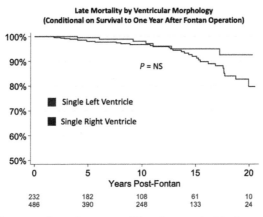

**Fig. 7.** Kaplan-Meier curves for outcome conditional on survival to 1 year after Fontan operation. Survival for single RV, which is predominantly HLHS, is approximately 80% at 20 years. There is no statistical difference between these long-term outcomes for single RV versus single LV. (*From* Downing TE, Allen KY, Glatz AC, et al. Long-term survival after the Fontan operation: Twenty years of experience at a single center. *J Thorac Cardiovasc Surg.* 2017;154(1):243–253.e2. doi:10.1016/j.jtcvs.2017.01.056; with permission.)

flow is passive, and, therefore, delivered under unique conditions. This leads to sustained abnormal elevations in central venous pressure and decreased cardiac output, which in turn result in venous congestion and decreased systemic perfusion. This physiology is believed to be one of the root causes of impairments in the Fontan patient.

Several Fontan patients develop evidence of heart failure. These patients may demonstrate evidence of exercise intolerance, poor growth, and general fatigue. In HLHS, the RV is the sole systemic ventricle. From a biological perspective, the RV in HLHS functions very differently at the molecular level than does the normal LV or RV.[28] In addition to the morphologic challenges the RV faces in playing this role, it also is subject to severely abnormal hemodynamic demands. These abnormalities predispose the ventricle to both systolic and diastolic dysfunctions. Circulatory failure remains an important cause of death in this patient population, and, in a report from the Dutch CONCOR registry, estimated mortality in a Fontan circulation patient admitted with heart failure was 24% at 1 year and 35% at 3 years from presentation.[29]

Hemodynamic and morphologic abnormalities in the Fontan circulation also may affect the performance of the AVV. AVV regurgitation potentially can develop at any stage of HLHS palliation, and it can vary in its degree of severity. AVV regurgitation can result in volume overload and ventricular dilation, which may compromise the performance of the ventricle and worsen cardiac output. A severity of moderate or greater AVV regurgitation is a significant risk factor for long-term mortality after Fontan operation.[30]

There typically is a mild degree of cyanosis in all patients with Fontan circulatory physiology. This may be due to a patent fenestration, which results in shunting of deoxygenated blood from the Fontan baffle to the right atrium. Additionally, coronary sinus blood, which normally is significantly desaturated, returns to the heart on the pulmonary venous side. Due to better aeration at upper aspects of the lung and in the absence of a subpulmonary ventricle, better perfusion due to gravity at lower segments of the lung, some degree of lung ventilatory-perfusion mismatch also may occur. With exercise, oxygen saturations often drop further due to exaggerations in these mechanisms for cyanosis. And over time, cyanosis may progress due to the development of venovenous collaterals, which serve as a decompression pop-off from the congested systemic venous system to the lower pressure pulmonary venous system. Another variable may be the development of pulmonary arteriovenous malformations that lead to intrapulmonary shunting. Because of cyanosis, hemoglobin levels often are elevated. In a healthy HLHS patient with a saturation of 90% to 93%, a hemoglobin level of 14 g/dL to 17 g/dL should be anticipated. Population-based normal levels of 12 g/dL to 13 g/dL may reflect relative anemia in a child with HLHS and may require pursuit of increased iron stores. A rising hemoglobin level may be an early indicator of worsening progressive hypoxemia.

Patients with Fontan circulation are at risk for thromboembolic events.[31] Low-velocity blood flow and stasis, as well as a possible inherent mild congenital coagulopathy[32] in the face of right-to-left shunting, leads to risks of stroke. Anticoagulation primarily through antiplatelet activity with daily low-dose aspirin is the most common approach. Warfarin is reserved for the high-risk patient who may have prior evidence of a thrombus or history of thrombo-embolic event or have evidence for protein-losing enteropathy (PLE), although this requires frequent blood check for international normalized ratio, and chronic therapy can further lead to bone demineralization. Individuals at very high risk or those who may recently have had catheter-based device or stent implantation may benefit from enoxaparin therapy for short periods of time until new endothelial cell generation takes place (up to 6 months after intervention).

### Organ System Consequences in a Fontan Circulation

Individuals with HLHS exist with a single RV and a Fontan circulation. The obligatory physiologic features of elevated systemic venous pressure and relatively low cardiac output can exert deleterious influences on organ function over time. Furthermore, organ injury may occur as a consequence of hypoperfusion or moderate hypoxia and cyanosis that exists prior to the Fontan operation. Finally, congenital differences in organ structure and function may be present as part of the inherent substrate, thus uniquely defining HLHS as more than just a cardiac anomaly but perhaps a more systemic difference in biological composition in comparison to others.

Several organs are affected. Liver fibrosis is prevalent in all individuals with a Fontan circulation.[33] The degree of fibrosis is highly variable and is not demonstrated to be directly related to elevated central venous pressures, although venous congestion likely plays an important role. Hemodynamics or flow kinetics through the Fontan pathway was not associated with degree of fibrosis either.[34] The authors found that time of duration with a Fontan circulation (age at evaluation) was the most significant factor associated with quantitative degree of liver fibrosis. Fibrogenesis in general may be promoted by the Fontan circulation, with renal as well as myocardial fibrosis also seen. Although liver fibrosis is universal, liver function remains within normal capacity in the vast majority. It is unclear as yet whether or not the degree of liver fibrosis is linearly progressive and will result in crossing the threshold for dysfunction as time goes on. The presence of fibrosis has increased the risk of hepatocellular cancer at a young age, although fortunately this is a rare occurrence.[35]

Bone health is impaired in many children with HLHS and Fontan circulation.[36] Bone mineral density scans show poor mineralization. Vitamin D levels are low in many, with elevation in parathyroid levels and secondary hyperparathyroidism common. Mild changes in renal blood flow with hypoperfusion and gut malabsorption may play a role in dysregulating calcium metabolism. Practitioners should be aware of these risks and measure vitamin D levels and supplement as necessary.

Chronic venous congestion leads to lymphatic congestion, which now is recognized as an important contributor to complications in a Fontan circulation. Venous congestion leads to increased organ lymph production, while drainage is impaired by connection into the high-pressure venous system, leading to lymphatic engorgement and a stressed lymphatic circulatory system.[37] In some individuals, congested lymphatic vessels connect to low pressure external sites, such as the airway or gastrointestinal system. Although finding a pathway of least resistance with attempts to decompress lymphatic congestion simply is the body obeying the laws of biophysics, such decompression can lead to clinical disasters. An abundance of lymph can accumulate in the airways leading to plastic bronchitis, a condition that can obstruct airways and lead to acute asphyxiation. Similarly, lymphatic decompression into the gut lumen can lead to chronic lymph leakage with loss of substantial amounts of protein-rich lymph, resulting in PLE. These lymphatic insufficiency syndromes of plastic bronchitis and protein losing enteropathy occur in 5% to 7% of patients with Fontan circulation.[26] Chronic cough, cyanosis, and atelectasis with expectoration of bronchial casts are seen in plastic bronchitis. Hypoalbuminemia, hypogammaglobulinemia with peripheral edema, and ascites are the hallmarks of PLE. Novel techniques for imaging the lymphatic system as well as interventional strategies for embolization and occlusion of offending lymphatic vessels has been lifesaving for many patients.[38–40] Lymphatic congestion in the absence of decompression may play a role in promoting fibrogenesis and also is a contributor to the interesting finding of lymphopenia in many patients. Immunodeficiency typically is not seen, although children with Fontan circulation have an increased predilection toward warts and molluscum, which may be due to an imbalance in lymphocyte subtypes due to loss.[41]

### Neurocognitive deficits

With the advent of increasing survival for HLHS has come the capacity to focus attention on functional outcomes for this population. To a degree, many of these children are under a microscope of observation, with little that goes undiscovered, yet here is what is found. Neurocognitive deficits are common[42] and often manifest as a child enters school-age years.[43] Individuals with HLHS can exhibit a somewhat lower IQ, lower academic achievement in reading and math, and issues with visual-spatial skills, working memory, and processing speed compared to the general population. Increasingly recognized are high rates of attention-deficit disorder and hyperactivity. Executive function challenges and social cognition problems also are common, which can limit a successful school experience. It is essential to point out the wide variability in these findings within the population. Early recognition of those at risk with proper neuropsychological and educational testing is mandatory because early intervention can make an important positive difference. Although there is a natural reluctance on the part of practitioners to use stimulant agents in the treatment of children with congenital heart disease, there is no evidence to support a contraindication in this population. To the contrary, many children with HLHS exhibit very good and safe benefit from the use of agents, such as methylphenidate, atomoxetine, and others, and these drugs should be high on the list of consideration for therapy, if indicated based on proper testing and diagnosis.

The etiology of these neurocognitive deficits is an area of significant research at this time and most likely multifactorial. Although previously attributed to the effects of heart surgery and CPB early in life, evidence suggests this is not the case. Central nervous system development is different from normal in HLHS, with unique structural abnormalities, such as open operculum and brain immaturity.[44] Postnatal but preoperative brain imaging with magnetic resonance imaging (MRI) reveals white brain matter injury and other abnormalities.[45] Whether or not these are inherent congenital structural and functional abnormalities tightly associated with HLHS or perhaps acquired prenatally as a consequence of altered blood flow patterns and variability in oxygen delivery is yet unclear.[46] Recent interest is focused on the role of the placenta and placental vascular dysfunction as a contributor to poorer oxygenation in the fetus with HLHS relative to normal, because placental structural abnormalities are common.[47]

Despite these concerns, many adolescents and adults with HLHS are doing very well with reasonable quality of life. Some now are achieving higher levels of education with accomplishments, such as PhD work and medical degrees, as evidence of a wide spectrum of outcome possibilities. Nevertheless, when the adult HLHS population overall is studied as a group, there are issues that certainly stand out for focus and attention. Approximately two-thirds of young adults with single-ventricle/Fontan circulation have disorders of behavior, psychiatric morbidity, and attention-deficit disorder. Brain MRI studies show injury in regions that control cognition, anxiety, and depression.[48,49] Anxiety and depression are extremely common and have an impact on employment opportunities and quality of life. Ironically, it is these noncardiac consequences of HLHS perhaps more so than the cardiac that have an impact on overall outcomes and quality of life.[50] Recognition of these potential challenges early in life can allow for initiation of strategies to mitigate and modify some of these outcomes.

### Clinical Surveillance and Well-Being in Hypoplastic Left Heart Syndrome and Fontan Circulation

Now that survival is possible for most individuals with HLHS, there is no doubt these individuals are at risk for a host of challenges. The American Heart Association has released a consensus statement on the child and adult with Fontan circulation, which includes a suggested protocol for cardiovascular and end-organ surveillance, as part of good health care maintenance practice. Although ambitious, it does lay out a plan for approaching complications in a proactive as opposed to reactive manner.[26]

Physical and mental health wellness also is gaining focused attention, with several single-ventricle–Fontan circulation specialty clinics established at a variety of centers in North America. These specialized Fontan clinics focus on the unique complications seen and bring together multidisciplinary specialty teams to include hepatologists; endocrinologists; neurologists; exercise, nutrition, and mental health specialists; and others. Specialized resources can be provided more efficiently to patients and provider knowledge gained more quickly by the cohorting of patients and increasing health care provider exposure through creation of dedicated teams. Importantly, promotion of exercise, in particular aerobic (cardio) exercise and lower extremity muscle strengthening, is demonstrated to be of value.[51] Concerns about sudden events in this population are not evidence based, and the authors' patients with HLHS and Fontan circulation are highly deconditioned. A lifestyle that is active and filled with exercise is of tremendous merit and should be promoted. Finally, mental and behavioral health care should be made available to patients with HLHS and their families to manage the burden of anxiety and depression that exists. Pediatricians play an important role in identifying these concerns and in directing patients to proper diagnostic and treatment services.

### SUMMARY AND FUTURE DIRECTIONS

There is room for an optimistic future for HLHS; as the number of survivors continues to increase, research endeavors improve and knowledge gaps narrow. Because much is still unknown, however, uncertainty about the future dominates. Patients, families, and their primary health care providers need to appreciate the importance of research, with encouragement to patients and families to participate in clinical trials and other investigational activities. Pharmacologic therapies may play a role in favorably manipulating the cardiovascular physiology, as recently demonstrated by a randomized clinical trial of phosphodiesterase-5 inhibition (udenafil), which improved some aspects of exercise capacity.[52] Novel agents to prevent or perhaps reverse fibrosis may be possible, as are the development of new and safer anticoagulants. Strategies to strengthen RV myocardial performance through stem cell therapy[53] or even creation of a mechanical or biomechanical subpulmonary pump to replace the missing ventricle are possible and under development.[54] A pathway for survival for HLHS is possible, for what otherwise is a lethal birth defect of the heart. Much amazing work has been accomplished to date, but for next steps, much more needs to be done for this fragile and unique condition in order to achieve the promise of a fully normal quality and duration of life.

### ACKNOWLEDGEMENTS

Dr. Rychik's efforts in single ventricle and Fontan circulation research is supported by the Robert & Dolores Harrington Endowed Chair in Pediatric Cardiology at The Children's Hospital of Philadelphia.

## REFERENCES

1. Feinstein JA, Benson DW, Dubin AM, et al. Hypoplastic left heart syndrome: current considerations and expectations. J Am Coll Cardiol 2012;59:S1–42.
2. Rychik J, Rome JJ, Collins MH, et al. The hypoplastic left heart syndrome with intact atrial septum: atrial morphology, pulmonary vascular histopathology and outcome. J Am Coll Cardiol 1999;34:554–60.
3. Glatz JA, Tabbutt S, Gaynor JW, et al. Hypoplastic left heart syndrome with atrial level restriction in the era of prenatal diagnosis. Ann Thorac Surg 2007;84: 1633–8.
4. Rychik J, Szwast A, Natarajan S, et al. Perinatal and early surgical outcome for the fetus with hypoplastic left heart syndrome: a 5-year single institutional experience. Ultrasound Obstet Gynecol 2010;36:465–70.
5. Liu MY, Zielonka B, Snarr BS, et al. Longitudinal assessment of outcome from prenatal diagnosis through fontan operation for over 500 fetuses with single ventricle-type congenital heart disease: the philadelphia fetus-to-fontan cohort study. J Am Heart Assoc 2018;7:e009145.
6. Jantzen DW, Moon-Grady AJ, Morris SA, et al. Hypoplastic left heart syndrome with intact or restrictive atrial septum: a report from the international fetal cardiac intervention registry. Circulation 2017;136:1346–9.
7. Norwood WI, Kirklin JK, Sanders SP. Hypoplastic left heart syndrome: experience with palliative surgery. Am J Cardiol 1980;45:87–91.
8. Ohye RG, Sleeper LA, Mahony L, et al. Comparison of shunt types in the Norwood procedure for single-ventricle lesions. N Engl J Med 2010;362:1980–92.
9. Newburger JW, Sleeper LA, Gaynor JW, et al. Transplant-free survival and interventions at 6 years in the SVR trial. Circulation 2018;137:2246–53.
10. Ohye RG, Schranz D, D'Udekem Y. Current therapy for hypoplastic left heart syndrome and related single ventricle lesions. Circulation 2016;134:1265–79.
11. Report of the new england regional infant cardiac program. Pediatrics 1980;65: 375–461.
12. Mascio CE, Irons ML, Ittenbach RF, et al. Thirty years and 1663 consecutive Norwood procedures: Has survival plateaued? J Thorac Cardiovasc Surg 2019;158: 220–9.
13. Tabbutt S, Ghanayem N, Ravishankar C, et al. Risk factors for hospital morbidity and mortality after the norwood procedure: a report from the pediatric heart network single ventricle reconstruction trial. J Thorac Cardiovasc Surg 2012; 144:882–95.
14. Hehir DA, Dominguez TE, Ballweg JA, et al. Risk factors for interstage death after stage 1 reconstruction of hypoplastic left heart syndrome and variants. J Thorac Cardiovasc Surg 2008;136(94-9):99.e1-3.
15. Anderson JB, Beekman RH 3rd, Kugler JD, et al. Improvement in interstage survival in a national pediatric cardiology learning network. Circ Cardiovasc Qual Outcomes 2015;8:428–36.
16. Anderson JB, Brown DW, Lihn S, et al. Power of a learning network in congenital heart disease. World J Pediatr Congenit Heart Surg 2019;10:66–71.
17. Gardner MM, Mercer-Rosa L, Faerber J, et al. Association of a home monitoring program with interstage and stage 2 outcomes. J Am Heart Assoc 2019;8: e010783.
18. Brown DW, Mangeot C, Anderson JB, et al. Digoxin use is associated with reduced interstage mortality in patients with no history of arrhythmia after stage i palliation for single ventricle heart disease. J Am Heart Assoc 2016;5:e002376.

19. Jacobs ML, Rychik J, Rome JJ, et al. Early reduction of the volume work of the single ventricle: the hemi-Fontan operation. Ann Thorac Surg 1996;62:456–61 [discussion: 461–2].

20. Mott AR, Spray TL, Gaynor JW, et al. Improved early results with cavopulmonary connections. Cardiol Young 2001;11:3–11.

21. LaPar DJ, Mery CM, Peeler BB, et al. Short and long-term outcomes for bidirectional glenn procedure performed with and without cardiopulmonary bypass. Ann Thorac Surg 2012;94:164–70 [discussion: 170–1].

22. Hijazi ZM, Fahey JT, Kleinman CS, et al. Hemodynamic evaluation before and after closure of fenestrated Fontan. An acute study of changes in oxygen delivery. Circulation 1992;86:196–202.

23. Mavroudis C, Zales VR, Backer CL, et al. Fenestrated Fontan with delayed catheter closure. Effects of volume loading and baffle fenestration on cardiac index and oxygen delivery. Circulation 1992;86:II85–92.

24. Rychik J, Fogel MA, Donofrio MT, et al. Comparison of patterns of pulmonary venous blood flow in the functional single ventricle heart after operative aortopulmonary shunt versus superior cavopulmonary shunt. Am J Cardiol 1997;80: 922–6.

25. Gewillig M, Brown SC, van de Bruaene A, et al. Providing a framework of principles for conceptualising the Fontan circulation. Acta Paediatr 2020;109:651–8.

26. Rychik J, Atz AM, Celermajer DS, et al. Evaluation xthe American Heart Association. Circulation 2019. https://doi.org/10.1161/CIR.0000000000000696. CIR0000000000000696.

27. Downing TE, Allen KY, Glatz AC, et al. Long-term survival after the Fontan operation: Twenty years of experience at a single center. J Thorac Cardiovasc Surg 2017;154:243–253 e2.

28. Miyamoto SD, Stauffer BL, Polk J, et al. Gene expression and beta-adrenergic signaling are altered in hypoplastic left heart syndrome. J Heart Lung Transplant 2014;33:785–93.

29. Zomer AC, Vaartjes I, van der Velde ET, et al. Heart failure admissions in adults with congenital heart disease; risk factors and prognosis. Int J Cardiol 2013; 168:2487–93.

30. King G, Ayer J, Celermajer D, et al. Atrioventricular valve failure in fontan palliation. J Am Coll Cardiol 2019;73:810–22.

31. Coon PD, Rychik J, Novello RT, et al. Thrombus formation after the Fontan operation. Ann Thorac Surg 2001;71:1990–4.

32. Odegard KC, McGowan FX Jr, Zurakowski D, et al. Procoagulant and anticoagulant factor abnormalities following the Fontan procedure: increased factor VIII may predispose to thrombosis. J Thorac Cardiovasc Surg 2003;125:1260–7.

33. Goldberg DJ, Surrey LF, Glatz AC, et al. Hepatic fibrosis is universal following fontan operation, and severity is associated with time from surgery: a liver biopsy and hemodynamic study. J Am Heart Assoc 2017;6:e004809.

34. Trusty PM, Wei Z, Rychik J, et al. Impact of hemodynamics and fluid energetics on liver fibrosis after Fontan operation. J Thorac Cardiovasc Surg 2018;156: 267–75.

35. Egbe AC, Poterucha JT, Warnes CA, et al. Hepatocellular carcinoma after fontan operation: multicenter case series. Circulation 2018;138:746–8.

36. Avitabile CM, Goldberg DJ, Zemel BS, et al. Deficits in bone density and structure in children and young adults following Fontan palliation. Bone 2015;77:12–6.

37. Biko DM, DeWitt AG, Pinto EM, et al. MRI evaluation of lymphatic abnormalities in the neck and thorax after fontan surgery: relationship with outcome. Radiology 2019;291:774–80.

38. Dori Y, Keller MS, Rome JJ, et al. Percutaneous lymphatic embolization of abnormal pulmonary lymphatic flow as treatment of plastic bronchitis in patients with congenital heart disease. Circulation 2016;133:1160–70.

39. Itkin M, Piccoli DA, Nadolski G, et al. Protein-losing enteropathy in patients with congenital heart disease. J Am Coll Cardiol 2017;69:2929–37.

40. Rychik J, Dodds KM, Goldberg D, et al. Protein losing enteropathy after fontan operation: glimpses of clarity through the lifting fog. World J Pediatr Congenit Heart Surg 2020;11:92–6.

41. Morsheimer MM, Rychik J, Forbes L, et al. Risk factors and clinical significance of lymphopenia in survivors of the fontan procedure for single-ventricle congenital cardiac disease. J Allergy Clin Immunol Pract 2016;4:491–6.

42. Tabbutt S, Nord AS, Jarvik GP, et al. Neurodevelopmental outcomes after staged palliation for hypoplastic left heart syndrome. Pediatrics 2008;121:476–83.

43. Marino BS, Lipkin PH, Newburger JW, et al. Neurodevelopmental outcomes in children with congenital heart disease: evaluation and management: a scientific statement from the American Heart Association. Circulation 2012;126:1143–72.

44. Glauser TA, Rorke LB, Weinberg PM, et al. Congenital brain anomalies associated with the hypoplastic left heart syndrome. Pediatrics 1990;85:984–90.

45. Mahle WT, Tavani F, Zimmerman RA, et al. An MRI study of neurological injury before and after congenital heart surgery. Circulation 2002;106:I109–14.

46. Sun L, Macgowan CK, Sled JG, et al. Reduced fetal cerebral oxygen consumption is associated with smaller brain size in fetuses with congenital heart disease. Circulation 2015;131:1313–23.

47. Rychik J, Goff D, McKay E, et al. Characterization of the placenta in the newborn with congenital heart disease: distinctions based on type of cardiac malformation. Pediatr Cardiol 2018;39:1165–71.

48. Bellinger DC, Watson CG, Rivkin MJ, et al. Neuropsychological status and structural brain imaging in adolescents with single ventricle who underwent the fontan procedure. J Am Heart Assoc 2015;4(12):e002302.

49. Singh S, Roy B, Pike N, et al. Altered brain diffusion tensor imaging indices in adolescents with the Fontan palliation. Neuroradiology 2019;61:811–24.

50. Goldberg CS, Hu C, Brosig C, et al. Behavior and quality of life at 6 years for children with hypoplastic left heart syndrome. Pediatrics 2019;144.

51. Cordina R, d'Udekem Y. Long-lasting benefits of exercise for those living with a Fontan circulation. Curr Opin Cardiol 2019;34:79–86.

52. Goldberg DJ, Zak V, Goldstein BH, et al. Results of the FUEL trial. Circulation 2020;141:641–51.

53. Burkhart HM, Qureshi MY, Rossano JW, et al. Autologous stem cell therapy for hypoplastic left heart syndrome: Safety and feasibility of intraoperative intramyocardial injections. J Thorac Cardiovasc Surg 2019;158:1614–23.

54. Rodefeld MD, Marsden A, Figliola R, et al. Cavopulmonary assist: Long-term reversal of the Fontan paradox. J Thorac Cardiovasc Surg 2019;158:1627–36.

# Outcomes in Adult Congenital Heart Disease

## Neurocognitive Issues and Transition of Care

Roni M. Jacobsen, MD*

## KEYWORDS

- Congenital heart disease • Adult congenital heart disease • Neurodevelopment
- Neurocognitive • Transition • Transfer

## KEY POINTS

- Improvements in care for patients with congenital heart disease (CHD) has resulted in a greater than 90% survival into adulthood, now with more adults than children living with CHD.
- Neurocognitive issues are common in patients with CHD and can lead to neurocognitive decline in adults with CHD, although there may be some modifiable variables.
- Comprehensive care in adolescents and adults with CHD is critical. It should not only include cardiac concerns but also address neurocognitive and mental health issues as a standard of care.
- An individualized approach is necessary for effective transition and transfer of care from pediatric to adult congenital cardiology care.
- Successful transition and transfer of care can decrease morbidity and mortality and improve long-term outcomes in adults with CHD.

## INTRODUCTION

The number of patients with congenital heart disease (CHD) reaching adulthood is rapidly growing because of advances in diagnostic, therapeutic, and clinical care. The improved survival of this patient population has provided a complex new frontier, challenging health care providers to not only care for these patients' CHD but also to consider their neurocognitive, mental, emotional, and physical health as significant aspects of their lifelong care and overall quality of life. Thus, comprehensive care is imperative for this patient population, particularly as it relates to their ability to transition to and function in adulthood.

Pediatric and Adult Congenital Cardiology, University of Colorado School of Medicine, Children's Hospital Colorado, University of Colorado Hospital, Aurora, CO, USA
* Department of Pediatrics, Division of Pediatric Cardiology, 13123 East 16th Street, B100, Aurora, CO 80045.
E-mail address: roni.jacobsen@childrenscolorado.org

Pediatr Clin N Am 67 (2020) 963–971
https://doi.org/10.1016/j.pcl.2020.06.009

## CONTENT

### Adults with Congenital Heart Disease: Why Care Is Becoming a Bigger Issue

Survival for patients born with moderate to complex CHD has significantly improved, now greater than 90% of infants born with CHD survive to adulthood, leading to a rapidly growing population of adults with CHD. It is estimated that more than 2.4 million people currently live with CHD in the United States, including more than 1.4 million adults and 1 million children.[1,2] As this patient population continues to age, a more comprehensive and innovative approach is required to provide their care, with a shift from survival to a focus on improving their quality of life. It has become apparent that successful transition from pediatric and adolescent care to adult care is quite involved, including assessment of their CHD, which encompasses anatomic and electrical issues, genetic syndromes, neurocognitive function, mental illness, physical capabilities, and psychosocial constraints.

### Current Knowledge of Neurocognitive Development and Decline in Congenital Heart Disease

Although neurocognitive development in infants, children, and adolescents with CHD has been studied extensively, data regarding neuropsychological functioning in adults with CHD are scarce. It is well known that children and adolescents with CHD are at increased risk of neurocognitive, socioemotional, and mood and anxiety problems. These deficits can lead to greater difficulty in adaptation to educational and occupational success over time, which affects the patients and society.[2–6] Several variables have been studied in an attempt to identify modifiable risk factors to help predict and improve neurocognitive outcomes in children and adolescents with CHD. However, instead of a single or even a few specific key elements, these variables seem to be interrelated, cumulative, and likely synergistic over time.[3]

Data suggest that patient and preoperative factors, such as low birth weight, gestational age, and altered fetal cerebral perfusion, play a role in neurocognitive outcomes, because it seems the developing brain acquires characteristic patterns of white matter injury.[3,7] Similar to preterm infants, recent literature suggests that the selective brain vulnerability seen in newborns with CHD is primarily a problem with dysmaturation, which is failure of oligodendrocyte progenitor cells to differentiate into myelin-forming oligodendrocytes.[3,7–17] In addition, in contrast with normal newborn infants, newborns with CHD have an immature pattern of brain microstructure and metabolism, less mature morphologic structure, and smaller brain volumes.[3,14–16] This combination of white matter injury and brain immaturity predisposes infants with CHD to postnatal injury and is an important antecedent of adverse developmental outcomes.[3,8–17] Thus, patients with CHD are at risk for further neurodevelopmental comorbidities related to treatment and postoperative complications over time.

On average, school-aged children with critical CHD have lower scores on intelligence and achievement scores; worse fine and gross motor function; higher likelihood of learning disabilities and use of special services; and abnormalities of speech, language, and behavior.[2,18–24] Executive dysfunction is associated with worse psychosocial health status and quality of life in patients with CHD, particularly as it relates to their ability to function in everyday life. Ongoing medical variables and social constraints may exacerbate these underlying deficits as children age, including impaired adherence to medical recommendations and follow-up, particularly during the adolescent and transition phase.[23,25]

Adults with CHD have an increased risk of deficits in multiple cognitive domains. On a screening questionnaire, 34% reported difficulty in areas of mathematics, memory, and attention.[26] Formal neuropsychological testing has shown a higher prevalence of executive dysfunction (problem solving, planning), lower scores on cognitive screening, poorer memory performance, slower psychomotor or processing speeds, and weaker attention.[25–28]

However, in the mid-20s to late 20s, the most important developmental changes to the brain cease, shifting from abnormal neurodevelopment to increasing burden of neurologic injury and potential neurocognitive decline.[3,25] Dementia is a primary predictor of mortality in adults with CHD. The risk of all-cause dementia is increased by 60% in individuals with CHD, with at least a 2 times increased risk of early-onset dementia (before 65 years of age) in this patient population.[25,28,29]

### Prevalence of Mental Illness in Patients with Congenital Heart Disease

Mental illness is common and multifactorial in patients with CHD. Children with CHD are at increased risk of having attention-deficit/hyperactivity disorder (ADHD) and autism spectrum disorder.[5,25,30–33] Attention-deficit disorder; executive dysfunction; and mood, language, and social cognition issues may manifest as inappropriate behavior, limiting relationships.[3–6] In the general population, patients with ADHD have a higher risk for impaired mental health, work performance, and financial stress scores, which can likely be extrapolated to adults with CHD.[25,33] Adults with neurocognitive impairment have a 3 to 4 times increased risk of comorbid psychiatric disorders.[3,25,32] A recent study by Khanna and colleagues[6] showed a 20% risk of mental illness in adolescents and a 33% risk in adults with CHD living in Colorado over a 3-year surveillance period. In addition, specific genetic disorders commonly associated with CHD also carry an increased risk of mental illness. For example, patients with 22q11.2 deletion have an increased risk of schizophrenia.

Mood disorders are commonly associated with cognitive difficulties. Although underrecognized, adolescents and adults with CHD have a higher rate of anxiety and depression, including generalized anxiety, heart-related anxiety, and depressed mood, which often correlates with a fear of physical activity, loneliness, and perceived health status that contributes to poor transition, nonadherence to medical advice, and denial of illness effects.[6,25,30–38] Attention, conduct, behavior, and impulse control disorders occurred in 6.0% of adolescents, but only in 1.3% of adults with CHD living in Colorado.[6] However, this may represent an underdiagnosis and undertreatment in the adult CHD population.

Adults with CHD are also at increased risk for posttraumatic stress disorder (PTSD) symptoms related to medical therapies in childhood.[25,30–32,34,35] Self-reported PTSD symptoms has been described in 11% to 21% of adults with CHD; however, less than 5% of these patients have a formal diagnosis and fewer than half are receiving mental health care.[35] However, despite the increased prevalence of mental health in adolescents and adults with CHD, the rate of substance abuse, including smoking and alcohol, are similar to or lower than in age-matched peers. Khanna and colleagues[6] reported alcohol and substance-related disorders in 6.2% of adults with CHD living in Colorado.

In addition, all age groups of patients with CHD have reduced quality of life compared with their peers.[4] Thus, patients with CHD require comprehensive cardiac and mental health care throughout their lifetimes.

### Effects of Acquired Adult Risk Factors on Neurocognitive Decline in Congenital Heart Disease

Although patients born with CHD seem to have an innate vulnerability to insults with resultant neurocognitive issues, there are also acquired risk factors that may contribute to neurocognitive decline as this patient population ages.[3] Traditional risk factors for neurocognitive decline in adults with CHD include depression, low educational attainment, hypertension, obesity, impaired glucose tolerance or diabetes mellitus, and likely physical inactivity.[25] Associations between vascular risk factors and compromises in cognitive health begin to appear in midlife or earlier.[28,39,40] Yaffe and colleagues[28] showed worse cognition as a result of cumulative exposure to cardiovascular risk factors from early to middle adulthood in normal adults, which may be even more pronounced in adults with CHD.

Atherosclerotic coronary artery disease is associated with an increased risk of Alzheimer disease and vascular dementia. Moons and colleagues[40] reported that at least 80% of adults with CHD have at least 1 coronary artery disease risk factor. Adults with CHD have been reported to have an increased risk of hypertension, stroke, and chronic kidney disease compared with age-matched peers.[27] Hypertension is common in patients with CHD. Obesity is estimated to affect 31% of the adult congenital population.[25] Patients with CHD also seem to have a higher risk of diabetes mellitus as a result of abnormal glucose metabolism, caused by suppression of insulin because of high circulating levels of norepinephrine, excessive clearance of insulin in lung caused by left to right shunt, and hypoxia of liver and/or pancreas in those with cyanotic heart disease or congestive heart failure.[40,41] These atherosclerotic risk factors can contribute to stroke risk, vascular dementia, and cognitive decline. Brain hypoperfusion, as seen in heart failure and atrial fibrillation, which are common in adults with CHD, has also been associated with cognitive decline, including memory and executive function.[25,28,29,39,40,42–44] In addition, most patients with CHD do not meet the physical activity recommendations for the general population, and lack of physical activity has been linked to cognitive decline.

Thus, it seems there are some modifiable risk factors, including poor diet, physical and mental inactivity, smoking, head trauma, and alcohol, which may be addressed to decrease the risk of, and possibly even prevent, neurocognitive decline.[25]

### Available Resources and Approaches to Care

The spectrum of neurodevelopmental and psychosocial dysfunction in patients with CHD is expected to have significant implications for life success and societal costs as the population continues to age.[2,3,6,27] Thus, there needs to be an openness to discussion regarding neurocognitive and mental health at regular clinic visits between physicians and patients, including lifelong surveillance and prevention.

Cohen and colleagues[37] showed that basic questionnaires may help identify high-risk adults with CHD, including point-of-care assessment with simple questions about anxiety and depression. Structured professional psychological evaluation has been shown to identify up to 50% more patients with mood disorders. Thus, implementation of such questionnaires as a standard of care may allow for timely and appropriate referral for formal neurocognitive evaluation, diagnosis, and therapy.[37,38] Preliminary studies have indicated psychotherapy is a feasible and valuable treatment in adults with CHD.[25] Weight management and physical activity promotion may also be an important strategy to help prevent progression to neurocognitive decline as this patient population ages.

Because adults with CHD have increased risk and potential lifelong implications of neurocognitive and mental health issues and early onset of neurocognitive decline, cognitive screening starting at 50 years of age has been proposed. However, the interplay of psychiatric disorders, underlying neurocognitive deficits, and long-term function in adults with CHD warrants further study.[3,25]

## Contributions to Difficulties with Transition

Improved survival in patients with CHD has led to a transformation from a life-threatening childhood illness to a chronic adult illness.[2,3,45] As a result of this alteration in care, gaps exist, particularly regarding transition of care. Neurocognitive issues become particularly important during the time of transition and transfer from pediatric-orientated to adult-orientated care. Everitt and colleagues[45] also described other perceived barriers that may limit or interfere with the transition and transfer of care (**Table 1**).[45]

The most common time for lapse in cardiology care occurs during late adolescent into early adulthood, when patients with CHD are expected to change from pediatric-orientated to adult-orientated care. It is estimated that between 21% and 76% of adolescents and young adults have a lapse in cardiology care.[46–48] This issue is important, because gaps in care can lead to increased morbidity and mortality in this patient population. Yeung and colleagues[47] showed that a lapse in care greater than or equal to 2 years between the last pediatric cardiology visit and obtaining adult CHD care was associated with a 3-fold increased need for catheter or surgical intervention within 6 months. Despite a high prevalence of complicated cardiac anatomy combined with significant adult comorbidities, fewer than 30% of adults and only 48% of adults with CHD are appropriately followed by specialists.[48] In addition, inadequate transition planning has adverse effects on patients, their families, and health care delivery systems, including delayed transfer to adult care, increased financial and emotional burden, and inappropriate care.[45]

Successful transition and transfer of care in this patient population is paramount to long-term outcomes and should be a standard of care. Transition from pediatric to adult care is defined as "the purposeful, planned movement of adolescents and young adults with chronic physical and medical conditions from child-centered to adult-orientated health care systems."[49] The transition process should start at 12 years of

**Table 1**
**Barriers perceived by patients, families, and health care providers to interfere with the transfer of adolescents with congenital heart disease from pediatric to adult care**

| Domain | Perceived Barriers |
|---|---|
| Structural[40–42] | Insurance availability |
| | Subspecialty health care training and education |
| | Interinstitutional transfer |
| | Lack of reimbursement for transition visits and care coordination |
| Institutional[30,54–56] | Lack of formal transition programs |
| | Lack of adult CHD provider availability and training |
| | Institutional aging-out policies |
| | Lack of primary care physicians and hospitalists comfortable caring for CHD |
| | Complex navigation |
| Social[17,52,57] | Provider-patient and provider-parent attachment |
| | Patient self-advocacy and knowledge |
| | Parental involvement |
| Neurocognitive[38] | Developmental delays |
| | Disability in social, emotional, executive function domains |

*From* Everitt IK, Gerardin JF, Rodriguez FH, Book WM. Improving the quality of transition and transfer of care in young adults with congenital heart disease. Congenital Heart Disease. 2017;12:242-250; with permission.

age and finish with transfer of care between 18 and 21 years.[42,45–47,50] Successful transition of care is maximization of lifelong functioning and well-being, with every patient having an individualized transition and transfer of care plan regardless of specific health care needs.[50] However, identification of individual components is crucial because resources and delivery methods may vary.[51]

An ideal transition program includes a comprehensive health care team, including nurses, social workers, care coordinators, and adult and pediatric physicians.[42,52,53] In a randomized controlled trial, Mackie and colleagues[46] showed that a nurse-led educational intervention directed at older adolescents with CHD decreased the likelihood of delay in obtaining adult CHD care and improved CHD management and self-management skills, which were sustained 18 months later. Recommendations and goals for transition education have been described and include verbal, written, and experimental efforts to teach patients and families about their specific heart disease, expectations, and concerns regarding CHD, as well as skills to navigate the health care system as adults.[42] Importantly, transition is a continual process, with the ultimate goal being patient autonomy when possible and successful transfer of care to an adult CHD provider.

## SUMMARY

The number of patients with CHD reaching adolescence and adulthood is increasing, now with more adults than children living with CHD. The health care team is often challenged with how to provide the most appropriate care to this aging patient population, particularly as new questions and concerns arise from a medical, emotional, social, and financial standpoint. Providers should encourage an open dialogue to discuss not only ongoing cardiac well-being but also physical, neurocognitive, and mental health issues, with the patients and families. Comprehensive patient-centered care is crucial to improved quality of life and successful transition and transfer of care into adulthood in this patient population.

## DISCLOSURE

The author has nothing to disclose.

## REFERENCES

1. Mazor Dray E, Marelli AJ. Adult congenital heart disease: scope of the problem. Cardiol Clin 2015;33:503–12, vii.
2. Gurvitz M, Khan A. Epidemiology of ACHD: what has changed and what is changing? Prog Cardiovasc Dis 2018;61:275–81.
3. Marelli AJ, Miller SP, Bradley SM, et al. Brain in congenital heart disease across the lifespan: the cumulative burden of injury. Circ 2016;133:1951–62.
4. Areias ME, Peixotoa B, Santos I, et al. Neurocognitive profiles in adolescents and young adults with congenital heart disease. Rev Port Cardiol 2019;37(11): 923–31.
5. Ilardi D, Ono KE, McCartney R, et al. Neurocognitive functioning in adults with congenital heart disease. Congenit Heart Dis 2016;12:165–74.
6. Khanna AD, Duca LM, Kay JD, et al. Prevalence of mental illness in adolescents and adults with congenital heart disease from the colorado congenital heart defect surveillance system. Am J Cardiol 2019;124:618–26.
7. Miller SP, Ferriero DM. From selective vulnerability to connectivity: insights from newborn brain imaging. Trends Neurosci 2009;32:496–505.

8. Buser JR, Maire J, Riddle A, et al. Arrested preoligodendrocyte maturation contributes to myelination failure in premature infants. Ann Neurol 2012;71:93–109.

9. Back SA, Miller SP. Brain injury in premature neonates: a primary cerebral dysmaturation disorder? Ann Neurol 2014;75:469–86.

10. Chau V, Synnes A, Grunau RE, et al. Abnormal brain maturation in preterm neonates associated with adverse developmental outcomes. Neurology 2013;81: 2082–9.

11. Dimitropoulos A, McQuillen PS, Sethi V, et al. Brain injury and development in newborns with critical congenital heart disease. Neurology 2013;81:241–8.

12. McQuillen PS, Goff DA, Licht DJ. Effects of congenital heart disease on brain development. Prog Pediatr Cardiol 2010;29:79–85.

13. Ball G, Pazderova L, Chew A, et al. Thalamocortical connectivity predicts cognition in children born preterm. Cereb Cortex 2015;25:4310–8.

14. Miller SP, McQuillen PS, Hamrick S, et al. Abnormal brain development in newborns with congenital heart disease. N Engl J Med 2007;357:1928–38.

15. Licht DJ, Shera DM, Clancy RR, et al. Brain maturation is delayed in infants with complex congenital heart defects. J Thorac Cardiovasc Surg 2009;137:529–36 [discussion: 536].

16. Limperopoulos C, Tworetzky W, McElhinney DB, et al. Brain volume and metabolism in fetuses with congenital heart disease: evaluation with quantitative magnetic resonance imaging and spectroscopy. Circulation 2010;121:26–33.

17. Andropoulos DB, Hunter JV, Nelson DP, et al. Brain immaturity is associated with brain injury before and after neonatal cardiac surgery with high-flow bypass and cerebral oxygenation monitoring. J Thorac Cardiovasc Surg 2010;139:543–56.

18. Wernovsky G. Current insights regarding neurological and developmental abnormalities in children and young adults with complex congenital cardiac disease. Cardiol Young 2006;16(suppl 1):92–104.

19. Bellinger DC, Wypij D, Rivkin MJ, et al. Adolescents with d-transposition of the great arteries corrected with the arterial switch procedure: neuropsychological assessment and structural brain imaging. Circulation 2011;124:1361–9.

20. Neal AE, Stopp C, Wypij D, et al. Predictors of health-related quality of life in adolescents with tetralogy of Fallot. J Pediatr 2015;166:132–8.

21. Brock LL, Brock CD, Thiedke CC. Executive function and medical nonadherence: a different perspective. Int J Psychiatry Med 2011;42:105–15.

22. Shillingford AJ, Glanzman MM, Ittenbach RF, et al. Inattention, hyperactivity, and school performance in a population of school-age children with complex congenital heart disease. Pediatrics 2008;121:e759–67.

23. Razzaghi H, Oster M, Reefhis J. Long-term outcomes in children with congenital heart disease.: National Health Interview Survey. J Pediatr 2015;166:119–24.

24. Bean Jaworski JL, Flynn T, Burnham N, et al. Rates of autism and potential risk factors in children with congenital heart disease. Congenit Heart Dis 2017;12: 421–9.

25. Keir M, Ebert P, Kovacs AH, et al. Neurocognition in adult congenital heart disease: how to monitor and prevent progressive decline. Can J Cardiol 2019;25: 1675–85.

26. Brunmeier A, Reis MP, earing MG, et al. Identifying self-reported neurocognitive deficits in the adult with congenital heart disease using a simple screening tool. Congenit Heart Dis 2019;13:728–73.

27. Billet J, Cowie MR, Gatzoulis MA, et al. Comorbidity, healthcare utilisation and process of care measures in patients with congenital heart disease in the UK:

cross-sectional, population-based study with case-control analysis. Heart 2008; 94:1194–9.

28. Yaffe K, Vittinghoff E, Pletcher MJ, et al. Early adult to midlife cardiovascular risk factors and cognitive function. Circulation 2014;129:1560–7.

29. Afilalo J, Therrien J, Pilote L, et al. Geriatric congenital heart disease: burden of disease and predictors of mortality. J Am Coll Cardiol 2011;58:150915.

30. Bromberg JI, Beasley PJ, D'Angelo EJ, et al. Depression and anxiety in adults with congenital heart disease: a pilot study. Heart Lung 2003;32:105–10.

31. Horner T, Lberthson R, Jellinek MS. Psychosocial profile of adults with complex congenital heart disease. Mayo Clin Proc 2000;75:31–6.

32. Kovac AH, Bendell KL, Colman J, et al. Adults with congenital heart disease: psychological needs and treatment preferences. Congenit Heart Dis 2009;4:139–46.

33. White KS, Prudue C, Ludbrook P, et al. Cardiac denial and psychological predictors of cardiac care adherence in adults with congenital heart disease. Behav Modif 2016;40:29–50.

34. Keir M, Bailey B, Lee A, et al. Narrative analysis of adults with complex congenital heart disease: childhood experiences and their lifelong reverberations. Congenit Heart Dis 2018;13:740–7.

35. Deng LX, Khan AM, Drajpuch D, et al. Prevalence and correlates of posttraumatic stress disorder in adults with congenital heart disease. Am J Cardiol 2016;117:853–7.

36. Stout KK, Daniels CJ, Aboulhosn JA, et al. 2018 AHAH/ACC guideline for management of adults with congenital heart disease. Circulation 2018;139(14):32–3.

37. Scott C, Ashley L, Reis M, et al. Neurocognitive impairment is common in the adult with congenital heart disease: identification using a novel clinical questionnaire. J Am Coll Cardiol 2017;69:11.

38. Tyagi M, Austin K, Stygall J, et al. What do we know about cognitive functioning in adult congenital heart disease? Cardiol Young 2014;24:13–9.

39. Viswanathan A, Rocca WA, Tzourio C. Vascular risk factors and dementia: how to move forward? Neurology 2009;72:368–74.

40. Moons P, Van Deyk K, Dedroog D, et al. Prevalence of cardiovascular risk factors in adults with congenital heart disease. Eur J Cardiovasc Prev Rehabil 2006;13: 612–6.

41. Hair G, Corpus M, Lamarre FR, et al. Alteration of glucose and insulin metabolism in congenital heart disease. Circulation 1972;46:333–46.

42. Bagge CN, Henderson VW, Lausen HB, et al. Risk of dementia in adults with congenital heart disease: population-based cohort study. Circulation 2018;137: 1912–20.

43. Kwok CS, Loke YK, Hale R, et al. Atrial fibrillation and incidence of dementia: a systematic review and meta-analysis. Neurol 2011;76:914–22.

44. Qui C, Winblad B, Marengoni A, et al. Heart failure and risk of dementia and Alzheimer disease: a population-based cohort study. Arch Intern Med 2006;166: 1003–8.

45. Everitt IK, Gerardin JF, Rodriguez FH III, et al. Improving the quality of transition and transfer of care in young adults with congenital heart disease. Congenit Heart Dis 2017;12:242–50.

46. Mackie AS, Rempel GR, Kovacs AH, et al. Transition intervention for adolescents with congenital heart disease. J Am Coll Cardiol 2018;71:1768–77.

47. Yeung E, Kay J, Roosevelt GE, et al. Lapse of care as a predictor for morbidity in adults with congenital heart disease. Int J Cardiol 2008;125:62–5.

48. Reid FJ, Irvine MJ, McCrindle BW, et al. Prevalence and correlates of successful transfer from pediatric to adult health care among a cohort of young adults with complex congenital heart defects. Pediatrics 2004;113(3 pT1):e197–205.

49. Blum RW, Nelson-Mmari K. The health of young people in a global context. J Adolesc Health 2004;35:402–18.

50. American Academy of Pediatrics, American Academy of Family Physicians, and American College of Physicians. Transitions Clinical Report Authoring Group. Supporting the health care transition from adolescence to adulthood in the medical home. Pediatrics 2011;128(1):182–200.

51. Landsberg MJ, Gurvitz M. Transition educations: formative steps, in need of direction. J Am Coll Cardiol 2018;71:1778–80.

52. Got Transition? Center for Health Care Transition Improvement National Alliance to Advance Adolescent Heath. Available at: http://www.gottransition.org.

53. Barbaresi WJ, Coligan RC, Weaver AL, et al. Mortality, ADHD, and psychosocial adversity in adults with childhood ADHD: a prospective study. Pediatrics 2013; 131:637–44.

54. Clarizia NA, Chahal N, Manlhiot C, et al. Transition to adult health care for adolescents and young adults with congenital heart disease: perspectives of the patient, parent and health care provider. Can J Cardiol 2009;25(9):e317–22.

55. Knauth A, Verstappen A, Reiss J, et al. Transition and transfer from pediatric to adult care of the young adult with complex congenital heart disease. Cardiol Clin 2006;24(4):619–29, vi.

56. Peter NG, Forke CM, Ginsburg KR, et al. Transition from pediatric to adult care: internists' perspectives. Pediatrics 2009;123(2):417–23.

57. Scal P, Evans T, Blozis S, et al. Trends in transition from pediatric to adult health care services for young adults with chronic conditions. J Adolesc Health 1999; 24(4):259–64.

# Innovations in Congenital Interventional Cardiology

Jenny E. Zablah, MD, FSCAI, FACC, FAAP*,
Gareth J. Morgan, MBBaO, BCH, MRCPCH, MPhil, MSCAI

## KEYWORDS

- Congenital interventional cardiology • Innovation • 3D rotational angiography
- Advanced imaging • New cardiac devices

## KEY POINTS

- Imaging in the catheterization laboratory has moved from 2-dimensional angiography to 3-dimensional fusion imaging and using virtual and augmented reality environments to plan and perform procedures.
- Fusion imaging has allowed the use of computed tomography and MRI images to guide procedures in the catheterization laboratory with decreased radiation and contrast doses.
- Development of new device technology has facilitated procedures at both ends of the spectrum of congenital heart disease, from patent ductus arteriosus closure in neonates weighing less than 700 g to percutaneous pulmonary valve replacement in older children and adults with hugely dilated right ventricular outflow tracts.
- Cardiac catheterization under MRI guidance is a promising approach that may increase diagnostic accuracy while decreasing patient and procedural team exposure to ionizing radiation.

## INTRODUCTION

The desire to avoid cardiopulmonary bypass, multiple redo sternotomies, and long hospital stays has fueled the development of techniques and technologies that allow excellent cardiovascular outcomes without the morbidity traditionally associated with cardiopulmonary bypass surgery. In the past 15 years, there have been major technological advancements in congenital interventional cardiology that have allowed progressive improvement in cardiac imaging in the catheterization laboratory, expansion of the variety of procedures and availability of different devices to overcome prior challenges in congenital patients.

This review aims to describe some of the latest advances in congenital interventional cardiology and capture the changes in the field in the past decade.

University of Colorado School of Medicine, Congenital Interventional Cardiology Attending, Children's Hospital Colorado, 13123 16th East Avenue, Box 100, Aurora, CO 80045, USA
* Corresponding author.
*E-mail address:* Jenny.zablah@childrenscolorado.org

Pediatr Clin N Am 67 (2020) 973–993
https://doi.org/10.1016/j.pcl.2020.06.012
0031-3955/20/© 2020 Elsevier Inc. All rights reserved.

pediatric.theclinics.com

## ADVANCES IN CATHETERIZATION LABORATORY IMAGING

We have come a long way in a short time. Many interventional cardiologists still in practice will remember the trials of sifting through reels of 8-mm cine-angiography film and using analogue mechanical projectors to display frames that had been painstakingly selected and indexed. Advances in image storage, retrieval, and visualization may be easily dismissed, but digital archiving probably represents the single biggest step forward for interventional practice.

### Three-Dimensional Printed Models

Three-dimensional (3D) printed models are increasingly used in cardiology and cardiac surgery, especially in congenital heart disease (CHD). They allow comprehensive spatial conceptualization of the cardiac anatomy and hence assist in preoperative planning as well as simulation of cardiac procedures in the catheterization laboratory (cath lab).[1] 3D printed models also have an important role in patient education as well as in medical training (**Fig. 1**).

Constant improvements in materials, processing times, and anatomic detail allied with decreasing costs continue to provide new opportunities for the use of 3D printed models in CHD.

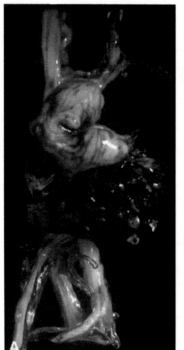
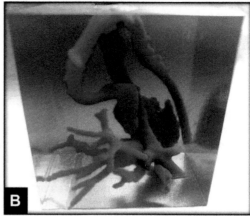

**Fig. 1.** Three-dimensional printed models. (*A*) Three-dimensional printed model from a 4D flow MRI showing flow dynamics on a single ventricle patient. (*B*) Three-dimensional printed model in a transparent cube to maintain the anatomic vascular and airway relationship. These images were printed from a 3DRA cath lab dataset.

## Virtual Reality

As a potentially new platform for advanced imaging in the cath lab, virtual reality (VR) is an exciting prospect. It facilitates the interaction between and manipulation of high-resolution representations of patient-specific imaging data.

VR has been used as a *surgical and interventional planning tool,* allowing physicians to navigate complex cardiac anatomy using datasets from computed tomography (CT), MRI, 3D echocardiography, or 3D rotational angiography (3DRA). VR is also used as a *distraction tool for patients,* allowing patients to have procedures that may otherwise need deep sedation or general anesthesia with minimal or no sedation. For example, we use VR distraction therapy during pulmonary hypertension or post-heart transplant evaluations, allowing these chronic patients to have shorter procedures with minimal or no sedation, hence a quicker post-catheterization recovery. As well as decreasing the risks of general anesthesia in this at-risk group, it also allows minimization of the physiologic disturbances to the pulmonary systemic vascular beds, improving the accuracy of the data acquired.

*Interventional guidance* is a growing benefit of VR. We are currently developing a VR software simulator that allows to virtually insert models of various percutaneously placed pulmonary valves within a 3D-reconstruction of the patient's pulmonary outflow tract, rendered from CT or MRI. This is unique, as the rendering is a beating heart model not a fixed, averaged reconstruction. This software helps with procedural planning and selecting the correct pulmonary valve type and size before the actual procedure and allows planning of valve positioning, anticipating any potential problems (**Fig. 2**).

## From 2-Dimensional to 3-Dimensional Angiography

Along with major developments in x-ray detector plate technology, which have allowed digital high-definition imaging to be available with lower ionizing radiation production, have come various platforms to allow 3D reconstruction of angiograms. Most manufacturers now offer 3DRA software on their imaging systems. 3DRA is intended

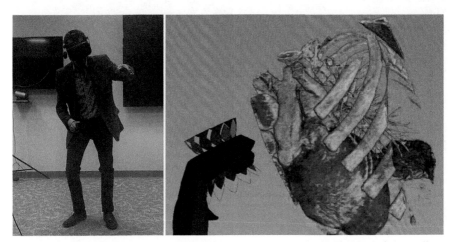

**Fig. 2.** VR simulation for percutaneous valve implantation. VR simulation software allows the interventional cardiologist to select the pulmonary valve that would be the best fit for an individual patient using a recent cardiac CT. This software allows assessment of the pulmonary artery in systole and diastole.

to provide high-speed and high-resolution 3D visualization of vascular anatomy. 3DRA generates a 3D reconstruction from multiple 2D radiographic images taken during a rotation of the imaging equipment around the patient. The rotation occurs over 5 to 20 seconds around an isocenter point and rotates between 200° and 360°, depending on the equipment manufacturer.

The associated software package then creates CT-like 3D volumes by stitching multiple images together.

3DRA was initially used to obtain better visualization of complex vascular anatomy and structural relationships, but with time, the technology has evolved allowing even more benefits, detailed as follows.

*Procedural guidance using image overlay.* Reconstructed images from 3DRA can be merged onto the imaging screen with live fluoroscopy to guide interventional procedures. 3DRA overlay with live fluoroscopy enhances the navigation of catheters and wires around complex heart anatomies, helps to identify the best imaging angles to visualize structures of interest, and aids the accurate placement of stents and occlusion devices.[2] With the right training, use of this technology can decrease overall procedural time and decrease contrast and radiation doses[3] (**Fig. 3**).

Assessing the relationship between *vascular structures and the airways*. This has become possible with newer generation 3DRA. As well as "CT-like" multiplanar reconstructions (MPR), newer generations of 3DRA now allow 3D reconstruction of the airway after a 3DRA with contrast injection in the neighboring vascular structures. For congenital cardiac interventions, this information is extremely important as it may predict and help to avoid airway compression during interventions such as pulmonary artery stenting. It may also be a useful modality in the diagnosis and management of airway compression caused by, for example, vascular rings, dilated pulmonary arteries, anomalous vascular courses, or dilated aorta[4] (**Figs. 4** and **5**).

Obtaining *reliable and reproducible measurements of cardiac and vascular structure* is a forgone expectation when angiography is performed as part of pre-procedural

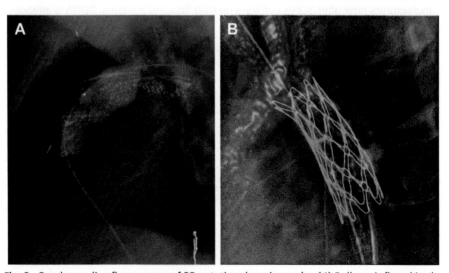

**Fig. 3.** Overlay on live fluoroscopy of 3D rotational angiography. (*A*) Balloon inflated in the RVOT with the narrow portion of the balloon matching the narrowest segment on the overlaid 3DRA. (*B*) Preintervention 3DRA overlaid on the postintervention live fluoroscopy, showing the improved diameter with the new stent placed.

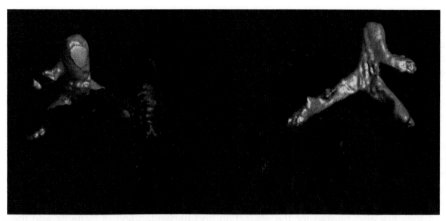

**Fig. 4.** Airway reconstruction from 3DRA using Philips Azurion System. 3D-airway reconstruction (*blue*) demonstrating an aberrant bronchus that supplies the right upper lobe. The relationship of the airway with the branch PAs is also demonstrated, with posterior flattening of the right bronchus secondary to extrinsic compression.

planning. This has produced some challenges when interpreting 3DRA imaging. As interventional cardiologists have developed practices and protocols to produce the highest spatial resolution 3DRA imaging, they have made compromises. A common practice is to use cardiac pacing during the 3DRA acquisition to decrease cardiac output and motion for the duration of the 3DRA acquisition spin. This maximizes the concentration of contrast medium within the vascular structure of interest for longer, helping to obtaining a better image. The downside of this is that the vessel

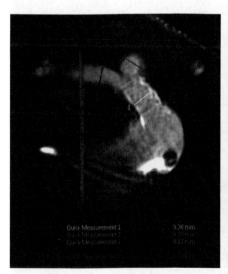
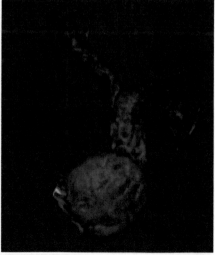

**Fig. 5.** MPR measurements. Measurements of the right ventricle to PA conduit were performed, after stent placement, using the XperCT tool from the Philips Azurion System. This tool allows us to process the 3DRA datasets from the cath lab in a similar way to a standard CT, measuring structures in multiple planes and obtaining snapshots and movies of the area of interest.

measurements are not accurate, as the sequence is obtained during a nonphysiological condition. It then becomes necessary to perform a standard biplane angiogram to obtain the measurements before an intervention, creating a redundancy of information that is far from the objective of the technology. In our center, we perform 3DRAs without pacing, obtaining a dynamic image with reliable measurements in systole and diastole. We have developed a protocol that allows both high-quality 3DRA pictures and reliable measurements, avoiding repeat angiography and resulting in an overall decrease in contrast volume and radiation dose (**Fig. 5**).

Another new application of 3DRA is the creation of *3D printed models* from 3DRA datasets. In Denver, we have developed a technique of importing the 3DRA images into a DICOM viewer that allows them to be processed in the same manner as images from a cardiac CT or MRI. This has allowed us to routinely print 3D models from the imaging acquired during the patient's cardiac catheterization. These models provide information for upcoming cardiac surgery planning or future cardiac catheterizations, but they are also printed for the education and understanding of patients and their families. Datasets from 3DRA give enough information to allow segmentation and 3D printing of the vessels and the airways, providing another option to practically assess the relationship between the vasculature and the airways in patients with complex anatomy (**Fig. 6**). Families and patients have consistently commented on an improvement in their understanding of cardiac anatomy since we started the routine

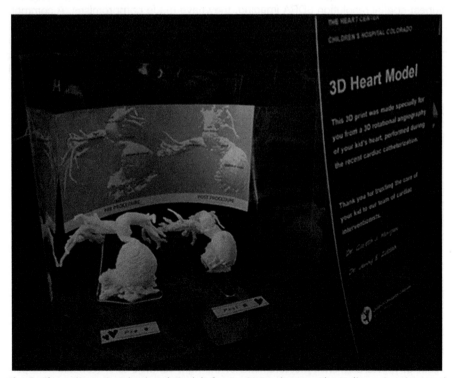

**Fig. 6.** Three-dimensional printed models from a 3DRA dataset. Three-dimensional printed models before and after intervention, printed from the 3DRA performed during the patient's cardiac catheterization. The total time of processing and printing was 10 hours. The family took these models home before discharge.

provision of 3D cardiac models, which we use for counseling, then proved to the patients with annotated diagrams and descriptions. These printed models have demonstrated not only a clinical application but also an educational and psychological use for patients, families, and trainee education.

*VR and augmented reality platforms* for procedural guidance from 3DRA datasets is now possible. On the same basis as 3D printed models from 3DRA datasets, we have processed these images and imported them to VR programs. These images are used to assess intracardiac anatomy in a VR environment, allowing interaction with the different structures, measurement of areas of interest, and procedural discussion and planning. The processing takes minutes and can be used during the same procedure in which the dataset is acquired without significant delay. This technology can change the approach to complex cases and decreases the need to repeat multiple angiograms and the need for complex offline image processing that may result in increased contrast volume, radiation dose, procedural delay, and procedural duration (**Fig. 7**).

As well as generating 3D data sets during catheterization procedures, for use during that procedure or to assist with subsequent procedural planning or patient and physician education, there have also been huge strides forward in the development and use of 3D models and online platforms from CT and MRI, which can either directly interact with fluoroscopic imaging or bring an extra dimension to image review as a method of determining the indication for a procedure as well as planning the most efficacious method to perform it.

### Three-Dimensional Image Fusion Technologies

CT and MRI can be very helpful in accurately defining cardiovascular anatomy and planning interventional procedures in the cath lab.[5] Several systems are available to allow multimodality image fusion in the cath lab.

- VesselNavigator (Philips Healthcare, Eindhoven, Netherlands):VesselNavigator is the most recently available 3D image fusion software that uses preregistered CT or MRI datasets to support device navigation during interventional procedures. It

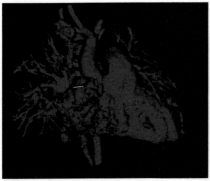 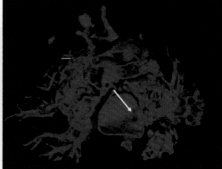

**Fig. 7.** VR for interventional planning. Using cardiac CT, MRI, or 3DRA datasets, VR assessment of key cardiac structures such as abnormal pulmonary veins is possible. This allows us to identify mechanisms of pulmonary vein stenosis and helps plan the intervention. In this patient, there was a history of left lower pulmonary vein stenosis. Using VR, we identified the problem as an acute angle at the insertion of the pulmonary vein into the left atrium.

facilitates the overlay of a 3D data set on top of live fluoroscopic imaging to create a 3D environment for the manipulation of diagnostic and interventional equipment through complex anatomy. The use of VesselNavigator fusion requires 4 steps: (1) SEGMENTATION: The pre-acquired MRI or CT dataset is processed to identify and highlight the anatomic areas of interest; (2) PLANNING: Markers are placed on the dataset which will appear fused onto the fluoroscopic image to highlight key anatomic locations (eg, the position of a coronary artery); (3) REGISTRATION: The 3D dataset and the live fluoroscopic image are brought into alignment in 3D space; (4) LIVE GUIDANCE. The procedure is conducted with the added advantage of a 3D dataset integrated into the fluoroscopic imaging, which maintains its orientation and alignment no matter at what angle the fluoroscopic image is acquired (**Fig. 8**).3D image fusion technology has been proven to decrease radiation exposure and contrast dose in complex procedures like percutaneous pulmonary valve replacement.[6] This technology is extremely useful, but like many other advances its effective application comes after a learning curve. We must recognize that poor understanding and application of such technology could decrease accuracy and expose the patient to excess risk. Widespread collaboration, training and proctoring is important.

- EchoNavigator (Philips Healthcare):Real-time fusion of live echocardiographic and radiographic images for procedural guidance is possible with this system. It differs from VesselNavigator, as both of the imaging modalities are acquired and fused simultaneously during the interventional procedure. The echocardiogram and radiographic images are synchronized and move together when the c-arm is repositioned. Changes in the echocardiographic modalities and planes can be effected by the interventional cardiologist at the table or by the cardiologist performing the transesophageal echocardiography (TEE) (**Fig. 9**).EchoNavigator requires teamwork and communication between the proceduralist and the imaging cardiologist to obtain the best outcomes. In patients with CHD, the technology is useful to create or close atrial septal defects or fenestrations in Fontan pathways. It is also used to guide procedures that require access to small perforations like patent foramen ovales (PFO), small Fontan fenestrations, or when accessing selective on of multiple holes present; as in fenestrated atrial or ventricular septal defects).Although EchoNavigator was not

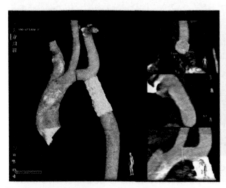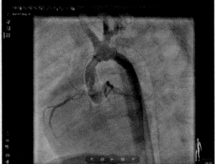

**Fig. 8.** VesselNavigator. VesselNavigator allows creation of a 3D anatomic representation of the area of interest from cross-sectional imaging, allowing us to obtain measurements and place markers on the imaging for guidance (*left*). It also has ability to overlay the processed cross-sectional imaging onto live fluoroscopy for procedural guidance (*right*).

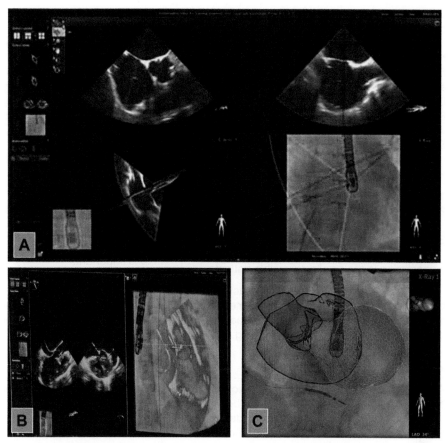

**Fig. 9.** EchoNavigator. EchoNavigator allows a multiplanar view of the heart using transesophagic echocardiogram (*A*). After registering the TEE probe with the fluoroscopic system, markers can be placed in targets of interest for the interventional cardiologist and help guide the intervention (*B*). The newest version of EchoNav allows a combination of fusion imaging with machine learning and automated heart model generation (*C*). (*Courtesy of Philips Healthcare, Netherlands.*)

created for interventions in patients with CHD, our practice has demonstrated its feasibility and efficacy in complex pediatric and adult patients with CHD; reduces overall radiation doses without affecting procedural times. For example, our experience demonstrated that performing a right heart catheterization using EchoNavigator in patients undergoing atrial septal defect (ASD) closure can decrease the total Air Kerma to <1 mGy.[7]

## DEVICES AND TECHNOLOGY
### *Transcatheter Patent Ductus Arteriosus Closure on Very Low Weight Patients*

Transcatheter patent ductus arteriosus (PDA) closure has for many years been the procedure of choice for children >6 kg due to the low rate of adverse events and high efficacy. Historically, this procedure was rarely performed in premature neonates because of concerns regarding vascular access, patient fragility, contrast effects in these patients, and most importantly, the lack of suitable PDA closure device.

Several devices have been adapted to be used in this population with acceptable results, but in 2014, the first paper by Bass and Wilson[8] showed the feasibility and efficacy of implanting a new miniaturized nitinol device to occlude the PDA in newborn animal model. This device was released in Europe as the "Amplatzer Ductal Occluder II Additional Sizes" (ADO II AS) (St Jude Medical, St Paul, MN); it was approved by the Food and Drug Administration (FDA) in the United States in 2019 for premature infants weighing more than 700 g and renamed AMPLATZER PICCOLO OCCLUDER (Abbott, Santa Clara, CA).

The success rate in infants weighing less than 2 kg has been partly due to several key design characteristics, including the following:

1. Extremely low-profile delivery catheter (4F).
2. Procedural flexibility: It can be deployed using venous access only, avoiding arterial access in small infants.
3. Appropriate range of device sizes: The device is available in a range of lengths and diameters, which allows a predictable intraductal deployment and effective shunt occlusion in the smallest possible patients.

This device has shifted the current practice of PDA surgical ligation in premature neonates of very low weight to transcatheter PDA closure with improved recovery time and decreased post-procedural complications.[9] There are case reports of this device being used in patients as small as 500 g when clinically indicated.[10] (**Fig. 10**).

### Atrial Septal Defect Closure Devices

ASDs are commonly closed percutaneously. Newer technology has allowed us to expand the range of patients who may benefit from this approach.

Until 2019, the only FDA-approved devices for ASD closure were the Amplatzer Septal Occluder and the Gore Septal Occluder. The "Amplatzer" was the only device that was capable of closing larger defects but has had a small but appreciable incidence of erosion through cardiac tissue, which has encouraged caution in practice. Device erosion has been more frequent with larger implants and in patients with

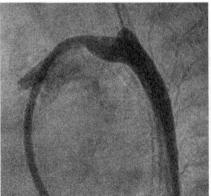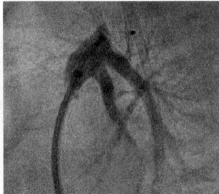

**Fig. 10.** Device occlusion of a PDA on a 690 g ex-24-week neonate. The PDA was closed via a 4-French sheath in the femoral vein. A large PDA was seen on angiography (*left*) with complete occlusion after placement of a Piccolo (*right*).

particular anatomic features. In an effort to allow closure of large defects with minimal risks of erosion, the new GORE CARDIOFORM ASD Occluder (GCA; W.L. Gore and Associates, Flagstaff, AZ) became commercially available. This device has a large diameter central waist and an expanded range of diameters. The GCA allows the closure of larger defects thanks to the self-centering design and the softer more flexible construct should protect against the long-term risk of erosion (**Fig. 11**).[11]

The complete closure of an ASD in patients with pulmonary hypertension can be detrimental due to the potential risk of a pulmonary hypertensive crisis not being ameliorated by the presence of a potential R-L shunt. Approximately 8% to 10% of patients with ASD can develop pulmonary hypertension (PH), a severe chronic condition with progressive increase in right ventricular (RV) pressure and pulmonary vascular resistance (PVR), associated with secondary right heart failure, and high mortality rates. ASD-associated PH (ASDAPH) is usually independent of the degree, duration of shunting, and defect size. In these cases, a fenestrated closure of the ASD may be preferable. A residual restrictive interatrial shunt in these patients may enhance systemic output at the expense of some potential for systemic desaturation. The availability of an ASD closure device with a "built-in" fenestration to allow intermittent decompression of the RA is a potentially large step forward for patients with PH. The Occlutech Fenestrated ASD device (Occlutech, Helsingborg, Sweden) is already available on a compassionate use basis and will hopefully soon be available for regular clinical use, with a growing literature of device safety and efficacy in this complex patient population[12] (**Fig. 12**).

On a related theme, there are some patient groups who require the creation of an atrial-level shunt due to dysfunction of either their left ventricle or pulmonary circulation. Devices such as the Occlutech Atrial Flow Regulator (AFR) (Occlutech) are

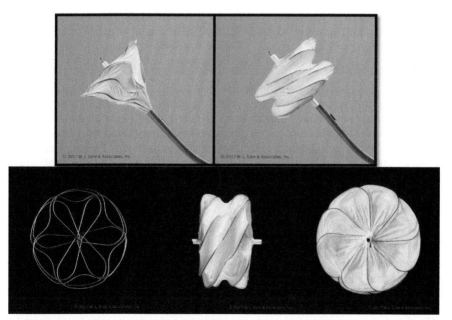

**Fig. 11.** GCA occluder. The GCA has an adaptable waist, which fills and conforms to ASDs from 8 to 35 mm. The device is made of expanded polytetrafluoroethylene (ePTFE) that has low thrombogenicity produces a minimal inflammatory response. (*Courtesy of* W.L. Gore and Associates, Flagstaff, AZ.)

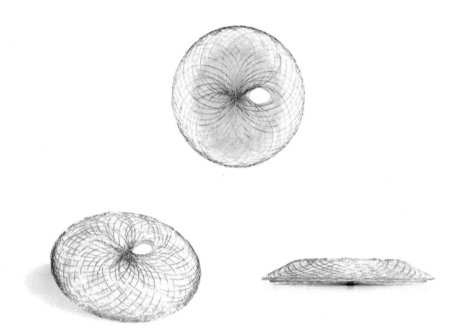

**Fig. 12.** Occlutech Fenestrated ASD device. This device allows partial closure of an ASD, maintaining a predictable restrictive atrial communication in patients with ASDs and PH. (*Courtesy of* Occlutech, Helsingborg, Sweden.)

designed to maintain a permanent interatrial communication with a predetermined diameter. The resulting decompression of the dysfunctional circulation may to lead to reduced symptoms and improved exercise tolerance and quality of life (**Fig. 13**). In patients with CHD, the AFR has also been used in patients with functional single ventricle circulations, to allow accurately sized decompressing fenestrations in Fontan circuits. This can benefit patients who have chronically failing Fontan physiology as well as those who require staged closure of a surgically placed fenestration[11]

The AFR design includes a double-disc, circular device made of self-expanding, nitinol wire mesh. A flexible waist in the center connects the 2 discs and has a centrally located hole or tunnel. A welded ball structure located on the right atrial disc which serves as the attachment and release point for the delivery system. The deployment technique across the atrial septum of this device is like the commercially available ASD devices and positioning is confirmed using TEE or intracardiac echocardiography.

### Biodegradable Technology in the Catheterization Laboratory

Replacing the current materials used for implants in the cath lab with biodegradable materials has obvious benefits and is seen by many as a final common pathway for all future device development. Current technological concepts can be broken into 2 major categories based on their material composition:

*Bioabsorbable polymers:* Polymers, for example, poly L-lactic acid, break down by hydrolysis into inert organic chemicals which confer an excellent safety profile. From the interventional cardiologists' perspective, poor predictability of degradation and a lack of inherent x-ray visibility are drawbacks for this group of materials.

A

B

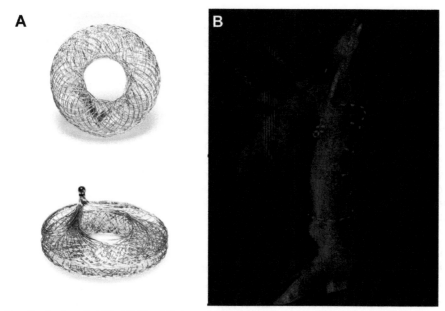

**Fig. 13.** Occlutech AFR. (*A*) The AFR is a nitinol-based device created to maintain a permanent communication between cardiac chambers (atrial septal defect or Fontan fenestration). (*B*) 3DRA of a patient with single ventricle physiology following a Fontan procedure with a large fenestration. An AFR was placed across the fenestration to decrease its size, but maintain a reliable and predictable flow across it. (*Courtesy of* Occlutech, Helsingborg, Sweden.)

*Biocorrodible metals*: Metals such as zinc or magnesium break down by biocorrosion, which is potentially inflammatory or toxic at the cellular or tissue level, although some research indicates zinc may suppress inflammation at the cellular level. This may be beneficial in lowering rates of neointimal proliferation, which is problematic for current small and medium diameter bare metal stents.[13]

Publications about biodegradable devices have been around for more than 15 years. The *BioSTAR device* was introduced in 2007 (CE Mark in European community and HPB in Canada) for ASD and PFO closure. It consists of a metal framework covered by a biodegradable membrane generated from a layer of acellular porcine collagen that is, broken down and absorbed over time. This implant achieved comparable closure rates to commercially available ASD occluders in small-to-moderate ASDs with only a minimal skeleton of foreign material remaining after 6 months.[14] The late complications seen with the BioSTAR device (severe fever episodes, severe headache, and malaise that subsequently subsided after device removal) might be attributable to specific material and immunologic properties of the partially biodegradable device.[15]

The Carag bioresorbable septal occluder (CBSO) (CARAG AG, Baar, Switzerland) is a self-centering ASD occluder, without any metal framework, composed of polylactic-co-glycolic acid. This device received CE mark across Europe in mid-September 2017. Preliminary data showed an excellent efficacy of CBRO with successful outcome in all 10 patients, 4 with small ASDs and 6 with patent foramen ovale.[16]

The experience with bioabsorbable stents is slightly different. The Absorb GT1 Bioresorbable Vascular Scaffold (BVS) stent (Abbott Vascular, Abbott Park, IL) was the first commercially approved bioabsorbable stent that became available in July 2016 in the United States. This is a bioabsorbable polymer stent made of poly-ʟ-lactic acid that was thought to be promising for use in coronary artery disease during the initial ABSORB trials. It was compared directly to a commercially available bare metal coronary stent; unfortunately, the device was removed from the market in mid-2017. Although the BVS proved noninferior to metal drug-eluting stents for target lesion failure, there was higher stent thrombosis, ischemia-driven target lesion revascularization, and non-periprocedural myocardial infarction from the ABSORB IV clinical trial.[17] This stent was promising for several categories of patients with CHD, like neonates with pulmonary artery or pulmonary vein stenosis or those for who nonsurgical treatment of coarctation of the aorta may be considered. The technological principle would allow placement of stents in neonates through tiny delivery systems, without the foreboding prospect of leaving a small nondilatable metal stent in the vessel in the long term. Further work in development of similar devices will hopefully provide these options for pediatric patients.

## PROCEDURES
### Percutaneous Closure of Ventricular Septal Defects

Ventricular septal defects (VSDs) are one of the most common congenital heart defects, with spontaneous closure rate of approximately 45% when found in isolation. For patients with moderate to large defects, surgery has long been the preferred approach for VSD closure, particularly in health systems in which access to excellent congenital surgery is de rigueur.

The successful transcatheter closure of a VSD was described more than 30 years ago in 1987. Since then, this method has become a common practice, especially in parts of Asia. In the United States, it has been adopted less commonly and used preferably in patients that are at high surgical risk or whose indications for surgery are borderline.

With the development of muscular and perimembranous VSD devices, and availability of a variety of suitable devices originally designed for closure of PDAs, this procedure has become more attractive with decrease in complications like device embolization, device-related aortic insufficiency, heart block, and tricuspid valve disruption (**Fig. 14**).

### Percutaneous Pulmonary Valve Replacement

Since the initial development of the Melody valve, the congenital community has relied on technological advances from transcatheter aortic valve replacement community to expand the applications for patients with congenital pulmonary valve diseases. Newer valve platforms, designed specifically for dilated right ventricular outflow tracts (RVOT) are currently in clinical trials in the United States, Europe, and Asia. These new devices should allow a significant expansion of the range of patients who can benefit from percutaneous rather than surgical implantation of prosthetic pulmonary valves.

The Edwards SAPIEN S3 valve (Edwards Lifesciences LLC, Irvine, CA) is a balloon-expandable valve with an extremely tough, cobalt-chromium frame protecting a trileaflet bovine pericardial tissue valve. This valve is currently under a clinical trial in the United States for use in the pulmonary position (COMPASSION S3), but in reality, it has become an off-label standard for pulmonary valve replacement. The available sizes are 20 mm, 23 mm, 26 mm, and 29 mm. This range of valve sizes has allowed percutaneous valve implantation in many patients who could not be treated with the Melody valve.

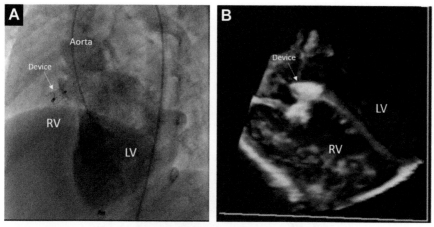

**Fig. 14.** VSD device closure. (*A*) Left ventricular angiogram after device release across a perimembranous VSD with minimal residual shunting. (*B*) Three-dimensional transesophageal echocardiogram demonstrating the device in good position across the VSD.

For patients whose RVOTs are too big for treatment with the Edwards SAPIEN valve, the company designed the Alterra Adaptive Prestent. This is a self-expanding, partially covered stent that was designed to internally reconfigure large, compliant, and irregular outflow tracts. The Alterra Adaptive Prestent is to be used as a docking adaptor for the 29-mm SAPIEN S3 transcatheter heart valve within the RVOT.[18] Although this technology has many advantages, including providing a rigid predictable landing zone for a percutaneous pulmonary valve and potentially allowing multiple, future re-valving procedures, the device is not a "one-size-fits-all" and may be limited by the gross anatomic variations seen in these outflow tracts (**Fig. 15**).

The Harmony Transcatheter Pulmonary Valve (TPV) (Medtronic, Minneapolis, MN) is a porcine pericardial tissue valve mounted on a self-expanding nitinol frame. The device is hourglass shaped, has a central diameter of 23.5 mm at the valve, and is approximately 55 mm in length. This is the only TPV device designed specifically for the native RVOT that has undergone an early feasibility clinical trial in the United States and Canada so far. Three-year results from the Native TPV early feasibility study revealed excellent safety and clinical efficacy outcomes[19] (**Fig. 16**).

Several other valves are under trial in Asia and Europe. These include the Venus p-valve (MedTech, Shanghai, China), a trileaflet porcine pericardial tissue valve. Sticking with the hourglass shape of most innovative valve platforms, the central valve diameter ranges from 22 to 36 mm. Proximal and distal flared portions help to stabilize the valve in the RVOT and main pulmonary artery. Early experience has been encouraging, suggesting that the Venus P-valve can be implanted safely, with good results with follow-up over 5 years in some patients.[20,21]

The Pulsta TPV (TaeWoong Medical Co, Gyeonggi-do, South Korea) is a self-expandable valve with flared-ends to adapt to the larger native RVOT delivered via a relatively low-profile delivery catheter. The stent is 38 mm long and is made from knitted nitinol wire with the leaflets made from treated porcine pericardial tissue.[22] The outer diameter of the valve ranges from 18 to 28 mm. There is currently a large multicenter study ongoing in South Korea. There are currently no plans for a large-scale study for this valve to seek FDA approval in the United States.

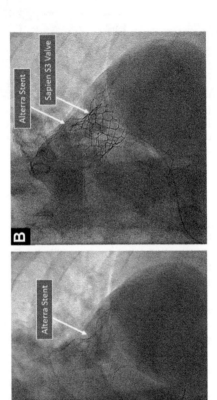

**Fig. 15.** Adaptive prestent. (*A*) Fluoroscopy of the prestent in place in a dilated RVOT. (*B*) A 29-mm SAPIEN S3 implanted inside the prestent with angiogram demonstrating no residual pulmonary insufficiency.

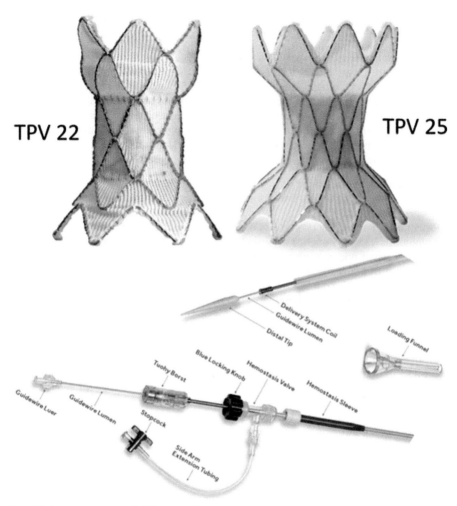

**Fig. 16.** Harmony TPV and delivery catheter system. The Harmony TPV is a porcine pericardial tissue valve designed specifically for the native RVOT. This is the only valve of this type that has undergone an early feasibility clinical trial in the United States and Canada. (*Courtesy of* Medtronic, Minneapolis, Minnesota.)

The Alterra Adaptive Prestent, the Harmony valve, the Venus P-valve and the Pulsta valve are all examples of innovative technologies that should change the face of percutaneous pulmonary valve implantation over the next 5 years. They are leading a practice change that may see percutaneous valve implantation being feasible in more than 75% of patients with dysfunctional RVOTs.

### Hybrid Procedures

The concept of hybrid procedures, which typically describe joint working between surgeons and interventionists to facilitate improved outcomes in high-risk patients, started in the late 1990s and now challenges many of the traditional approaches to congenital intervention and surgery from neonates to adult congenital patients. It is an important mindset for young practitioners to comprehend as hybrid approaches are associated with decreased hospital stay, morbidity, and need for intensive care.

### Periventricular ventricular septal valve closure

This approach allows direct access to the heart following surgical sternotomy for direct placement of a closure device across the VSD, without the need for cardiopulmonary bypass or radiation. Although this approach has been primarily performed in small infants who were too small for traditional transcatheter closure, had poor vascular access or poor ventricular function, there have been reports of the approach being used in adult patients with postinfarct VSDs and iatrogenic postoperative VSDs. The results with this technique are still limited but encouraging.[23]

### Pulmonary valve replacement

Patients in different clinical scenarios may benefit from a hybrid approach for pulmonary valve replacement:

Patients with *extremely dilated RVOTs* that exceed the range of currently available percutaneous valves. Patients with multiple comorbidities may benefit from an "off-pump" operation and a minimal sternotomy. After opening the chest, the surgeon can use one of many methods to decrease the circumference of the outflow tract. The method chosen by our team has been to suture 2 parallel 5-cm-long Teflon strips along the length of the main pulmonary outflow tract approximately 10 to 15 mm apart. A continuous suture is then used through these strips to draw them together, like a corset, producing a smaller waist to allow secure implantation of the pulmonary valve via a standard transcatheter approach.[24]

In small patients, manipulating catheters and large delivery systems around the right heart and through the tricuspid valve may produce significant hemodynamic instability. This can be avoided by directly accessing the right ventricle and inserting the delivery system.[25] After performing a limited lower sternotomy, and placing a purse-string on the antero-inferior surface of the RV, the selected delivery system and the corresponding percutaneous pulmonary valve can be placed with fluoroscopic guidance.

### Hybrid approach for hypoplastic left heart syndrome

The first complete hybrid palliative approach for hypoplastic left heart syndrome (HLHS) was described by Gibbs and colleagues[26] in 1993, with surgical banding of the branch pulmonary arteries (PAs) and percutaneous stenting of the arterial duct. After initial reports showed a high mortality in these patients, the technique was briefly abandoned, but the method evolved and was refined and redescribed by the group in Columbus, OH, in 2005. In this model, the surgeon and interventionalist work side-by-side to band the PAs and stent the arterial duct through direct access to the PA, with further transcatheter intervention to the atrial septum performed as a separate procedure, only if necessary.[27] Over the years, the hybrid approach to HLHS has evolved into a recognized management strategy. Recent studies comparing the hybrid approach with the Norwood procedure demonstrated comparable outcomes through stage II palliation[28] (**Fig. 17**).

### MRI-Guided Cardiac Catheterizations

MRI guidance tantalizingly offers the interventionist the prospect of performing procedures without radiation exposure, and also could exploit the additional flow modalities available through MRI technology. First-in-man MRI-guided cardiac catheter interventions have been possible due to the development of MRI-compatible guidewires. Improvements in hardware and software have increased image quality and

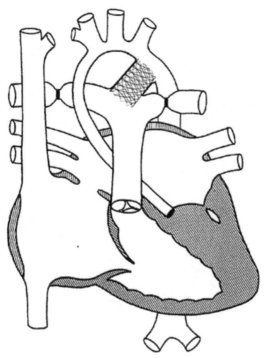

**Fig. 17.** Hybrid approach for HLHS. Diagram demonstrating banding of both branch PAs, PDA stent, and a wide-open atrial septum.

scanning times with better interactive tools for the operator in the MRI catheter suite to navigate through the anatomy as required in real time.[29]

The perfect setting for MRI-guided cardiac catheterizations is limited to a small number of centers, and clinical translation has been hindered by a lack of suitable CMR-compatible catheters and guidewires and by the limited capabilities of current visualization techniques.

Even without MRI-guided catheter manipulation, combining conventional MRI flow assessments with pressure measurements obtained by contemporaneous cardiac catheterization allows more accurate cardiac output, pulmonary blood flow, and PVR calculations than traditional cardiac catheterization, using Fick calculation or thermodilution. Although the procedural time may be increased, the radiation dose is significantly decreased, and accuracy of the data obtained is increased.[30]

## ACKNOWLEDGMENTS

The authors thank Nick Jacobson, Inworks/University of Colorado, for helping to develop the tool in **Fig. 2**, along with a multidisciplinary team of physicians.

## DISCLOSURE

Consultant for Abbott.

## REFERENCES

1. Sun Z, Lau I, Wong YH, et al. Personalized three-dimensional printed models in congenital heart disease. J Clin Med 2019;8(4):522.
2. Fagan TE, Truong UT, Jone PN, et al. Multimodality 3-dimensional image integration for congenital cardiac catheterization. Methodist Debakey Cardiovasc J 2014;10(2):68–76.
3. Minderhoud SCS, van der Stelt F, Molenschot MMC, et al. Dramatic dose reduction in three-dimensional rotational angiography after implementation of a simple dose reduction protocol. Pediatr Cardiol 2018;39(8):1635–41.
4. Truong UT, Fagan TE, Deterding R, et al. Use of rotational angiography in assessing relationship of the airway to vasculature during cardiac catheterization. Cathet Cardiovasc Intervent 2015;86:1068–77.
5. Chenier M, Tuzcu EM, Kapadia S, et al. Multimodality imaging in the cardiac catheterization laboratory: a new era in sight. Interv Cardiol 2013;5(3):335–44.
6. Goreczny S, Moszura T, Dryzek P, et al. Three-dimensional image fusion guidance of percutaneous pulmonary valve implantation to reduce radiation exposure and contrast dose: A comparison with traditional two-dimensional and three-dimensional rotational angiographic guidance. Neth Heart J 2017;25(2):91–9.
7. Jone PN, Zablah JE, Burkett DA, et al. Three-dimensional echocardiographic guidance of right heart catheterization decreases radiation exposure in atrial septal defect closures. J Am Soc Echocardiogr 2018;31(Issue 9):1044–9.
8. Bass JL, Wilson N. Transcatheter occlusion of the patent ductus arteriosus in infants – Experimental testing of a new Amplatzer device. Catheter Cardiovasc Interv 2014;83:250–5.
9. Alban-Elouen B, William R, Benbrik N, et al. Improved ventilation and hospital stay in premature babies after transcatheter closure of patent ductus arteriosus as compared to surgical ligation: a multi-center comparative study. Arch Cardiovasc Dis 2019;11(Issue 4):e380.
10. Taylor R, Forbes MJ, Kobayashi D. Transcatheter closure of patent ductus arteriosus in a tiniest baby – 510 grams. Prog Pediatr Cardiol 2019;101189:1058–9813.
11. McLennan D, Ivy D, Morgan GJ. Transvenous implantation of the occlutech atrial flow regulator: preliminary results from swine models. Congenit Heart Dis 2019. https://doi.org/10.1111/chd.12816.
12. Kaley V, Dahdah N, El-Sisi A, et al. Atrial septal defect–associated pulmonary hypertension: outcomes of closure with a fenestrated device. Adv Pulm Hypertens 2019;18(1):4–9.
13. Zampi J, Whiteside W. Innovative interventional catheterization techniques for congenital heart disease. Translational Pediatrics. 2018. Available at: http://tp.amegroups.com/article/view/18175. Accessed: February 25, 2020.
14. Morgan G, Lee K-J, Chaturvedi R, et al. A biodegradable device (BioSTAR™) for atrial septal defect closure in children. Cathet Cardiovasc Intervent 2010;76:241–5.
15. Happel CM, Laser KT, Sigler M, et al. Single center experience: Implantation failures, early, and late complications after implantation of a partially biodegradable ASD/PFO-device (BioStar®). Cathet Cardiovasc Intervent 2015;85:990–7.
16. Söderberg B, Vaskelyte L, Sievert K, et al. TCT-826 Prospective single center First In Human (FIH) clinical trial to evaluate the safety and effectiveness of a septal occluder with bioresorbable framework in patients with clinically significant atrial septum defect (ASD) or patent foramen ovale (PFO). J Am Coll Cardiol 2016;68(18 Supplement):B334.

17. Stone GW, Ellis SG, Gori T, et al. on behalf of the ABSORB IV Investigators. Blinded outcomes and angina assessment of coronary bioresorbable scaffolds: 30-day and 1-year results from the ABSORB IV randomized trial. Lancet 2018; 392:1530–40.

18. Zahn EM, Chang JC, Armer D, et al. First human implant of the Alterra Adaptive Prestent™: A new self-expanding device designed to remodel the right ventricular outflow tract. Catheter Cardiovasc Interv 2018;91:1125–9.

19. Benson LN, Gillespie MJ, Bergersen L, et al. Three-year outcomes from the harmony native outflow tract early feasibility study. Circ Cardiovasc Interv 2020;13: e008320.

20. Garay F, Pan X, Zhang YJ, et al. Early experience with the Venus P-valve for percutaneous pulmonary valve implantation in native outflow tract. Neth Heart J 2017;25:76–81.

21. Morgan G, Prachasilchai P, Promphan W, et al. Medium-term results of percutaneous pulmonary valve implantation using the Venus P-valve: international experience. EuroIntervention 2019;14:1363–70.

22. Kim GB, Kwon BS, Lim HG. First in human experience of a new self-expandable percutaneous pulmonary valve implantation using knitted nitinol-wire and trileaflet porcine pericardial valve in the native right ventricular outflow tract. Catheter Cardiovasc Interv 2017;89:906–9.

23. Butera G, Lovin N, Chessa M. Hybrid muscular ventricular septal defect closure: literature and results. In: Butera G, Cheatham J, Pedra C, et al, editors. Fetal and hybrid procedures in congenital heart diseases. Cham (Switzerland): Springer; 2016. p. 93–8.

24. Morgan GJ. Pulmonary regurgitation- is the future percutaneous or surgical? Front Pediatr 2018;6:184.

25. Gupta A, Kenny D, Caputo M, et al. Initial experience with elective periventricular Melody valve placement in small patients. Pediatr Cardiol 2017;38:575–81.

26. Gibbs JL, Wren C, Watterson KG, et al. Stenting of the arterial duct combined with banding of the pulmonary arteries and atrial septectomy or septostomy: a new approach to palliation for the hypoplastic left heart syndrome. Br Heart J 1993;69:551–5.

27. Galantowicz M, Cheatham JP. Lessons learned from the development of a new hybrid strategy for the management of hypoplastic left heart syndrome. Pediatr Cardiol 2005;26(3):190–9.

28. Cao JY, Lee SY, Phan K, et al. Early outcomes of hypoplastic left heart syndrome infants: meta-analysis of studies comparing the hybrid and Norwood procedures. World J Pediatr Congenit Heart Surg 2018;9(2):224–33.

29. Kuberan P, Henry C, Reza R. MR-guided cardiac interventions. Top Magn Reson Imaging 2018;27(3):115–28.

# The Next Frontier in Pediatric Cardiology
## Artificial Intelligence

Sharib Gaffar, MD[a,1], Addison S. Gearhart, MD[b,1],
Anthony C. Chang, MD, MBA, MPH, MS[c,*,2]

### KEYWORDS

- Artificial intelligence • Machine and deep learning • Cognitive computing
- Natural language processing • Robotic process automation

### KEY POINTS

- Physicians can combine clinical expertise with artificial intelligence (AI) information to provide high-level surveillance, prevention, predictive intervention, and health maintenance to the pediatric population.
- Clinical decision support with data mining and AI offers further insight into patient behaviors and health trends, but ultimately requires physician insight for final judgment.
- AI significantly augments the value of cardiac MRI, CT, radiographs, and echocardiograms, providing higher levels of specificity for physicians to increase their diagnostic acumen.
- Applications of AI include patient risk stratification, education, and training in congenital heart disease through augmented and virtual reality, robotic automation minimizing redundant workflow tasks, and individualized patient management plans developed with precision medicine.
- Data access and ownership for pediatric patients are the rate-determining factors for widespread AI integration with pediatric cardiology in the coming decade.

### INTRODUCTION

The past decade has ushered artificial intelligence (AI) into the clinical realm with improvements in technology, the development of sophisticated machine learning, and

[a] UC Irvine Pediatrics Residency Program, Choc Children's Hospital of Orange County, 757 Westwood Plaza, Ste 5235, Los Angeles, CA 90095-8358, USA; [b] Boston Children's Hospital Heart Center, 300 Longwood Avenue, Boston, MA 02115, USA; [c] The Sharon Disney Lund Medical Intelligence and Innovation Institute (MI3), Children's Hospital of Orange County, 1120 W La Veta Ave, STE 860, Orange, CA 92868, USA
[1] Co-first authors.
[2] Senior author.
* Corresponding author.
*E-mail address:* achang007@aol.com

Pediatr Clin N Am 67 (2020) 995–1009
https://doi.org/10.1016/j.pcl.2020.06.010
0031-3955/20/© 2020 Elsevier Inc. All rights reserved.

the widespread collection of data accompanying the early 2010s transition to electronic health records (EHRs). With more advanced computer hardware and software, more refined iterations of machine learning, and more diverse and expansive patient data, physicians are now seeing clinical medicine and informatics merge to provide optimum patient management. Over the next decade, further improvements can be expected in these 3 areas, with future physicians practicing medicine in conjunction with AI, rather than adapting to the growing pains of its rapid introduction. Pediatrics and pediatric cardiology in the 2020s will likely benefit the most of all medical specialties from adoption and manipulation of AI to treat patients.

Pediatrics is a specialty focused on primary prevention and health surveillance, with an appreciation for the long-standing negative effects on population health following early intervention failures. AI can benefit pediatrics further than internal medicine because of the decreased future burden on clinics, hospitals, and insurance companies if these young patients maintain their health. It is no coincidence that the same benefits machine learning provides to clinical decision support (promoting health maintenance, health surveillance, and preventive strategies) are also the main reasons pediatrics has improved the health and wellness of children worldwide, especially over the past 40 years.[1] Machine learning, deep learning, and reinforcement learning can facilitate health surveillance and maintenance, allowing pediatricians to better anticipate their patients' health needs and target their discussions throughout childhood visits.

## HOW DOES ARTIFICIAL INTELLIGENCE INTEGRATE INTO CLINICAL PRACTICE?

The data-to-intelligence pyramid characterizes how pediatricians and pediatric cardiologists can view AI as an evolutionary adjunct to their clinical practices (**Fig. 1**). Robust AI in health care relies on accurate, high-quality health care data. Large volumes of patient health data are processed and interpreted to obtain the next level of the pyramid: meaningful patient information (see **Fig. 1**). Although machine learning requires vast sums of data, physicians require only the distilled relevant information to make clinical decisions. By applying their experience and analysis of the relevant information, physicians are able to attain knowledge (see **Fig. 1**). Intelligence is therefore the ability to acquire and apply this knowledge. As AI becomes commonplace, physicians will be expected to interpret this new insight for more sound clinical decision making. This physician expertise, or wisdom, is likely to gain value over the next decade as future physicians are trained to incorporate AI into their medical management. Wisdom is the accumulated knowledge and experience that gives the ability to discern or judge. The increase in robotic process automation will allow AI to offload time-intensive mundane repetitive tasks such as billing and documentation. This process may give physicians increased job satisfaction, returning their career to one focused on applying wisdom to patient care, and strengthening the patient-physician relationship.[2]

## CLINICAL DECISION SUPPORT

Decision making in pediatric cardiology is often multifaceted and vulnerable to many heuristics and biases.[3] The integration of AI, imaging, and clinical information shows promise to generate new diagnostic insights through interpretation of large reservoirs of data that remove many inherent biases in cardiology. In the Multi-Ethnic Study of Atherosclerosis (MESA), Ambale-Venkatesh and colleagues[4] showed the feasibility of machine learning paired with clinical information and data from deep cardiac imaging phenotyping to design a cardiovascular risk prediction tool with greater accuracy

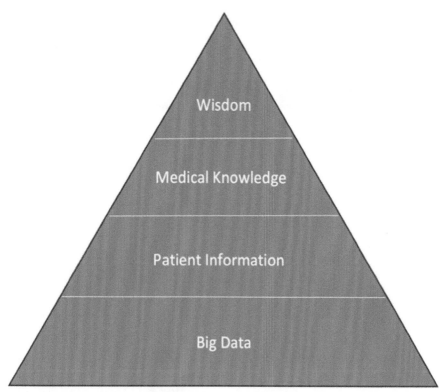

**Fig. 1.** The data-to-intelligence pyramid shows how AI increases physician wisdom. AI interprets large volumes of data to provide meaningful, relevant patient information, which the physician combines with experience to attain knowledge. Accumulated knowledge and experience eventually leads to physician wisdom for sound clinical decisions.

than standard methods. Similarly, the recent development of a machine learning algorithm trained on demographics, electrocardiography, and cardiac MRI patient data successfully identified baseline imaging and clinical variables lost to regression analysis for the prediction of deterioration in patients with repaired tetralogy of Fallot.[5] A deep-learning algorithm called deep learning–based early warning system proved able to detect patients who underwent cardiac arrest using 4 vital signs.[6]

The emergence of increased data volume, sophistication of data, and proliferation of data streaming sources increases the risk of clinicians missing markers that indicate significant patient health changes. As a result, there is increased physician recognition of machine learning's utility as a clinical decision support system because of its ability to isolate clinically important values from continual data streams (**Fig. 2**).

Deep reinforcement learning has proved adept at interpreting relevant data for complex decision making in the intensive care, hospital, or outpatient setting. Researchers at the Children's Hospital Los Angeles pediatric intensive care unit (PICU) leveraged recurrent neural networks on patient data collected over a 10-year span to generate a dynamic real-time PICU mortality prediction risk score that achieved significantly higher accuracy than the standard clinical mortality scoring systems.[7]

Although these studies highlight the power of AI predominantly in intensive care, they can be easily modified for outpatient clinical implementation to yield more

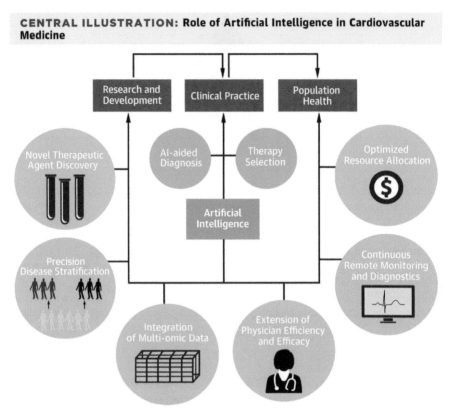

**CENTRAL ILLUSTRATION: Role of Artificial Intelligence in Cardiovascular Medicine**

**Fig. 2.** In the next decade, AI will be integrated into the 3 major areas of pediatric cardiology: clinical practice, pediatric cardiology research, and population studies. AI can analyze large sums of data from all 3 sectors to provide the most comprehensive and up-to-date clinical evaluation of a patient at each office visit. (*From* Johnson KW, Torres SJ., Glicksberg BS., et al. Artificial intelligence in cardiology. Journal of the American College of Cardiology, 71(23), 2668-2679. doi:S0735-1097(18)34408-5; with permission.)

therapeutic power to pediatric cardiologists. Because of the rapid acceptance of wearable devices in the pediatric community, the next decade will provide outpatient pediatric cardiologists with a wealth of continual patient data streams from wearables. These continual data allow outpatient health monitoring of patients with congenital heart disease (CHD) in much the same way as they were acutely monitored in the intensive care unit. Deep learning–based early warning algorithms can be modified to provide cardiologists with a predictive tool determining when their patients may require hospital admission.

## CARDIAC IMAGING

Radiology was one of the first medical fields to showcase deep learning's diagnostic capability, and often superiority, in detecting subtleties in medical imaging. Pediatric cardiology is also especially rich in imaging, lending itself well to increasing AI applications. Convolutional neural networks (CNNs) are deep-learning neural networks with 1 or more convolutional layers followed by 1 or more fully connected layers, or hidden layers, of networks with unique applications in discovering and merging local image input features with increasing levels of abstraction for prediction of clinical outcomes (**Fig. 3**).[8,9] CNNs, and deep learning in general, understandably require large training datasets to establish predictive accuracy. Unlike echocardiography, cardiac MRIs are novel to pediatric cardiology, and there is a general dearth of single-center large-data cardiac MRI training sets. However, studies such as that done by Slomka and colleagues[10] prove that multicenter registries collectively contributing deidentified data can effectively overcome the data scarcity of each individual institution and establish AI training sets.

AI has allowed various stages of cardiac MRI to become automated. Deep-learning techniques applied to adult cardiac MRI can automate chamber segmentation, view planning for cardiac MRI acquisition, and cine MRI analysis.[11–13] These same techniques can also be applied to pediatric cardiology in the future for further analysis of each sequence. In addition, deep learning has enabled reconstruction of images from cardiac MRI to achieve quality similar to gold-standard breath-hold cine techniques for children unable to hold their breath.[14] Faster image acquisition is ideally suited for irritable or critically ill pediatric patients, and higher-quality images can potentially decrease the need for sedation or invasive diagnostic catheterizations. All of these AI developments mean that turnaround time for cardiac MRI reads is minimized, allowing earlier diagnosis and faster onset of appropriate therapy.

Early AI work in echocardiography showed successful automated quantification of left ventricular function and assessment of valvular disease.[15] More recently, Zhang and colleagues[16] described their work using a CNN for automated real-time standard view classification, image chamber segmentation, and automated ejection fraction and strain measurements to improve workflow (**Fig. 4**). Nath and colleagues[17] designed a natural language processing algorithm capable of large-scale, automated, accurate extraction of structured to unstructured data from echocardiography reports stored within the EHR. Taken together, both studies hint at the future clinical practice composed of automated normal echocardiograms. CNNs will be able to read normal echocardiograms and notify the cardiologist for any borderline or abnormal cases requiring further evaluation. Each incorrect diagnostic read teaches the CNN, and improves its ability to make complex reads. At the same time, the clinical cardiologist is spared from the mundane time constraints of reading large volumes of entirely normal echocardiograms. This ability improves efficiency, with decreased dispatch times for diagnostic reports, and repurposes most of the time cardiologists spend reading echocardiograms to scrutinize abnormal or equivocal scans.

The value of AI in cardiac imaging may eventually extend beyond the rudimentary assessment of normal versus abnormal reads. Deep-learning algorithms applied to cardiac MRI proved superior to clinicians' assessment in the detection of pulmonary hypertension.[18] Similar advancements with AI in echocardiography include algorithms capable of differentiating constrictive from restrictive pericarditis and hypertrophic cardiomyopathy from physiologic cardiomyopathy seen in athletes.[19,20] A trained CNN was able to detect hypertrophic cardiomyopathy, cardiac amyloidosis, and pulmonary arterial hypertension, laying the foundation for automated interpretation support in the future.[18] The trend in cross-institutional expansion of imaging databases also enables future deep-learning strategies to detect subtleties that predict the likelihood and time frame for clinical deterioration of patients, allowing more sophisticated treatment strategies.[18] Development of algorithms tailored to specific diseases could determine the optimal frequency of surveillance echocardiograms, reducing health care expenditure and time burdens on families without compromising the detection rate of clinical decompensation.

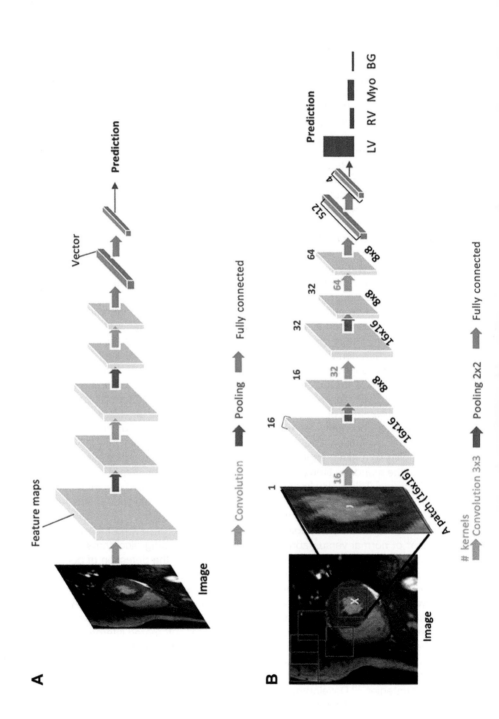

## PRECISION MEDICINE

Precision medicine refers to a comprehensive approach to disease treatment and prevention that takes into account each individual's genetics, anatomy, physiology, and environment to promote a patient-specific treatment strategy. Growing recognition for this field suggests it will be the cornerstone of pediatric cardiology in the near future. Pediatric cardiology is particularly rich with heterogeneous sources of data, ranging from imaging to clinical data. There are also continually expanding volumes of patient-specific data, including social determinants of health, surgical and interventional history, laboratory findings, implantable remote monitors, and biosensors.[2,21] These seemingly disparate sources of data are rarely interpreted together, making it difficult for pediatric cardiologists to obtain a full clinical picture of the patient's health at a single point in time (**Fig. 5**).[21] It is this disparity that makes pediatric cardiology a natural launching point for multidimensional AI integration and disruptive technologies.

Successful development of AI-enabled individualized medicine platforms will rely on neural networks interpreting the clinical significance of subtle relationships between the many layers of nonlinear data surrounding each patient with CHD (see **Fig. 5**).[2,21] These subtleties can then be monitored in a clinic setting, allowing milder medical management before patient decompensation. In addition, AI algorithms developed from abstracted data have shown increased accuracy in prediction and disease classification because they rely less on classic statistical assumptions required to make conjectures from the usual collected data in typical scientific research (see **Fig. 2**).[2] These algorithms are especially helpful in pediatric cardiology because of the rarity of certain diseases and general reluctance to perform large-scale prospective trials on children. Artificial neural networks could uncover potentially hidden structure in pediatric cardiology big data to establish new targets for novel CHD therapies.

AI algorithms can improve diagnostic and predictive accuracy with both smaller patient populations focused on niche syndromes and larger, more common CHD populations. A recent study found that AI algorithms offer more precise classifications of CHD phenotypes, allowing narrowed predictive analytics for novel timely interventions.[22] Shah and colleagues[22] applied a machine learning algorithm to patients with heart failure with preserved ejection fraction and developed a new phenotypic risk assessment system for heart failure. Similarly, Wolf and colleagues[23] developed an AI-powered collaborative clinical decision support structure from multicenter data and found the duration of mechanical ventilation following infant cardiac surgery affects clinical outcomes. This multicenter study showcased the scalability of a single machine learning algorithm beyond single-institution implementation, with minimal detrimental effects to predictive accuracy.

◀——————————————————————————————————————

**Fig. 3.** (*A*) The various separate layers that make up a convolutional neural network. Multiple convolutions and poolings are completed to learn specific hierarchical maps of certain aspects of the image. The maps are eventually converted into a vector of choice using fully connected layers, and the vectors can represent different criteria, such as statistical values, calculations, or labels. (*B*) Vectors in this case labeled the center pixel of each input patch of this cardiac MRI scan to eventually create a predictive patch segmentation map. Myo, left ventricular myocardium; BG, background; RV, right ventricle cavity; LV, left ventricle cavity. (*From* Chen C, Qin C, Qiu H, et al. Deep learning for cardiac image segmentation: a review. *Front. Cardiovasc. Med.*, 7(25), 1-33. https://doi.org/10.3389/fcvm.2020.00025; with permission.)

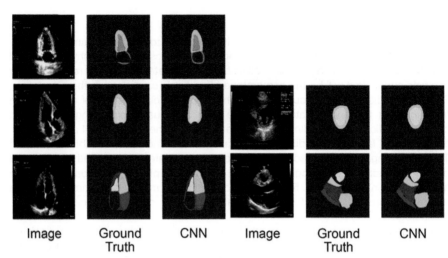

| Image | Ground Truth | CNN | Image | Ground Truth | CNN |

**Fig. 4.** CNNs were able to effectively map different cardiac chambers across 5 different sonographic views after completing the training dataset. The image is the original echocardiogram image, the ground truth details the training image, and CNN shows the performance of the automated segmentation algorithm in mapping each individual cardiac chamber. (*From* Zhang J, Gajjala S, Agrawal P. et al. Fully automated echocardiogram interpretation in clinical practice. Circulation, 138(16), 1623-1635. https://doi.org/10.1161/CIRCULATIONAHA.118.034338 [doi]; with permission.)

By extension, Ruiz-Fernandez and colleagues[24] optimized 4 AI-based algorithms in a clinical decision support system for estimating risk in congenital heart surgery. These risk indices and predictive algorithms highlight the benefits of AI in a clinical setting, where pediatric cardiologists can minimize patient risk with medical therapies and potentially increase the time between invasive reparative interventions. With accurate predictive risk calculators continually monitoring each patient at every visit, pediatric cardiologists can trend patient decompensation with more precision, offering timely medical management.

Recent expansion of augmented reality (AR) and virtual reality (VR) into pediatric cardiology revitalizes the prospect of personalized precision medicine. Improving software can now build virtual hearts that can be deconstructed in layers to clearly visualize both CHD lesions and their prospective repairs.[25] Further VR is currently underway to visualize blood flow through these lesions, allowing surgeons to anticipate potential complications or barriers to different surgical approaches.[26] AR and VR are also capable of improving patient and family understanding of complex congenital cardiac lesions. The three-dimensional (3D) rotatable images can clarify structural defects to patients' families quickly and with less confusion from medical jargon. These same 3D structures can be used by surgeons to simulate rare procedures, minimizing skills atrophy, and for medical students, residents, and fellows to provide exposure and understanding of rare CHD lesions.

## FUTURE APPLICATIONS FOR ARTIFICIAL INTELLIGENCE

The most prominent application of AI currently involves wearable technology, or wearables. Medical wearables in the past decade have evolved into unobtrusive multipurpose devices that travel and interface with their users, tracking continuous health

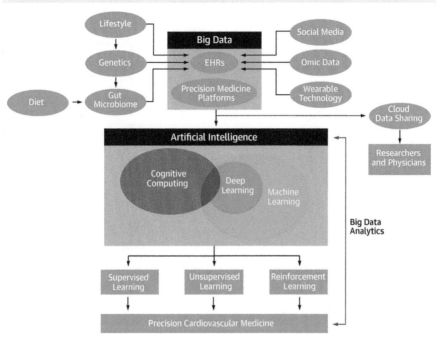

**CENTRAL ILLUSTRATION: Artificial Intelligence in Precision Cardiovascular Medicine**

**Fig. 5.** Big data include the sum of social, environmental, and medical data, among others, all securely stored in EHRs or a separate platform for physician application when the patients arrive for their visits. AI and supervised, unsupervised, and reinforcement learning access big data for each patient before the physician encounter to generate a clinical picture of the patient's health status. The physician then uses this clinical picture to deliver precision care. (*From* Krittanawong, C., Zhang, H., Wang, Z., et al. (2017). Artificial intelligence in precision cardiovascular medicine. *Journal of the American College of Cardiology, 69*(21), 2657-2664. doi:S0735-1097(17)36845-6 [pii]; with permission.)

information, such as heart rate, blood pressure, oxygen saturation, or heart rhythm, and transmitting it to a remote server for further health analysis (**Fig. 6**).[27] Because of their rapid acceptance, especially in the pediatric community, they may become an additional source of health information in the next 10 years that pediatric cardiologists can analyze to better manage their patients.[28] Wearables provide a continuous stream of patient-level information that will soon be available in voluminous quantities never before seen in health care, and represent a new aspect of health information for which physicians have had no prior access (see **Fig. 6**).

Commercially available wearables are increasing in sophistication, and some now have the ability to detect physiologic markers at rates comparable with or better than medical-grade technology.[29] Devices such as the Apple Watch have proved to be as sensitive as 12-lead clinical electrocardiograms (ECGs) in detecting arrhythmias, and have shown a high positive predictive value for tachyarrhythmias such as atrial fibrillation.[29] In addition, photoplethysmography, which is used by multiple wearable devices, has repeatedly proved reliable for pulse detection.[30] As these monitoring devices gain embedded AI, they will transform from strictly data streaming sources to

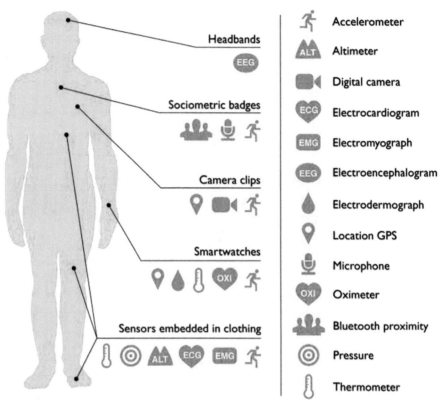

**Fig. 6.** Modern wearables interface with consumers in various ways (headbands, clothing, smartwatches) to measure different physiologic markers of the user's health. These wearables can provide real-time feedback of the user's health status, or alert others for concerning physiologic markers. Embedded AI will allow faster and more in-depth interpretation of user wellness. ECG, electrocardiogram; EEG, electroencephalogram; EMG, electromyogram; GPS, global positioning system; OXI, oximetry. (*From* Piwek L, Ellis DA, Andrews S, et al. The rise of consumer health wearables: Promises and barriers. *PLoS Medicine, 13*(2), e1001953. https://doi.org/10.1371/journal.pmed.1001953 [doi]; with permission.)

diagnostic or predictive devices. Without advanced embedded AI, these current wearables could remain relegated to predominantly monitoring devices.

However, even in their current forms, these wearables can act as potentially life-saving monitors in the outpatient setting for children with CHD. Postoperative arrhythmia detection can be vital in decreasing the risk of complications for patients who have undergone reparative surgery of their CHDs, especially because arrhythmias are the third most common cause of postoperative mortality in surgically repaired patients.[31] One of the benefits of managing pediatric populations is their adeptness at accommodating disruptive technology; they are more willing to both trial new technology and embrace new devices, and are currently one of the largest contributors to the wearable device sector growth.[27] In the coming decade, medical-grade wearable heart rhythm monitors may become obsolete, paralleling the increased popularity of purchasing medical-grade consumer wearables capable of automatically interpreting and transmitting ECGs of arrhythmias, as well as alerting cardiologists in real-time when harmful arrhythmias develop.

## IMPORTANT ISSUES IN ARTIFICIAL INTELLIGENCE

Amid the progressive integration of AI into clinical practice lies the controversial topic of who has the rights to patient health information. Physician buy-in is crucial for complete integration of AI projects in health care, and there rightfully remain concerns regarding the level of data transparency following private acquisition of large volumes of patient information. Does the wearable company, who invested in and designed the AI and hardware that both tracks health data and packages it into discrete understandable information, deserve permanent ownership of each users' most private information? Should insurance companies have access to this type of data if they may be used against the patient to deny coverage when they miss an appointment or forget to take their medication? Do businesses dealing with EHRs have an ethical responsibility to share deidentified patient data if these data may improve the wellness and health of children worldwide?

### Ethics

Pediatric cardiologists' reluctance in trusting unfamiliar technology stems from AI's theoretic direct impact on the clinical trajectory of their fragile patient population. Physicians sworn to the Hippocratic oath must protect their patients above all else, which in the modern era also includes protecting their digital rights.[32] The business of medicine further clouds ethical considerations of AI, because questions regarding adequate patient compensation for their health data currently remain unanswered. In pediatrics, these topics should remain at the forefront of all discussions because of the vulnerability of the patient population and their inability to advocate for themselves. Concerns for confidentiality and inequities regarding the extent of shared patient health information are further exacerbated in pediatric cardiology because of the smaller patient population, sometimes with characteristic CHDs that remain identifiable despite the best efforts to maintain privacy.

### Access

At the same time, a cloud-based system of worldwide publicly available deidentified health data would allow AI to work with the least biased, most comprehensive information with which to offer large-scale health surveillance and prevention strategies. Globally obtained, freely accessible encrypted data increase the power of big data and machine learning, and could provide more reliable analyses of even rare congenital diseases, offering physicians the clearest picture of how to manage their patients. In pediatrics especially, proper management strategies can reap significant benefits on patient lifespan as these children develop. With more adults currently living with CHD than afflicted neonates, proper health maintenance can both extend and improve these patients' quality of life.[33] Further extending the lifespan of this patient population with AI machine learning requires widespread unrestricted access to vast sums of global health data.

### Ownership

Different private companies developing AI systems may collaborate with hospitals or EHRs to analyze patient data, especially in intensive care units. When predictive indices allow for appropriate intervention on a decompensating patient, does the patient, hospital, or private company own the data that the AI system analyzed? The answer to this question may ultimately address how AI is monetized. On a similar note, wearable devices have seen increased adoption, especially in patients less than 18 years of age, and the time is fast approaching when physicians will need to advocate for their pediatric patients' protected health information.[27] A consensus regarding the value of data, their access, how they may be used, and their final ownership should be reached sooner rather than later to avoid creating a fragmented and walled cloud that prevents AI in health care from reaching its potential to provide the best management of the health of children.

### Bias

Despite what AI may provide to clinicians, it is essential for physicians and high-stakes specialties such as pediatric cardiology to remember that AI is an adjunct, rather than the final word, in clinical decision making. As AI standardizes global management of common CHDs, pediatric cardiologists must remain cognizant of the heuristics and biases embedded in data that initially seem impartial.[3] For example, although AI may determine that a specific surgical procedure is the best overall management for the patient, in reality the best procedure may be the one that the institution's surgeon has the most technical proficiency in performing. AI can assist the pediatric cardiologist to make more informed clinical decisions only if the cardiologist ask the right questions and appropriately frames the clinical problem.[3] The pediatric cardiologist's wisdom attained from a combination of knowledge, experience, and care for their patients will frequently lead to the best available management.

### Regulation

Pediatric cardiologists worldwide may soon need to come to a consensus regarding how AI is used for their patient population. Cardiologists must develop a system addressing the ethics of AI, the level of information access available globally, and the terminal ownership of the collected data. These 3 large categories control the extent of reach of AI in a clinical setting, and, without a unified stance on standardized regulation of health data, cardiologists could directly and indirectly place their patients' health at risk. Both private AI companies and insurance companies stand to financially benefit significantly from access to these data, with potential negative repercussions to patients if their health is continually monitored for profit.

## SUMMARY

The gold-standard AI system would provide physicians instantaneous access to their patients' updated portfolio of protected health information, complete with surveillance and health prevention recommendations, before entering the examination room. A wireless cloud-based platform would store this protected health information, composed of continual data from wearable technology, family history, genetic testing, demographics, past medical history, past medications, and more. The same platform would compare the patient's data against global databases of deidentified, encrypted, aggregate patient information to offer smart recommendations, prediction of future risk of disease, and preventive treatment plans. Notes are composed before exiting the room, synced to the platform, and simultaneously sent to an app on the patient's mobile device for review, with further explanation by a virtual assistant. Fully automated systems would manage billing, arrange follow-up appointments, order appropriate tests discussed during the visit, and complete school forms or work excuses.

After the visit, physicians and patients could monitor treatment goal progress through wearable devices, laboratory results, AR and VR models, follow-up imaging studies, and visit information from other specialty clinics. Devices could send informative warnings when progress is not met as expected or medications are not taken as prescribed. Such failures would interpret the severity of the transgression to determine whether an immediate alert to the physician is warranted, or whether smart virtual assistants could schedule a nonurgent appointment. This picture represents a new sector of training for physicians: every physician, current and future, should be trained in data science and AI to better prepare them for the incoming integration of this technology in their practices. Physicians commit to a career of lifelong learning by virtue of their job, and this learning should not be constrained to purely medicine because physicians can improve their patients' lives in more ways than solely medical treatment.

AI is ultimately an adjunct for physicians, rather than a replacement. AI provides deeper clinical decision support and maximizes the value of cardiac imaging with consistent attention to details. AI automation also minimizes redundant workflow tasks and allows for precision medicine with the help of predictive indices and analysis of new continual streams of data, such as those provided by wearables. Clinicians are closer to achieving individualized patient care with AI, but must be wary of the ethical considerations regarding access, ownership, and bias of medical data.

## DISCLOSURE

The authors have no funding or conflicts of interest to disclose related to this publication.

## REFERENCES

1. Shu LQ, Sun YK, Tan LH, et al. Application of artificial intelligence in pediatrics: Past, present and future. World J Pediatr 2019;15(2):105–8.
2. Johnson KW, Torres Soto J, Glicksberg BS, et al. Artificial intelligence in cardiology. J Am Coll Cardiol 2018;71(23):2668–79.
3. Ryan A, Duignan S, Kenny D, et al. Decision making in paediatric cardiology. are we prone to heuristics, biases and traps? Pediatr Cardiol 2018;39(1):160–7.
4. Ambale-Venkatesh B, Yang X, Wu CO, et al. Cardiovascular event prediction by machine learning: The multi-ethnic study of atherosclerosis. Circ Res 2017; 121(9):1092–101.
5. Samad MD, Wehner GJ, Arbabshirani MR, et al. Predicting deterioration of ventricular function in patients with repaired tetralogy of fallot using machine learning. Eur Heart J Cardiovasc Imaging 2018;19(7):730–8.
6. Kwon JM, Lee Y, Lee Y, et al. An algorithm based on deep learning for predicting in-hospital cardiac arrest. J Am Heart Assoc 2018;7(13):e008678.
7. Aczon M, Ledbetter D, Ho L, et al. Dynamic Mortality Risk Predictions in Pediatric Critical Care Using Recurrent Neural Networks. ArXiv170106675 Cs Math Q-Bio Stat. 2017. Available at: http://arxiv.org/abs/1701.06675. Accessed January 18, 2020.
8. LeCun Y, Bengio Y, Hinton G. Deep learning. Nature 2015;521(7553):436–44.
9. Chen C, Qin C, Qiu H, et al. Deep learning for cardiac image segmentation: a review. Front Cardiovasc Med 2020;7(25):1–33.
10. Slomka PJ, Betancur J, Liang JX, et al. Rationale and design of the REgistry of fast myocardial perfusion imaging with NExt generation SPECT (REFINE SPECT). J Nucl Cardiol 2018. https://doi.org/10.1007/s12350-018-1326-4.
11. Avendi MR, Kheradvar A, Jafarkhani H. A combined deep-learning and deformable-model approach to fully automatic segmentation of the left ventricle in cardiac MRI. Med Image Anal 2016;30:108–19.
12. Lu X, Jolly MP, Georgescu B, et al. Automatic view planning for cardiac MRI acquisition. Med Image Comput Comput Assist Interv 2011;14(Pt 3):479–86.

13. Tao Q, Yan W, Wang Y, et al. Deep learning-based method for fully automatic quantification of left ventricle function from cine MR images: A multivendor, multicenter study. Radiology 2019;290(1):81–8.

14. Hauptmann A, Arridge S, Lucka F, et al. Real-time cardiovascular MR with spatiotemporal artifact suppression using deep learning-proof of concept in congenital heart disease. Magn Reson Med 2019;81(2):1143–56.

15. Gandhi S, Mosleh W, Shen J, et al. Automation, machine learning, and artificial intelligence in echocardiography: A brave new world. Echocardiography 2018; 35(9):1402–18.

16. Zhang J, Gajjala S, Agrawal P, et al. Fully automated echocardiogram interpretation in clinical practice. Circulation 2018;138(16):1623–35.

17. Nath C, Albaghdadi MS, Jonnalagadda SR. A natural language processing tool for large-scale data extraction from echocardiography reports. PLoS One 2016; 11(4):e0153749.

18. Dawes TJW, de Marvao A, Shi W, et al. Machine learning of three-dimensional right ventricular motion enables outcome prediction in pulmonary hypertension: A cardiac MR imaging study. Radiology 2017;283(2):381–90.

19. Mahmoud A, Bansal M, Sengupta PP. New cardiac imaging algorithms to diagnose constrictive pericarditis versus restrictive cardiomyopathy. Curr Cardiol Rep 2017;19(5):43.

20. Narula S, Shameer K, Salem Omar AM, et al. Machine-learning algorithms to automate morphological and functional assessments in 2D echocardiography. J Am Coll Cardiol 2016;68(21):2287–95.

21. Krittanawong C, Zhang H, Wang Z, et al. Artificial intelligence in precision cardiovascular medicine. J Am Coll Cardiol 2017;69(21):2657–64.

22. Shah SJ, Katz DH, Selvaraj S, et al. Phenomapping for novel classification of heart failure with preserved ejection fraction. Circulation 2015;131(3):269–79.

23. Wolf MJ, Lee EK, Nicolson SC, et al. Rationale and methodology of a collaborative learning project in congenital cardiac care. Am Heart J 2016;174:129–37.

24. Ruiz-Fernandez D, Monsalve Torra A, Soriano-Paya A, et al. Aid decision algorithms to estimate the risk in congenital heart surgery. Comput Methods Programs Biomed 2016;126:118–27.

25. Sacks LD, Axelrod DM. Virtual reality in pediatric cardiology: Hype or hope for the future? Curr Opin Cardiol 2020;35(1):37–41.

26. Updegrove A, Wilson NM, Merkow J, et al. SimVascular: An open source pipeline for cardiovascular simulation. Ann Biomed Eng 2017;45(3):525–41.

27. Piwek L, Ellis DA, Andrews S, et al. The rise of consumer health wearables: Promises and barriers. PLoS Med 2016;13(2):e1001953.

28. Mackintosh KA, Chappel SE, Salmon J, et al. Parental perspectives of a wearable activity tracker for children younger than 13 years: Acceptability and usability study. JMIR mHealth uHealth 2019;7(11):e13858.

29. Sadrawi M, Lin CH, Lin YT, et al. Arrhythmia evaluation in wearable ECG devices. Sensors (Basel) 2017;17(11). https://doi.org/10.3390/s17112445.

30. Paradkar N, Chowdhury SR. (2017). Cardiac arrhythmia detection using photoplethysmography. Conference Proceedings : Annual International Conference of the IEEE Engineering in Medicine and Biology Society. IEEE Engineering in Medicine and Biology Society. Annual Conference, July 11-15, 2017, p. 113–6. https://doi.org/10.1109/EMBC.2017.8036775.

31. McCracken C, Spector LG, Menk JS, et al. Mortality following pediatric congenital heart surgery: An analysis of the causes of death derived from the national death index. J Am Heart Assoc 2018;7(22):e010624.

32. Balthazar P, Harri P, Prater A, et al. Protecting your patients' interests in the era of big data, artificial intelligence, and predictive analytics. J Am Coll Radiol 2018; 15(3 Pt B):580–6.
33. Gilboa SM, Devine OJ, Kucik JE, et al. Congenital heart defects in the united states: Estimating the magnitude of the affected population in 2010. Circulation 2016;134(2):101–9.

# Statement of Ownership, Management, and Circulation
## UNITED STATES POSTAL SERVICE® (All Periodicals Publications Except Requester Publications)

| 1. Publication Title | 2. Publication Number | 3. Filing Date |
|---|---|---|
| PEDIATRIC CLINICS OF NORTH AMERICA | 424 – 66 | 9/18/2020 |

| 4. Issue Frequency | 5. Number of Issues Published Annually | 6. Annual Subscription Price |
|---|---|---|
| FEB, APR, JUN, AUG, OCT, DEC | 6 | $240.00 |

7. Complete Mailing Address of Known Office of Publication (Not printer) (Street, city, county, state, and ZIP+4®)

ELSEVIER INC.
230 Park Avenue, Suite 800
New York, NY 10169

Contact Person
Malathi Samayan

Telephone (Include area code)
91-44-4299-4507

8. Complete Mailing Address of Headquarters or General Business Office of Publisher (Not printer)

ELSEVIER INC.
230 Park Avenue, Suite 800
New York, NY 10169

9. Full Names and Complete Mailing Addresses of Publisher, Editor, and Managing Editor (Do not leave blank)

Publisher (Name and complete mailing address)

TAYLOR BALL, ELSEVIER INC.
1600 JOHN F KENNEDY BLVD. SUITE 1800
PHILADELPHIA, PA 19103-2899

Editor (Name and complete mailing address)

KERRY HOLLAND, ELSEVIER INC.
1600 JOHN F KENNEDY BLVD. SUITE 1800
PHILADELPHIA, PA 19103-2899

Managing Editor (Name and complete mailing address)

PATRICK MANLEY, ELSEVIER INC.
1600 JOHN F KENNEDY BLVD. SUITE 1800
PHILADELPHIA, PA 19103-2899

10. Owner (Do not leave blank. If the publication is owned by a corporation, give the name and address of the corporation immediately followed by the names and addresses of all stockholders owning or holding 1 percent or more of the total amount of stock. If not owned by a corporation, give the names and addresses of the individual owners. If owned by a partnership or other unincorporated firm, give its name and address as well as those of each individual owner. If the publication is published by a nonprofit organization, give its name and address.)

| Full Name | Complete Mailing Address |
|---|---|
| WHOLLY OWNED SUBSIDIARY OF REED/ELSEVIER, US HOLDINGS | 1600 JOHN F KENNEDY BLVD. SUITE 1800 PHILADELPHIA, PA 19103-2899 |

11. Known Bondholders, Mortgagees, and Other Security Holders Owning or Holding 1 Percent or More of Total Amount of Bonds, Mortgages, or Other Securities. If none, check box ▸ ☐ None

| Full Name | Complete Mailing Address |
|---|---|
| N/A | |

12. Tax Status (For completion by nonprofit organizations authorized to mail at nonprofit rates) (Check one)
The purpose, function, and nonprofit status of this organization and the exempt status for federal income tax purposes:
☒ Has Not Changed During Preceding 12 Months
☐ Has Changed During Preceding 12 Months (Publisher must submit explanation of change with this statement)

PS Form 3526, July 2014 (Page 1 of 4 (see instructions page 4)) PSN: 7530-01-000-9931   PRIVACY NOTICE: See our privacy policy on www.usps.com.

---

| 13. Publication Title | 14. Issue Date for Circulation Data Below |
|---|---|
| PEDIATRIC CLINICS OF NORTH AMERICA | JUNE 2020 |

15. Extent and Nature of Circulation

| | | Average No. Copies Each Issue During Preceding 12 Months | No. Copies of Single Issue Published Nearest to Filing Date |
|---|---|---|---|
| a. Total Number of Copies (Net press run) | | 568 | 483 |
| b. Paid Circulation (By Mail and Outside the Mail) | (1) Mailed Outside-County Paid Subscriptions Stated on PS Form 3541 (Include paid distribution above nominal rate, advertiser's proof copies, and exchange copies) | 276 | 264 |
| | (2) Mailed In-County Paid Subscriptions Stated on PS Form 3541 (Include paid distribution above nominal rate, advertiser's proof copies, and exchange copies) | 0 | 0 |
| | (3) Paid Distribution Outside the Mails Including Sales Through Dealers and Carriers, Street Vendors, Counter Sales, and Other Paid Distribution Outside USPS® | 220 | 180 |
| | (4) Paid Distribution by Other Classes of Mail Through the USPS (e.g., First-Class Mail®) | 0 | 0 |
| c. Total Paid Distribution (Sum of 15b (1), (2), (3), and (4)) | ▸ | 496 | 444 |
| d. Free or Nominal Rate Distribution (By Mail and Outside the Mail) | (1) Free or Nominal Rate Outside-County Copies included on PS Form 3541 | 51 | 22 |
| | (2) Free or Nominal Rate In-County Copies Included on PS Form 3541 | 0 | 0 |
| | (3) Free or Nominal Rate Copies Mailed at Other Classes Through the USPS (e.g., First-Class Mail) | 0 | 0 |
| | (4) Free or Nominal Rate Distribution Outside the Mail (Carriers or other means) | 0 | 0 |
| e. Total Free or Nominal Rate Distribution (Sum of 15d (1), (2), (3) and (4)) | ▸ | 51 | 22 |
| f. Total Distribution (Sum of 15c and 15e) | ▸ | 547 | 466 |
| g. Copies not Distributed (See Instructions to Publishers #4 (page #3)) | ▸ | 21 | 17 |
| h. Total (Sum of 15f and g) | ▸ | 568 | 483 |
| i. Percent Paid (15c divided by 15f times 100) | | 90.67% | 95.27% |

* If you are claiming electronic copies, go to line 16 on page 3. If you are not claiming electronic copies, skip to line 17 on page 3.

16. Electronic Copy Circulation

| | Average No. Copies Each Issue During Preceding 12 Months | No. Copies of Single Issue Published Nearest to Filing Date |
|---|---|---|
| a. Paid Electronic Copies ▸ | | |
| b. Total Paid Print Copies (Line 15c) + Paid Electronic Copies (Line 16a) ▸ | | |
| c. Total Print Distribution (Line 15f) + Paid Electronic Copies (Line 16a) ▸ | | |
| d. Percent Paid (Both Print & Electronic Copies) (16b divided by 16c × 100) ▸ | | |

☒ I certify that 50% of all my distributed copies (electronic and print) are paid above a nominal price.

17. Publication of Statement of Ownership

☒ If the publication is a general publication, publication of this statement is required. Will be printed ☐ Publication not required.
in the OCTOBER 2020 issue of this publication.

18. Signature and Title of Editor, Publisher, Business Manager, or Owner

Malathi Samayan - Distribution Controller    *Malathi Samayan*    Date 9/18/2020

I certify that all information furnished on this form is true and complete. I understand that anyone who furnishes false or misleading information on this form or who omits material or information requested on the form may be subject to criminal sanctions (including fines and imprisonment) and/or civil sanctions (including civil penalties).

PS Form 3526, July 2014 (Page 2 of 4)   PRIVACY NOTICE: See our privacy policy on www.usps.com

Printed and bound by CPI Group (UK) Ltd, Croydon, CR0 4YY

12/10/2024

01773490-0001